DAMS

BEAT THE

NEET

PG MEDICAL ENTRANCE EXAM WITH EXPLANATORY ANSWERS

Edited and Concept by

DR. SUMER K. SETHI

PEEPEE
PUBLISHERS AND DISTRIBUTORS (P) LTD.

Published by
Pawaninder P. Vij and Anupam Vij

Peepee Publishers and Distributors (P) Ltd.
Head Office: 160, Shakti Vihar, Pitam Pura, Delhi 110 034 (India)

Correspondence Address:

7/31, First Floor, Ansari Road, Daryaganj
New Delhi-110002 (India)
Ph: 65195868, 23246245, 9811156083
e-mail: peepee160@yahoo.co.in
e-mail: peepee160@rediffmail.com
e-mail: peepee160@gmail.com
www.peepeepub.com

First Edition: **2015**

ISBN: 978-81-8445-144-3

CONTENTS

1 A25-year-old woman complains of **intermittent vague right upper quadrant (RUQ) pain. She has been on oral contraceptive tablets for 6 years.** ACT scan of her abdomen shows multiple lowdensity solid masses **occupying the entire right lobe of her liver as well as most of the left lobe.** What is the best treatment for this patient?
a. Hepatic embolization
b. Discontinuation of oral contraceptives and a repeated CT scan of her abdomen in 3–6 months
c. CT-guided percutaneous needle biopsy of several liver masses
d. Laparoscopic biopsy of the liver masses and cholecystectomy

2 A 76-year-old woman undergoes **successful endoscopic stenting of the common bile duct (CBD) for obstructive jaundice secondary to an inoperable cholangiocarcinoma**. Two weeks later, she consults her physician because of a fever of 102 °F, **general malaise, nausea, and RUQ discomfort. On physical examination, icteric sclera and RUQ tenderness** are noted. Laboratory test results show leukocytosis, anemia, **and an elevated serum bilirubin level. Chest** x-ray shows no acute infiltrate, but the right diaphragm is elevated. What is the most likely diagnosis?
a. Cholangitis
b. Liver abscess
c. Acute calculous cholecystitis
d. Liver metastasis

3 A78-year-old woman develops a **liver abscess following stent drainage of jaundice**. What is the preferred therapy?
a. Oral administration of antibiotics
b. Aspiration of abscess
c. CT-guided percutaneous drainage alone
d. Administration of antibiotics and CT-guided percutaneous drainage

4 The most likely cause of the **finding pictured in Fig. in a patient who has undergone** no procedures is:

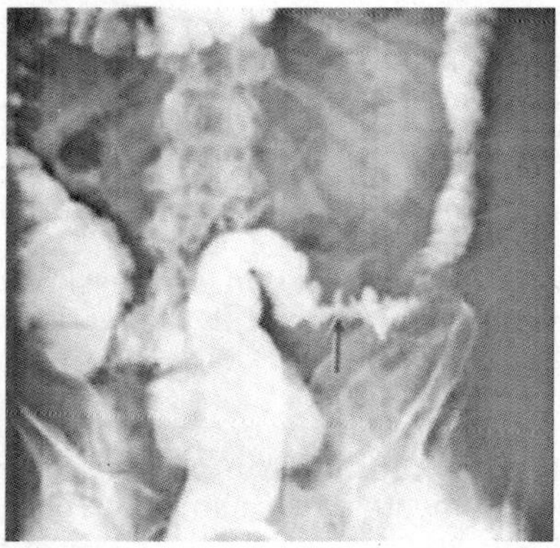

Barium enema x-ray.
a. Renal stone
b. Bladder tumor
c. Motion artifact
d. Sigmoid diverticulitis

5 **Assertion A**: Type 1 (autoimmune) diabetes mellitus is associated with MHC genes on more than one haplotype.
Reason R: The presence of both the DR3 and DR4 haplotypes in one individual confers a 20-fold increased risk for type 1 diabetes
a. Both A and R are true and R is correct explanation of A
b. Both A and R are true and R is not correct explanation of A
c. A is true but R is false
d. A is false but R is true

6 **Assertion A**: **Any gene defect that interferes with T cell development will also compromise antibody production**
Reason R: T cells are required for B cell responses
a. Both A and R are true and R is correct explanation of A
b. Both A and R are true and R is not correct explanation of A
c. A is true but R is false
d. A is false but R is true

7 **Assertion A**: Rheumatoid nodules are usually on extensor surfaces
Reason R: Areas subjected to mechanical pressure are at maximum risk
a. Both A and R are true and R is correct explanation of A
b. Both A and R are true and R is not correct explanation of A
c. A is true but R is false
d. A is false but R is true

8 A 35-year-old man presents with a **bleeding duodenal ulcer documented by endoscopy**. The patient is somewhat unstable, and bleeding does **not stop despite transfusing 8 U of blood.**What is the most appropriate surgical therapy?
a. Oversewing the ulcer alone
b. Oversewing the ulcer and performing a gastrojejunostomy
c. Oversewing the ulcer and performing a vagotomy and pyloroplasty
d. Oversewing the ulcer and performing a proximal gastrectomy

9 After undergoing a gynecologic **operation, a 36-year-old patient developed b-streptococcal septicemia**. Which is true of b-streptococcal infection?
a. It does not spread rapidly along lymphatic channels
b. It is mainly resistant to penicillin
c. It may spread rapidly through tissue planes
d. It is unlikely to cause overwhelming infection from an intravenous site

10 A 44-year-old man develops intra-**abdominal sepsis after undergoing difficult bowel resection and anastomosis.** He is initially given **ceftizoxime sodium (Cefizox),** which is in effective because of overgrowth of which of the following?
a. Pseudomonas
b. Staphylococcus aureus
c. Neisseria gonorrhoeae
d. Bacteroides fragilis

11 A64-year-old man is noted **on CT scan to have a liver abscess**. He is diagnosed as more likely to have a pyogenic than **amebic liver abscess. Why?**
a. Jaundice is absent
b. He has associated diarrhea

c. He has a history of biliary tract disease
d. There is a rapid response to metronidazole

12 What is true **of Candida sepsis**?
a. It carries a relatively low mortality risk
b. It is treated with actinomycin
c. It can be partly prevented by ketoconazole
d. It is caused by spore-forming organisms

13 A 43-year-old man had a **previous injury to his wrist. The ulnar nerve was severed**, as indicated by which of the following?
a. Claw hand involving the ring and little fingers
b. Claw hand involving the index and middle fingers
c. Atrophy of the thenar muscles
d. Absent sensation in the index finger

14 After falling on the **pavement, a 72-year-old woman is found to have a fracture of the radius and ulna (Colles' fracture).** What is true of this fracture?
a. The fall occurs on the dorsum of the wrist
b. Open reduction is most commonly indicated
c. Younger men are generally affected
d. The distal radial metaphysis is displaced dorsally

15 Optimal treatment for the patient whose chest x-ray is depicted below would be:

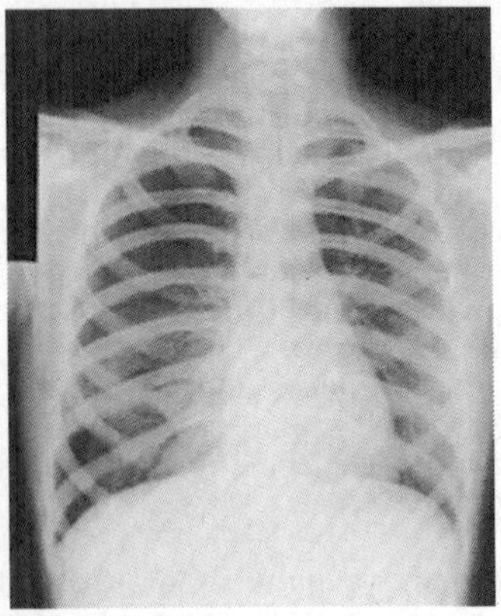

a. Diuretics
b. Metered dose inhalers using bata agonist drugs
c. IV antibiotics
d. Needle decompression

16 You will be required to select one answer for each item in the set.
a. Glucagonoma
b. Insulinoma
c. Zollinger-Ellison syndrome (ZES)
d. Watery diarrhea, hypokalemia, and achlorhydria (WDHA) syndrome
e. Somatostatinoma
f. Multiple endocrine neoplasia type-1 (MEN)-1
g. MEN-2A
h. MEN-2B

For each patient below, select the most likely diagnosis.
1. A 50-year-old woman complains of **weakness, profuse watery diarrhea and crampy** abdominal pain. She reports a 10-lb weight loss. Her serum potassium is 2.8 mEq/L.
2. A 45-year-old man presents with an upper **gastrointestinal bleed. An upper endoscopy reveals multiple duodenal ulcers and an enlarged stomach.**
3. A 35-year-old woman with epigastric pain,which did not improve on ranitidine, is found to have a nonhealing pyloric channel ulcer on **upper endoscopy. Her serum calcium level is 12 mg/dL.**

Option:
a. 1-d; 2-c; 3-f
b. 1-a; 2-h; 3-f
c. 1-d; 2-f; 3-c
d. 1-b; 2-h; 3-a

17 A 60-year-old man with a history of **alcoholism complains of intermittent chest pain**. A CT scan of the abdomen is **shown below**. What is the most likely diagnosis?

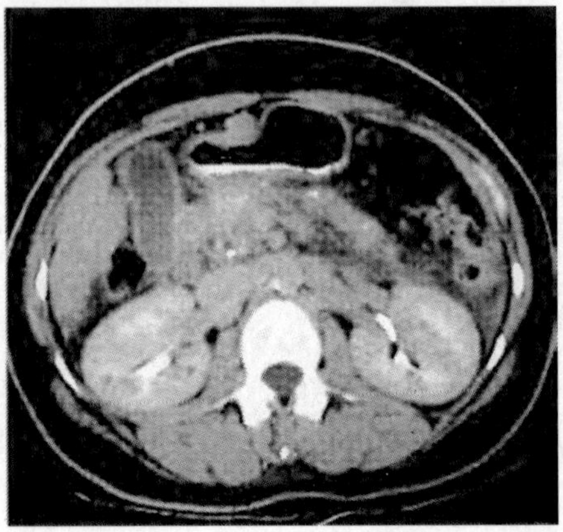

a. Gastric carcinoma
b. Chronic pancreatitis
c. Renal cell carcinoma
d. Aortic aneurysm

18 A 3-year-old boy presents to the emergency department with **cough and difficulty breathing.** The mother reports that he has **had a fever to 100°F and a barking cough since the night before. A chest radiograph is ordered.** Which radiologic sign is most useful in making **the diagnosis?**
a. Foreign body in the airway
b. The steeple sign
c. Deviated trachea
d. Unilateral lucent hemithorax

19 Regarding the shoulder joint:
a. CT arthrography is of little value in the assessment of the glenoid labrum
b. T2-W images and STIR (short tau inversion recovery) sequences with fat suppression can identify tears in the supraspinatus tendon
c. On ultrasound, the supraspinatus tendon is echobright
d. In anterior dislocation of the shoulder, cortical defects may occur in the anterior aspect of the head of the humerus

20 A 43-year-old woman presents for the **evaluation of bleeding gums**. The patient reports that for the past 2 months, her gums have bled more easily when she brushes her teeth. Physical examination reveals palatal petechiae **and scattered petechiae over the lower extremities bilaterally.** Which of the following laboratory tests is most likely to identify the abnormality responsible **for this patient's bleeding disorder?**
a. Prothrombin time (PT) and international normalized ratio (INR)
b. Complete blood count (CBC)
c. Partial thromboplastin time (PTT)
d. A mixing study

21 A 54-year-old man presents with **fatigue, weakness, and dyspnea on exertion. Physical examination reveals conjunctival pallor, palatal petechiae, and splenomegaly. A CBC reveals profound anemia and thrombocytopenia**. A bone marrow biopsy reveals agnogenic myeloid metaplasia (myelofibrosis). The patient's **splenomegaly is attributed to increased production of blood cells in the spleen.**Which of the following terms indicates blood cell production outside the bone marrow in the **spleen,liver, and other locations**?
a. Adjunctive hematopoiesis
b. Remote hematopoiesis
c. Accessory hematopoiesis
d. Extramedullary hematopoiesis

22 A 55-year-old man with **type 1 diabetes undergoes dialysis** three times a week for end-stage renal disease.You recently started **him on erythropoietin injections for chronic anemia (hematocrit, 25%)**.Which of the following is the best test to determine whether this patient will respond to the **erythropoietin treatment**?
a. Erythropoietin level b. Hematocrit
c. Creatinine level d. Reticulocyte count

23 You will be required to select one answer for each item in the set.
Thalassemia
Hereditary spherocytosis
Sickle cell disease
Idiopathic autoimmune hemolytic anemia
Thrombotic thrombocytopenic purpura
Idiopathic thrombocytopenic pupura
Systemic lupus erythematosus
Myeloid metaplasia
Non-Hodgkin's lymphoma
Felty's syndrome
1. A30-year-old man is noted to be anemic, with clinical jaundice and a palpable spleen on abdominal exam. Splenectomy is the only treatment for this patient's automsomal dominant disorder.
2. The peripheral smear of a child with anemia shows hypochromic microcytic anemia with target cells. What is the child's diagnosis?
3. A woman with longstanding rheumatoid arthritis has neutropenia on routine labs and splenomegaly is noted on physical examination.Which is the most likely diagnosis?

Option:
a. 1-b; 2-a; 3-f b. 1-c; 2-h; 3-f
c. 1-b; 2-a; 3-j d. 1-b; 2-h; 3-a

24 You will be required to select one answer for each item in the set.
a. Nonparasitic cyst
b. Hydatid cyst
c. Hamartoma
d. Adenoma
e. Focal nodular hyperplasia
f. Hemangioma
g. Hepatocellular carcinoma
h. Metastatic carcinoma
Select the most likely diagnosis for the patients below:
1. A 50-year-**old woman underwent wide excision of a 2.5-cm infiltrating** ductal carcinoma of the breast with axillary **lymph node dissection followed by radiation and chemotherapy 2 years ago.The patient now complains of RUQ** abdominal pain. A CAT scan reveals two masses in the right lobe of the liver.
2. A 35-year-old woman complains of RUQ pain after meals with nausea and vomiting. An ultrasound reveals cholelitiasis **and an anechoic 3-cm mass on the inferior surface of the right lobe of the liver.**

Option:
a. 1-h; 2-a b. 1-c; 2-a c. 1-b; 2-a d. 1-b; 2-h

25 A newborn full-term baby boy with diagnosis of imperforate anus (Fig) is also at risk to have a
a. Dextrocardia
b. Rib cage anomaly
c. Tracheoesophageal fistula
d. Ulnar skeletal deformity

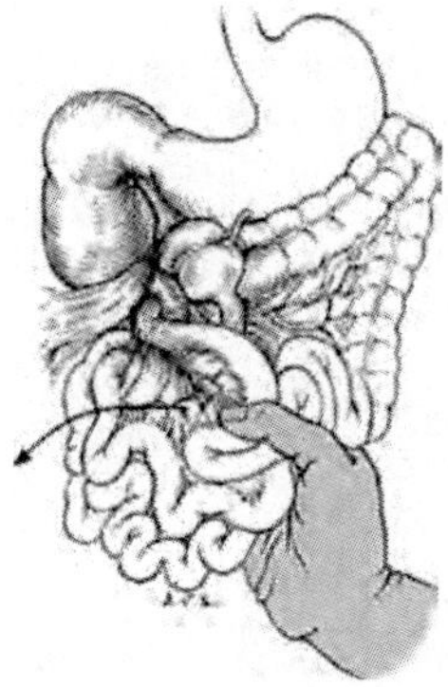

26 A 40-year-old man is involved in a car crash, **presenting with blood pressure of 80 mm Hg.** The patient is found to have subdural hematoma and a supracondylar fracture of the left femur FAST shows fluid within the abdomen. He is taken to the OR, where intra-**abdominal bleeding is controlled, and the subdural hematoma is drained.** The femur fracture (**Fig given below) should be treated by which of the following?**

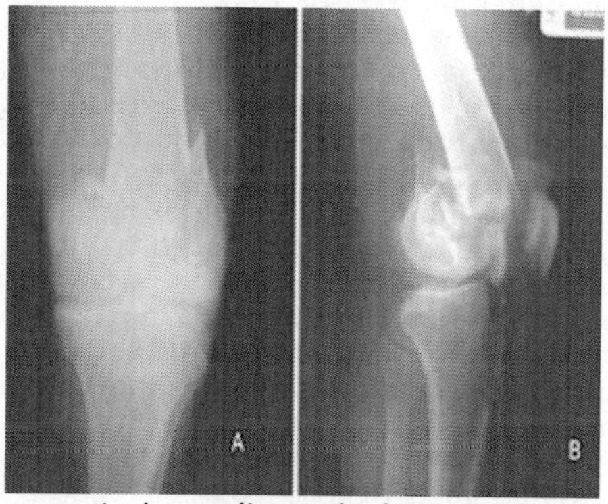

Anteroposterior radiograph demonstrating a comminuted supracondylar femur fracture with intra-articular extension.
a. Long-leg cast
b. Steinmann pin insertion and traction
c. Operative reduction and internal reduction
d. Aspiration of knee joint

27 An 18-year-old man is brought to the **emergency department with a stab wound just to the right of the sternum in the sixth intercostal space.** His blood **pressure is 80 mm Hg. Faint heart sounds and pulsus paradoxus are noted.**

Auscultation of the right chest revea is decreased breath sounds. The initial management of this patient should be which of the following?
a. Aspiration of the right chest cavity
b. Aspiration of the pericardium
c. Echocardiogram
d. Pericardial window

28 An 18-year-old man presents to the emergency **department with a gunshot wound to the left chest in the anterior axillary line in the seventh intercostal space**. A rushing sound is audible during inspiration. Immediate management is which of the following?
a. Exploratory laparotomy
b. Exploratory thoracotomy
c. Pleurocentesis
d. Closure of the hole with sterile dressing

29 A43-year-old man is hit in the face with a **baseball bat and presents to the emergency department** with massive facial swelling, **ecchymosis, and an elongated face. There is mobility of the middle third of the face on digital manipulation of the maxilla**. What is the likely diagnosis?
a. Lambdoid injury
b. Odontoid fracture
c. LeFort III fracture
d. Palatal split

30 A 34-year-old woman undergoes **chemotherapy for advanced-stage breast cancer. As expected, she develops pancytopenia.**Which cell line would you expect to be the last to recover in this patient?
a. Eosinophils
b. Platelets
c. Basophils
d. Monocytes

31 A 53-year-old woman is referred to your office by her **gynecologist for management of anemia**. She experienced menopause at 48 years of age and has had no **further vaginal bleeding. Two years ago, her hematocrit was 36%. During her last office visit, her hematocrit was 29%, and her MCV was 107 fl.** The patient is dependent on alcohol. She admits to drinking a pint of wine daily, and she engages in occasional binge drinking on weekends. She denies any other sources of blood loss or icterus. **She is apparently only mildly symptomatic with some fatigue. Which of the following statements regarding megaloblastic anemia** caused by folic acid deficiency is false?
a. Serum folic acid levels more accurately reflect tissue stores than do red blood cell folic acid levels
b. Folic acid deficiency can be differentiated from cobalamin deficiency by measuring methylmalonic acid and homocysteine levels; both are elevated in cobalamin deficiency, but only homocysteine is elevated in folic acid deficiency
c. Megaloblastic anemia caused by folic acid deficiency can be masked by concurrent iron deficiency anemia, but hypersegmented polymorphonuclear cells (PMNs) should still be present on the peripheral smear
d. Folinic acid can be used to treat patients with megaloblastosis and bone marrow suppression associated with the use of methotrexate

32 A 30-year-old woman presents **for evaluation. Over the past month, she has been experiencing increasing dyspnea with exertion.** She has otherwise been in good health and has no known cardiorespiratory problems. She has been consuming three or four alcoholic drinks an evening for the past 6 years. She is on no **medications. In giving her family history, she reports having a sibling with anemia. Her examination reveals normal vital signs and mild pallor in the conjunctiva. Her cardiorespiratory examination is normal.** A CBC reveals a WBC count of 3.5 × 103, a platelet count of **144,000, and a hemoglobin level of 8.4 g/dl, with a mean cell volume of 84 and a reticulocyte count of 0.8%.**What would be the most likely finding on this bone marrow examination?
a. Ringed sideroblasts and ineffective erythropoiesis
b. Hypercellularity of RBC precursors
c. Hypocellularity of the marrow blood-forming elements
d. Normal cellularity

33 In which age **group is the following injury** (Fig given below) most **likely to occur**?
a. 2 months b. 2 years c. 8 years d. 20 years

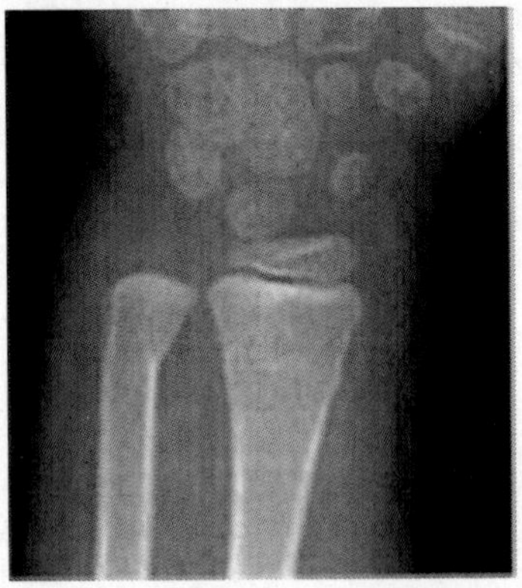

34 A 26-year-old man is stabbed in the **right intercostal space in the midclavicular line and presents to the emergency department**. On examination, subcutaneous **emphysema of the right chest wall, absent breath sounds, and a trachea shifted to the left are not**ed. What is the most likely serious diagnosis?
a. Pneumothorax
b. Tension pneumothorax
c. Massive hemothorax
d. Hemopneumothorax

35 A47-year-old woman involved in a skiing **accident suffered a severe blow to the** middle upper abdomen. Physical examination **revealed diffuse tenderness, but there was no evidence of rebound tenderness or guarding.** What test would be performed to rule out traumatic pancreatitis?
a. Peritoneal lavage
b. Serum amylase
c. CT scan with oral and intravenous contrast
d. Upper GI study

36 A 19-year-old man presents to the **emergency department with a gunshot wound through the umbilicus. The systolic blood pressure is 70 mm Hg** on palpation, and his abdomen is tightly

distended. Large-bore intravenous lines are **placed, and Ringer's lactate is infused. What should be the next step?**
a. Peritoneal lavage
b. CT scan of the abdomen
c. Exploratory laparotomy
d. PASG

37 A34-year-old man is brought into the emergency **department with a large open knife wound to the left thigh. The patient's systolic blood pressure is 90 mm Hg**. Blood is spurting from the wound. What is the initial management step?
a. Clamp the bleeding artery with a vascular clamp
b. Apply a tourniquet 7.5 cm above the wound
c. Apply direct pressure with sterile gauze
d. Apply PASG, and inflate both legs

38 A 40-year-old construction worker is **pulled from the rubble after a building collapses** and pins his right lower leg. X-rays in the emergency department reveal a comminuted fracture of the right tibia and fibula. The dorsal **pedis and posterior tibial pulses are palpable. The patient complains of severe pain that is accentuated with dorsiflexion of the foot**. The calf feels tense. What is the appropriate step?
a. ORIF of fracture
b. ORIF of fracture plus three-compartment fasciotomy
c. Closed reduction and observation
d. ORIF only if pulses become weak

39 An 18-year-old woman who is 8-**month pregnant is brought into the emergency** department. She was hit by a car and now complains of abdominal pain**. Her blood pressure is 80/60 mm Hg, pulse is 120 bpm, and respiration rate is 30 breaths per minute**. Large-bore intravenous lines are placed through the antecubital fossa. The fetal **heart rate is 160 bpm**. What is the next step?
a. Infuse 2000 mL of Ringer's lactate over 10–15 minutes
b. Apply a PASG, inflating only the legs
c. Displace the uterus to the left
d. Order an ultrasound of abdomen and pelvis to rule out free blood

40 A 60-year-old man is a front-seat **passenger in a car crash.** He is found to have three fractured ribs on the right, rupture of the liver, **pelvic fracture, right femoral fracture, and a left tibial fracture.** The patient is given broad-**spectrum antibiotics, and his injuries are managed by surgery, requiring 12 U of blood.** The patient improves initially, but on the third postoperative day, he develops **hypoxia (PaO_2, 55 mm Hg), with confusion, tachypnea, and petechia**. What is the most likely diagnosis?
a. Transfusion reaction
b. Antibiotic allergy
c. Fat embolus
d. Disseminated intravascular clotting (DIC)

41 A19-year-old man is brought to the **emergency department with a stab wound at the base of the neck (zone I**) (Fig).

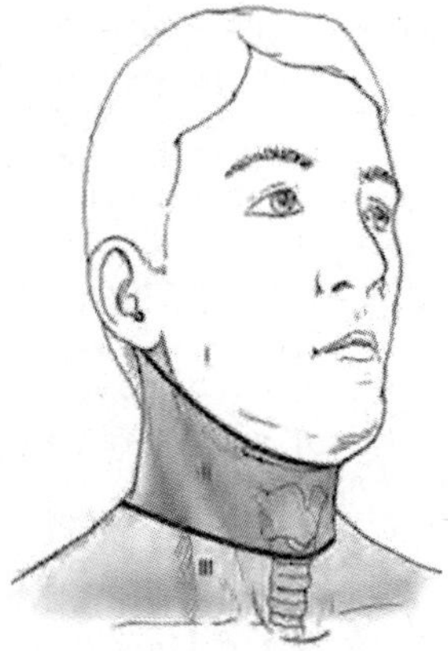

The most important concern for **patients with such injuries is which of the following**?
a. Upper extremity ischemia
b. Cerebral infarction
c. Exsanguinating hemorrhage
d. Mediastinitis

42 **You will be required to select one answer from each item in the set. For each patient with dyspnea, select the most likely diagnosis.**
a. Tension pneumothorax
b. Cardiac tamponade
c. Spontaneous pneumothorax
d. Open pneumothorax
e. Massive hemothorax
f. Flail chest
g. Rupture diaphram

1. A 23-year-old **man, tall and thin, was jogging** one evening when he suddently felt a sharp pain in the left chest, worse on taking **a deep breath and shortness of breath**.
2. A 45-year-old man was a passenger in a **car when he was T-boned by a truck at a high speed**. He is short in breath, complains of severe pain in the chest, and is hypoxic on the pulse oximeter. The breath sounds are diminished **on the left and the percussion note is completely dull. He rapidly becomes tachycardic and hypoten-sive.**
3. A 25-year-old woman was stabbed **by her boyfriend in the left chest. On** examination, she has a 1-cm stab wound just inferior to her left breast in **the mid-clavicular line.** There is jugular venous distension and breath sounds are completely absent **on the left side. She is becoming extremely dyspneic and hypoxic.**

Option:
a. 1-h; 2-e; 3-a
b. 1-c; 2-e; 3-a
c. 1-b; 2-a; 3-a
d. 1-b; 2-h; 3-a

43 **You will be required to select one answer from each item in the set. For each patient who was involved in a motor-vehicle crash, match the most likely injury.**
a. Diffuse axonal injury
b. Acute extradural hematoma
c. Acute subdural hematoma
d. Tentorial herniation
e. Flail chest
f. Posterior dislocation of the hip
g. Fracture of the pelvis
h. Diaphragmatic rupture

1. A 45-year-old man with a skull fracture of the temporal bone

2. A23-year-old man with a head-on collision, bent steering wheel and knee imprint on dashboard.
3. A 30-year-old with a side impact injury, has multiple rib fractures on the left side with pain and hypoxia.

Option:
a. 1-f; 2-e; 3-a
b. 1-b; 2-e; 3-a
c. 1-b; 2-f; 3-e
d. 1-f; 2-h; 3-a

44 A 47-year-old woman **presents to your office with a complaint of severe fatigue, weakness, and dyspnea on exertion.** She has had these symptoms for 2 days. The patient denies having fever, chills, weight changes, or **dysuria. Her medical history is significant for pernicious anemia and hypothyroidism.Results of thyroid studies were within normal limits 1 week ago. Her physical examination is positive for mild icterus and hepatosplenomegaly. CBC** is normal, with the exception of a hematocrit of 21%. Her hematocrit was **36% 3 months ago. Liver function tests show the total bilirubin level to be 4.6 mg/dl and the indirect bilirubin level to be 4.2 mg/dl. Other results are within normal limits.** A direct Coombs test is positive. Which of the following statements regarding **autoimmune hemolytic anemia is true?**
a. Autoimmune hemolytic anemia typically results in intravascular hemolysis
b. Autoimmune hemolytic anemia may be idiopathic or secondary to disorders such as systemic lupus erythematosus, chronic lymphocytic leukemia (CLL), HIV infection, or hepatitis C infection
c. Most patients with autoimmune hemolytic anemia are cured with steroid therapy
d. Splenectomy is curative for those patients who do not respond to simple steroid therapy

45 A 25-year-old black man comes for a **routine office visit. You have followed the patient for many years for his sickle cell disease.** The patient takes very good care of himself and has only required hospital admission four **times in the past 5 years. Two of these admissions occurred in the past 6 months.** You feel that the patient's clinical course is worsening. He has recently required the addition of **narcotics to his home regimen of nonsteroidal anti-inflammatory drug therapy. The patient states that he now has moderately severe pain in long bones two to three times monthly.** He has also developed worsening left hip pain over the past month. Which of the following statements **regarding sickle cell disease is true?**
a. In patients with homozygous sickle cell disease, roughly 50% of total hemoglobin is hemoglobin S
b. Risk factors that predispose to painful crises include a hemoglobin level greater than 8.5 g/dl, pregnancy, cold weather, and a high reticulocyte count
c. The most definitive test for the diagnosis of sickle cell anemia is the sodium metabisulfite test
d. Hydroxyurea has never been shown to be of benefit in the therapy of sickle cell disease

46 A 75-year-old man presents **complaining of headache and memory difficulties. He has lost 10 lb since his last office visit 6 months ago.** He smoked cigarettes for 40 years but was successful I quitting 10 years ago. He has a **history of deep vein thrombosis in his left leg, which was successfully treated by medication.His blood pressure is 135/85 mm Hg, and his temperature is 101°F (38.3°C). He complains of feeling flushed and of sweating. His laboratory values are as follows: Hct, 60%; WBC, 15,000/mm^3; platelets, 400,000/mm$_3$**; serum erythropoietin, 0.5 U/L. What is the most appropriate treatment for this patient?
a. Phlebotomy
b. Phlebotomy and hydroxyurea
c. Hydroxyurea
d. Anagrelide

47 A 21-year-old man presents to the emergency **department for evaluation of pain and fever. One week ago, the patient was involved in a head-on motor vehicle accident; he was not wearing a seat belt. At that time, the patient underwent an emergent resection of his spleen.** The patient states that for the past 2 days, he has been experiencing swelling and redness of his incision site, as well as fever. On physical examination, the **patient's temperature is 102 °F (38.9°C). Diffuse swelling and induration is noted at his incision site, and diffuse erythema surrounds the incision. Laboratory values are remarkable for a white blood cell (WBC) count of 26,000/mm^3** and a differential with 50% neutrophils and 22% band forms.Which of the following statements regarding **neutrophilia is true?**
a. Neutrophilia is usually defined as a neutrophil count greater than 1,000/mm^3
b. Thrombocytosis is commonly associated with splenectomy, but splenectomy has no association with neutrophilia
c. Serious bacterial infections are usually associated with changes in the number of circulating neutrophils, as well as the presence of younger cells, but they are not associated with changes in neutrophil morphology
d. With serious bacterial infections, characteristic morphologic changes of the neutrophils include increased numbers of band forms and increased numbers of cells with Dohle bodies and toxic granulations

48 A 59-year-old man complains of left-**sided weakness and recurrent headaches** for the past month, You order a **CT scan of the head, which is shown below.**What is the most likely diagnosis?

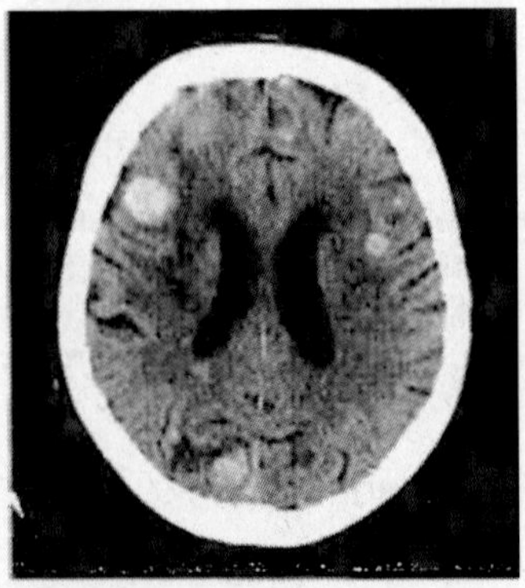

a. Intracerebral hematomas
b. Multiple Sclerosis
c. Metastases
d. Glioblastoma multiforme

49 **DIRECTIONS:** Each group of questions below **consists of lettered options followed** by a set of numbered items. For each numbered item, **select the one lettered option** with which it is most closely associated. Each lettered **option may be used once, more than once**, or not at all. Match the clinical description with **the most likely organism.**

a. Streptococcus pneumoniae
b. Staphylococcus aureus
c. Viridans streptococci
d. Providencia stuartii
e. Actinomyces israelii
f. Haemophilus ducreyi
g. Neisseria meningitidis
h. Listeria monocytogenes

1. A 30-year-old female with mitral **valve prolapse and mitral regurgitant murmur** develops fever, weight loss, and anorexia after **undergoing a dental procedure.** (CHOOSE 1 ORGANISM)
2. An 80-year-old-male, **hospitalized for hip fracture**, has a Foley catheter in place when he develops shaking chills, **fever, and hypotension.** (CHOOSE 1 ORGANISM)
3. A young man develops a painless, **fluctuant purplish lesion over the mandible**. Cutaneous fistula is noted after several weeks. (CHOOSE 1 ORGANISM)
4. A sickle cell anemia patient presents with high fever, **toxicity, signs of pneumonia, and stiff neck.** (CHOOSE 1 ORGANISM)

Option:
a. 1-f; 2-e; 3-a; 4-d
b. 1-c; 2-e; 3-a; 4-e
c. 1-c; 2-d; 3-e; 4-a
d. 1-f; 2-h; 3-a; 4-b

50 Match the clinical illness with the **appropriate opportunistic pathogen in patients with AIDS.**

a. Pneumocystis carinii
b. Toxoplasma gondii
c. Cryptosporidium
d. Cytomegalovirus
e. Salmonella

1. Pneumonia (CHOOSE 1 PATHOGEN)
2. Retinitis (CHOOSE 1 PATHOGEN)
3. Seizures (CHOOSE 1 PATHOGEN)
4. Bacteremia (CHOOSE 1 PATHOGEN)
5. Diarrhea diagnosed by direct examination of stool (CHOOSE 1 PATHOGEN)

Option:
a. 1-a; 2-d; 3-b; 4-e; 5-c
b. 1-a; 2-e; 3-b; 4-d; 5-c
c. 1-c; 2-d; 3-e; 4-a; 5-b
d. 1-c; 2-e; 3-a; 4-d; 5-b

51 A 34-year-old black female presents **with symptoms of cough, dyspnea, and lymphadenopathy. Physical exam shows cervical adenopathy and hepatomegaly**. Her chest radiograph is shown below. How should you pursue diagnosis?

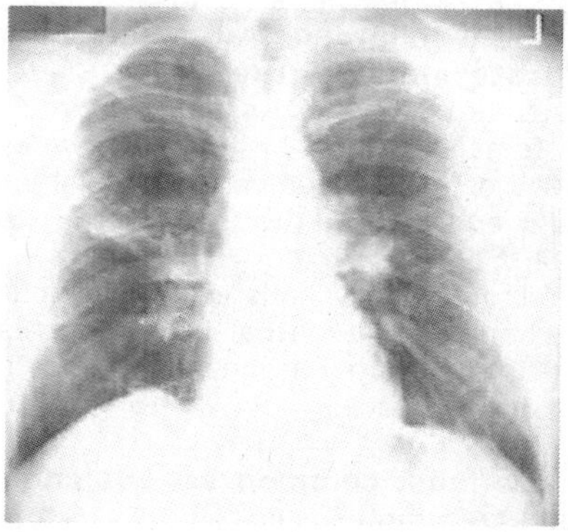

a. Open lung biopsy
b. Bronchoscopy and transbronchial lung biopsy
c. Scalene node biopsy
d. Serum angiotensin converting enzyme (ACE) level

52 The **most** common health problem of **aged** people is :

a. Visual impairment
b. Skin problems
c. Locomotor disorders
d. Psychiatric problems

53 If **mean, median and mode** are 10, 18, 26 respectively, the distribution is :

a. Symmetric
b. Normal
c. Positively skewed
d. Negatively skewed

54 Which nerve is **most at risk in the injury** in the **accompanying radiograph**?

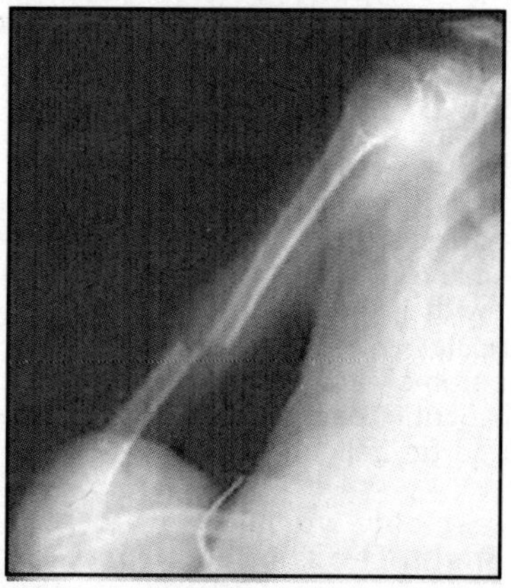

a. Median nerve
b. Radial nerve
c. Posterior interosseous nerve
d. Ulnar nerve

55 A 41-year-old man complains of **regurgitation of saliva and of ingested but undigested food. An esophagram reveals a "bird's beak" deformity**.Which of the following statements is true about this condition?

a. Chest pain is common in the advanced stages of this disease
b. More patients are improved by forceful dilation than by surgical intervention
c. Manometry can be expected to show high resting pressures of the lower esophageal sphincter
d. Surgical treatment primarily consists of resection of the distal esophagus with reanastomosis to the stomach above the diaphragm

56 Which of the following statements **concerning imperforate anus is true?**
a. Imperforate anus affects males more frequently than females
b. In 90% of males, but only 50% of females, the rectum ends below the level of the levator ani complex
c. The rectum usually ends in a blind pouch
d. The chance for eventual continence is greater when the rectum has descended to below the levator ani muscles

57 What is the **most common serious complication** of an end colostomy?
a. Bleeding
b. Skin breakdown
c. Parastomal hernia
d. Colonic perforation during irrigation

58 A 56-year-old man with a history of **coronary artery disease and a documented ejection fraction of 40% by echocardiography presents for further management**. At this visit, the patient denies having shortness of breath, dyspnea on exertion, **orthopnea, or lower extremity edema. He has never been admitted to the hospital for congestive heart failure (CHF).**According to the new American College of Cardiology/**American Heart Association (ACC/AHA)guidelines** for the evaluation and management of heart failure, in what stage of heart failure does this patient belong?
a. Stage A b. Stage B c. Stage C d. Stage D

59 A 56-year-old patient with **stage D ischemic cardiomyopathy comes to you for a second opinion. He is already receiving furosemide, an angiotensin**-converting enzyme (ACE) inhibitor, a beta blocker, and spironolactone. He has been told by a specialist that he needs a device to avoid dying from an irregular heart rhythm.What **nonpharmacologic treatments are available** for the prevention of sudden cardiac death in patients with ischemic cardiomyopathy?
a. Ventricular assist device (VAD)
b. Implantable cardioverter defibrillator (ICD)
c. Biventricular pacemaker
d. Intra-aortic balloon pump (IABP)

60 A 60-year-old woman with a **history of hypertension and mild chronic obstructive pulmonary disease (COPD) presents with a new complaint of progressive dyspnea**.Which of the following would best support a definite diagnosis of left-sided systolic heart failure as the cause of this patient's new **symptoms?**
a. Grade IV to VI murmur at the apex that radiates to the axilla
b. Fixed splitting of S2
c. Recumbent dyspnea
d. Pulsus alternans

61 A 54-year-old man presents to your clinic to establish primary care. He has a history **of diabetes, CHF,and hypertension. His blood pressure is 160/90 mm Hg, 2+ edema is present, and mild crackles are heard in the bases of his lungs. He takes no medications.** Which of the following statements incorrectly characterizes attributes of the medications to be considered for this patient?
a. Hydrochlorothiazide may exacerbate hyperglycemia
b. Without a loading dose, the blood level of digoxin will plateau in 7 days
c. Oral bioavailability of loop diuretics varies little from drug to drug
d. Spironolactone has been associated with gynecomastia

62 A 65-year-old woman with long-**standing hypertension has dyspnea associated with the classic symptoms and physical findings of CHF.** Her chest x-ray shows signs of pulmonary edema. Her echocardiogram,however, shows slightly **thickened myocardium and a normal left ventricular ejection fraction. A diagnosis of diastolic dysfunction is made**.Which of the following would improve this patient's symptoms?
a. Digoxin b. Furosemide
c. Enalapril d. Metoprolol

63 An 80-year-old man presents with **dyspnea and is found to have CHF caused by systolic** dysfunction. He also has mild renal **insufficiency, with a creatinine level of 1.4**.Which of the following statements is true regarding **ACE inhibitor therapy** in this patient?
a. It is contraindicated because of his age
b. It is contraindicated because of his renal insufficiency
c. Angiotensin II receptor blockers are preferred for CHF in elderly patients
d. ACE inhibitor therapy can be started, provided it is accompanied by careful monitoring of his creatinine and potassium levels

64 If the probability of **getting Rh +ve** is **0.9** and probability of newborn being **male is 0.5**, then the probability of new born being a **male with Rh +ve** is :-
a. 0.9 b. 0.5
c. 0.45 d. 1.3

65 A 26-year-old single woman complains of **recurrent periods of fatigue, irritability, crying spells, and insomnia, which last a few days and affect her work**.During the past year, the intensity of the symptoms has increased, but she has had these symptoms since her early 20s. She also reports sudden symptom relief at the onset of her **menses. Results of the physical examination and baseline laboratory work, including thyroid panel, are normal. Use of oral contraceptive (OC) pills has had little effect**. You suspect that this patient is suffering from premenstrual dysphoric disorder. What is the **next step in management**?
a. Ask the patient to keep a record for her physical discomfort and mood during the next 3 menstrual cycles
b. Discontinue her OC pills
c. Prescribe buspirone to relieve her anticipatory anxiety
d. Prescribe a low-dose selective serotonin reuptake inhibitor (SSRI) to be taken for 14 days during the luteal phase of her menstrual cycle for at least 6 months

66 An 18-year-old female presents with recent **weight gain,she has gained 19 lb since you last saw her 5 months ago**. Upon further inquiry, she discloses feeling out of control with food and admits to binge eating several times a day, mostly in the evening. She denies vomiting after her binges, stating that she tried **unsuccessfully. She also denies use of diet pills, laxatives, diuretics, or ipecac syrup. She is very depressed over this weight gain, feels unattractive, and tends to stay alone in her room, avoiding social contacts**. She started drinking alcohol. Her grades are poor as she has difficulty concentrating, her mind being absorbed by thoughts about food. She is desperate for a quick fix. What **would you do next?**

a. Refer her for cognitive behavioral therapy
b. Tell her that most college students gain weight in their first semester of college but that the weight gain will be temporary
c. Initiate a 6-week trial of fluoxetine and schedule follow-up visits
d. Prescribe sibutramine to suppress her appetite

67 A 40-year-old recreational tennis player **injures his left ankle.He has been applying ice and wearing an elastic wrap.** His medical history is suggestive of an inversion ankle injury. He reports that he continued **to play for 15 minutes after the injury but stopped because of increasing discomfort. Physical examination shows the lateral aspect of the ankle is swollen, with ecchymosis below the lateral malleolus.** Palpation reveals tenderness anterior to the lateral malleolus but no tenderness over the base of the fifth metatarsal. Anterior drawer and talar tilt tests are negative.Which of the **following approaches is the correct treatment?**

a. X-ray the ankle, elastic wrap, and crutches
b. X-ray the ankle and immobilize for 4 weeks
c. Early mobilization, air stirrup, strengthening, and proprioceptive exercises
d. None

68 The nurse calls you to evaluate a **23-year-old woman, gravida 3, para 2, who delivered an 4 kgs infant 3 hours ago.** She is having heavy vaginal bleeding and passing large clots. She required oxytocin for augmentation of **labor and had an epidural for labor. A second-degree laceration was repaired, and she was given an oxytocin infusion after delivery. The patient's BP is 110/74 mm Hg, and her pulse is 88 bpm**. What is the next appropriate step in management?

a. Have the nurse continue to monitor the amount of vaginal bleeding
b. Intramuscular injection of methylergonovine maleate (Methergine), 0.2 mg, and repeat in 5 minutes
c. Instruct the nurse to insert 2 large-bore IV lines, order type and crossmatch testing for administration of 2 units of packed red blood cells, and begin IV fluid resuscitation
d. Notify the operating room team to be prepared to perform dilation and curettage

69 A 32-year-old woman presents at **32 weeks' gestation for a routine prenatal** visit. Her pregnancy has been uncomplicated. Her only complaint is an occasional headache that is relieved with acetaminophen. **Fundal height is 31 cm, and fetal heart rate is 144 bpm. Her BP is 142/90 mm Hg, and she has 1+ protein on urine dipstick testing.** What is the next appropriate step in management?

a. Start treatment with oral methyldopa, 250 mg twice daily
b. Repeat BP measurement and urine dipstick testing at her next routine prenatal visit
c. Admit to the hospital for further evaluation
d. Order laboratory evaluation of complete blood cell (CBC) count; liver function tests; uric acid, BUN, and creatinine levels; 24-hour urine collection for determination of total protein level

70 2-month-old baby boy presents with vomiting **and diarrhea.** The diarrhea started today with 5 watery stools that **are yellow-green in color and foul smelling. His mother has noticed no blood or mucous in the stool.** Physical examination shows he is lethargic, with a respiratory rate of 50 breaths per minute and pulse of 160 **bpm. He weighs 6 kgs. He has a sunken fontanelle and the mucous membranes are dry. Capillary refill time is 3 seconds. After several attempts, an antecubital IV site is obtained.** What is the next appropriate step in management?

a. Obtain a chest x-ray and laboratory tests, including CBC count, measurement of electrolytes, stool and blood cultures, and urinalysis
b. Start an IV bolus of normal saline at 100 cc/h and reevaluate after the initial bolus
c. Place the infant on contact isolation precautions and start maintenance IV fluid administration of 5% dextrose in one-half strength normal saline at 20 cc/h
d. Start an IV fluid bolus of 5% dextrose in lactated Ringer's solution at 100 cc/h, then reevaluate

71 A 26-year-old woman comes in for a routine pelvic **examination and a Pap smear. She has had regular yearly Pap smears** since age 22, and they have all been normal.She has no known history of STDs. The result of this **Pap smear is atypical squamous cells of undetermined significance**. What is the appropriate next step?

a. Reassure the patient that, since all her previous Pap smears have been normal, she can have another Pap test in 1 year
b. Refer her for conization of the cervix because her history of multiple partners places her at increased risk for cervical cancer or precancerous changes
c. Perform colposcopy with fourquadrant biopsy and end. docervical curettage if no lesion is seen
d. Test for high-risk subtypes of human papillomavirus (HPV) and, if positive, perform colposcopy

72 The most practical clinical application of the Indocyanine Green Chorioangiography (ICG) is

a. Minimal classical CNV
b. Age related macular degeneration
c. Angioid streaks with CNV
d. Polypoidal choroidal vasculopathy

73 **Pain sensitive area of brain** are all of the following **except:**

a. Dural sinuses
b. Middle meningeal
c. Falx cerebri
d. Choroid plexus

74 Changes that **accompany normal aging with reference to the pulmonary system** include all of the following **except:**

a. Increased chest compliance
b. Decreased resting PO_2
c. Increased residual volume
d. Decreased lung elasticity

75 An **investigator studying the synthesis of thyroid hormones** has developed a transgenic animal deficient in **thyroid peroxidase**. Within the thyroid gland of this animal, which of the following is most likely **to be inhibited**?
a. Cleavage of iodine from iodinated tyrosines in the thyroid cell cytoplasm
b. Endocytosis of colloid from the follicle lumen into the thyroid cell
c. Iodide oxidation and binding to tyrosine in the follicle lumen
d. Movement of iodide from plasma into thyroid cells

76 A 30-year-old woman comes to the **emergency department because she thinks she has had a heart attack.** One hour ago, she had the sudden onset of chest pain, faintness, pounding heart, flushed **skin, and nausea that lasted 20 minutes.She now feels better**. She has limited her activity because she has had two similar **episodes over the past 2 weeks**. Medical evaluation is normal. Which of the following is the most **appropriate nonpharmacologic therapy**?
a. Assertiveness training
b. Cognitive behavioral therapy
c. Dynamic psychotherapy
d. Psychoanalysis

77 The diagram shows the equilibrium **between active and inactive forms of a receptor (R), its interaction with a drug (V)**, and the coupling of the active form of the receptor to a signal transduction pathway. Drug **W acts at site Y of the signal transduction pathway to diminish the physiologic effect of drug V.** Which of the following terms accurately describes the effect of drug W on the dose-response curve for drug V?

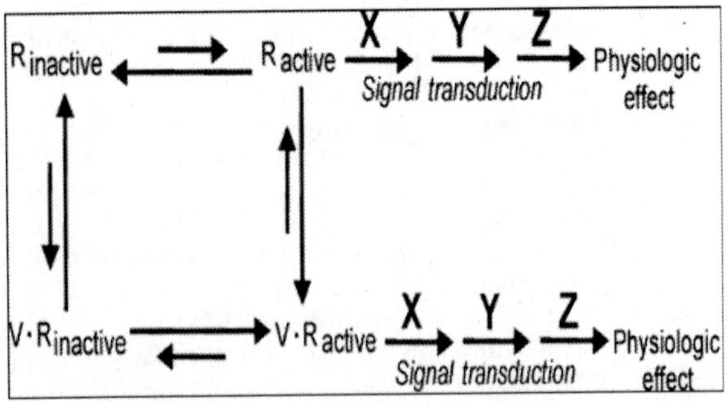

a. Competitive antagonism
b. Full agonism
c. Noncompetitive antagonism
d. Partial agonism

78 A 51-year-old woman with cancer is being **treated with a hematopoietic growth factor.** Leukocyte differentials before and **after treatment are shown:**

Before Treatment **After Treatment**
Leukocyte count 1000/mm^3
10,000/mm^3
Eosinophils 1%
1%
Lymphocytes 90%
9%
Neutrophils 9%
90%

The **growth factor** is most likely to be which of the following?
a. Granulocyte colony-stimulating factor
b. Transforming growth factor-β
c. Interleukin-6 (IL-6)
d. IL-8

79 All the **following phrases** correctly characterize **delusions except:**
a. False beliefs incongruent with an individual's experience
b. Common in schizophrenic disorders
c. Common in mania
d. Common in personality disorders

80 The circles represent the **size of a patient's pupils without treatment and following treatment with tyramine and with epinephrine.** Which of the following is compatible with the findings shown for the left eye?

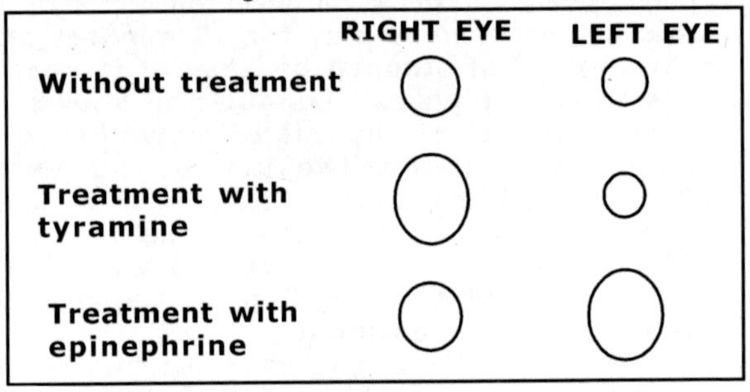

a. Blockade of α-adrenergic receptors
b. Blockade of β-adrenergic receptors
c. Blockade of muscarinic receptors
d. Sympathetic denervation

81 Which of the following **base pair sequences is palindromic**?
a. TCC
AGG
b. CCTAGG
GGATCC
c. CTCT
GAGA
d. CCAGGG
GGTCCC

82 **Recommended daily protein allowance for a 'Man' is:**
a. 40 g/d b. 50 g/d c. 60 g/d d. 15 g/d

83 **Phenytoin:**
a. Toxicity is associated with orchitis
b. Can be used in management of alcohol withdrawl syndrome
c. Is the drug of choice in absence seizures.
d. Is associated with red-green colour blindness

84 **Fish** is a **rich source of all of the following except:**
a. Unsaturated fatty acids
b. Vit A
c. Vit D
d. Phosphorus

85 A 50-year-old man being treated for increased **serum LDL concentration has muscle pain that has recently become more severe, especially with exercise.** He is most likely to be taking a

drug with which of the following **mechanisms of action**?
a. Decreasing binding of bile acids
b. Decreasing production of LDL
c. Decreasing the activity of lipoprotein lipase
d. Inhibiting the activity of 3-hydroxy-3-methylglutaryl (HMG) CoA reductase

86 A 74-year-old man has had confusion **for 2 weeks**. He has smoked **two packs of cigarettes** daily for 50 years. An x-ray of the chest **shows a 5-cm mass in the lung**. Laboratory studies of serum show:
Na^+ 110 mEq/L
Cl^- 72 mEq/L
K^+ 4.5 mEq/L
HCO_3^- 30 mEq/L
Glucose 200 mg/dL
Creatinine 1.4 mg/dL
Which of the following is the **most likely cause** of these findings?
a. Adenocarcinoma of the lung
b. Medullary carcinoma of the thyroid gland
c. Renal cell carcinoma
d. Small cell carcinoma of the lung

87 Which of the following diagnostic tests **is most likely to reveal osteomyelitis in a child** who stepped on a **nail 4 days ago**?
a. Roentgenogram of the foot
b. Technetium bone scan
c. Gallium bone scan
d. CT scan of the foot

88 A 29-year-old man has had malaise, **myalgias,and chills for 4 weeks**. On examination he is slightly jaundiced and has mild **rightupper-quadrant tenderness**. His SGOT, SGPT, and serum bilirubin levels are all twice **normal.Serum serologies are** as follows:
- Hepatitis B surface antigen—negative
- Hepatitis B e antigen—negative
- Antibody to hepatitis B surface antigen— negative
- Antibody to hepatitis B core antigen— positive

These results support the **conclusion that the man described**
a. Is in the incubation phase of hepatitis Binfection
b. Is a chronic carrier of hepatitis B virus
c. Has had a recent hepatitis B infection
d. Has never been exposed to hepatitis B virus

89 **A 22-year-old male fell on his** outstretched hand while running. He complains of severe pain in his right arm, which is swollen and tender**. The humeral shaft appears to be fractured. Clinical evidence of** associated nerve injury is present**. Which of the following is the nerve injury associated with this fracture?**
a. Axillary nerve
b. Median nerve
c. Ulnar nerve
d. Radial nerve

90 A 63-year-old woman with a history of ovarian cancer presents to the **emergency department with abdominal pain and nausea. Supine and upright abdominal films are shown below** (Fig). What is the most likely diagnosis?

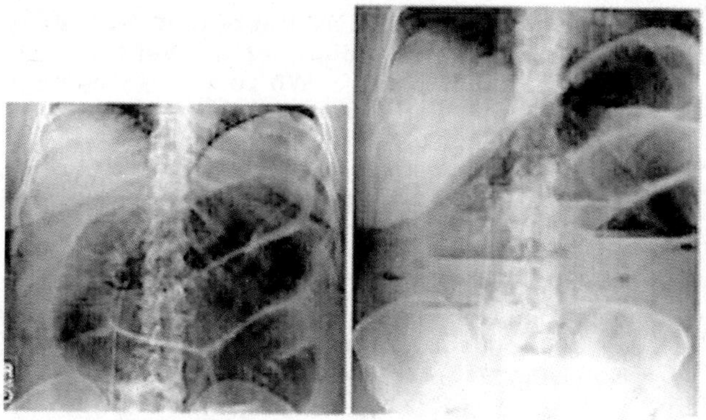

a. Paralytic ileus
b. Small bowel obstruction
c. Colonic obstruction
d. Pancreatitis with sentinel loop

91 **An afebrile 12-week-old infant presents with bilateral** conjunctivitis, cough, tachypnea, inspiratory rales, and scattered expiratory wheezing**. A complete blood count (CBC) reveals eosinophilia. The chest x-ray shows** hyperinflation and patchy interstitial infiltrates bilaterally. **Which of the following is the most likely diagnosis?**
a. Respiratory syncytial viral pneumonia
b. Bronchiolitis
c. Chlamydial pneumonia
d. Cystic fibrosis

92 **A 49-year-old man complains of a 6-**month history of worrying about his health, increased desire to sleep, demoralization, and difficulty focusing **attention on task. Which of the following is the most likely diagnosis?**
a. A manic episode
b. Somatization disorder
c. Generalized anxiety disorder
d. A depressive episode

93 **A 65-year-old woman presents with a** 2-day history of fever, chills, and a cough productive of purulent suputum**. She has a history of smoking two packs of cigarettes a day for the last 45 years. A chest x-ray shows a** right lower lobe consolidation**. Which of the following organisms is the most likely cause of her infection?**
a. Streptococcus pneumoniae
b. Haemophilus influenzae
c. Legionella pneumophila
d. Coccidioides immitis

94 **A 31-year-old woman, gravida 4 para 1,** aborta 2, presents for prenatal care in the middle of her second trimester. **She has a positive history of** substance abuse preceding and during this pregnancy. **On ultrasound examination, her singleton fetus is noted to have a limb** reduction defect of the right lower extremity**. Which of the following abused substances is most associated with** this fetal anomaly?
a. Tobacco b. Alcohol c. Narcotics d. Cocaine

95 **A 28-year-old female complains of numbness in** her fingertips and pain in her left hand that occasionally radiates up her arm**. She is often** awakened by the symptoms**. On physical**

examination, there is decreased sensation over the radial 3½ digits of the hand and the Phalen's test is positive. **Which of the following is the most likely diagnosis?**
a. Carpal tunnel syndrome
b. Pronator syndrome
c. Cubital tunnel syndrome
d. Ulnar nerve entrapment at the wrist

96 A female patient falls on an **icy sidewalk and complains of her thumb hurting. You take her x-ray and show her there are no fractures**. However, she asks what the small light circles (arrow) on the x-ray are. You explain they are **sesamoid bones in the tendon of the**

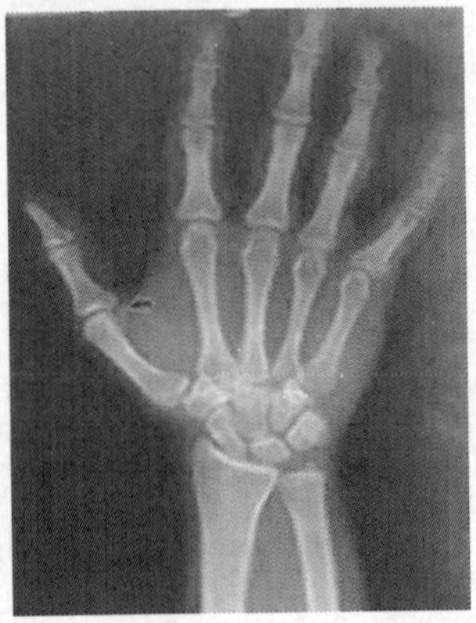

a. Flexor pollicis longus
b. Flexor pollicis brevis
c. Adductor pollicis
d. Abductor pollicis longus

97 Fig given below shows a **lead II electrocardiogram from a normal 30-year-old female** at rest. If a beta-adrenergic agonist such as **isoproterenol is administered intravenously** to this woman, what will be her resulting heart rate in beats per minute?

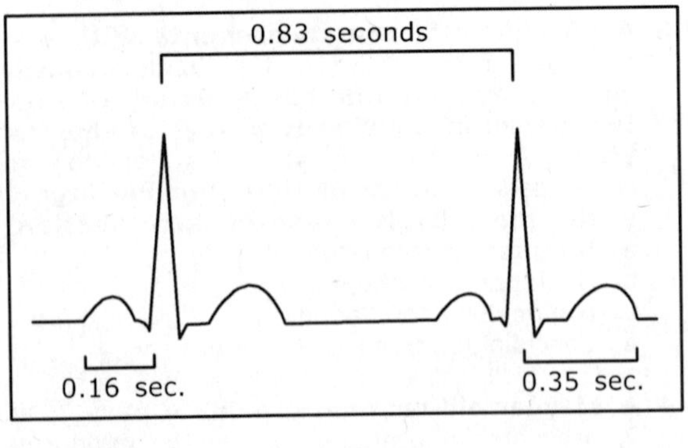

a. 55
b. 65
c. 70
d. 90

98 Hospital discharge of a 75-year-old man is delayed due to **unavailability of a bed in a nursing home. He is bedridden and unable to attend to his personal needs.** During a 3-day period, his pulse increases **from 82/min to 125/min, and blood pressure decreases from 124/72 mm Hg to 100/55 mm Hg**. Laboratory values include:

	Day 1	Day 3
Hemoglobin	16.4 g/dL	18.4 g/dL
Serum		
Urea nitrogen	18 mg/dL	56 mg/dL
Glucose	100 mg/dL	89 mg/dL
Na^+	135 mEq/L	151 mEq/L
Creatinine	1.1 mg/dL	1.2 mg/dL

Which of the following is the **most likely diagnosis**?
a. Acute renal failure
b. Dehydration
c. Diabetic ketoacidosis
d. Gastrointestinal hemorrhage

99 **Lipoprotein lipase deficiency** is associated with:
a. Abetalipoproteinaemia
b. Combined hyperlipidaemia
c. Familial combined hyperlipidaemia
d. Increased chylomicrons

100 **Reverse transcriptase-PCR** is used to ampify:
a. Antibodies b. DNA c. RNA d. Protein

101 Tumors of **acidophilic cells in the anterior pituitary of adults** are most likely to lead to:
a. Dwarfism
b. Acromegaly
c. Cushing's syndrome
d. Gigantism

102 The **most active form of thyroid hormone** in the stimulation **of oxygen use is:**
a. Thyroxine
b. Thyroglobulin
c. Triiodothyronine
d. Reverse triiodothyronine

103 In the **normal heart**, the major source of **energy for oxidative metabolism** is:
a. Glucose b. Lactate
c. Fatty acids d. Pyruvate

104 **Insulin deficiency** leads to which of the following phenomena?
a. Decreased glucose uptake by the brain
b. Inhibition of exercise-mediated increase in glucose uptake by skeletal muscle
c. Decreased catabolism of proteins
d. Increased glucagon secretion

105 **Many neurons in the basal ganglia** are: observed to begin to discharge
a. In association with somatosensory stimulation
b. At the onset of acoustic stimulation
c. Before the onset of slow movements
d. At a low rate that is independent of motor activity

106 Investigators are studying the use of a **new laboratory test to identify patients with a particular disease.** The table below summarizes the results of initial research **involving 200 subjects.**
Disease

Test Result	Present	Absent
Positive	60	40
Negative	20	80

Which of the following is the **approximate sensitivity** of a positive test result?

a. 0.30
b. 0.33
c. 0.60
d. 0.75

107 **Central value** of a set of **240** values can be obtained by:
a. 2nd quartile
b. 3rd quartile
c. 25th percentile
d. 1st quartile

108 Which of the following is **not true** about normal distribution curve:
a. Mean, median and mode coincide
b. Standard deviation is one
c. Mean is one
d. Total area of curve is one

109 The programme in which **Co-operative for assistance and relief every where (Care)** has provided maximum help in India is:
a. Immunization
b. Mid-day meal scheme
c. Family planning
d. Provision of medical equipments

110 The pulse of a group of normal healthy males was 72, **with the standard deviation of (2) What is the probability that a male chosen at random would be found to have a pulse of 80** or more. (The area of the normal curve corresponding to a deviate 4 = 0.49997)
a. 4 out of 100,000
b. 3 out of 100,000
c. 4 out of 1000
d. 3 out of 1000

111 A 25-year-**old black man presents to your office seeking to establish primary** care. The patient has no complaints and denies any **known medical history**. His blood pressure is noted to be 185/115; otherwise,his physical examination is normal. After measuring the patient's blood pressure a total of four times during **two office visits, you diagnose hypertension**. Which of the following statements regarding the initial evaluation of **hypertension in this patient is true**?
a. A retinal examination should now be performed on this patient
b. Because this patient has been diagnosed with hypertension, obtaining a family history of hypertension or early CV disease is no longer useful
c. During the initial examination, only a single careful blood pressure measurement is needed
d. This patient has no findings consistent with secondary hypertension

112 A 40-year-old white woman whom you have been **treating for resistant hypertension presents for routine follow-up. Laboratory results of screening tests were normal**. There is electrocardiographic evidence of LVH. The patient's lipid profile is normal. The patient has been receiving a thiazide diuretic, a calcium channel **blocker, and an ACE inhibitor at near maximal doses for several weeks. Her blood pressure today remains very elevated, at 175/100 mm Hg. She experienced a minimal response to titration of her antihypertensive medicines**. With the exception of elevated blood presure and a fourth heart sound, the patient's physical examinations have been consistently normal. **Today, the physical examination is unchanged, except that you notice a soft bruit in the left upper quadrant**. Which of the following statements regarding renovascular hypertension is true?
a. Renovascular hypertension is an exceptionally rare cause of hypertension in patients with treatment-resistant hypertension
b. Stenosing lesions of the renal circulation cause hypertension through ischemia-mediated activation of the renin-angiotensin-aldosterone system
c. Fibromuscular disease is an uncommon cause of renovascular hypertension in patients of this age
d. Atheromatous disease and fibromuscular disease are equally frequent causes of renovascular hypertension

113 A 72-year-old woman comes to see you **to establish care, after her previous physician retired. Her medical history is significant for diet-controlled diabetes and a myocardial infarction**. She is taking aspirin, simvastatin, and amlodipine. On examination, her blood pressure is **170/95 mm Hg. She has an S4 gallop and 1+ pretibial edema.** What should be the target blood pressure in the long term for this patient?
a. < 150/90 mm Hg
b. < 140/90 mm Hg
c. < 130/85 mm Hg
d. < 120/70 mm Hg

114 A previously healthy 47-year-old woman presents with **a complaint of palpitations of sudden onset. Her symptoms have been present for 12 hours.** Her evaluation includes an electrocardiogram, which reveals atrial fibrillation (AF) with a ventricular response of 135 beats/min. Her cardiac examination is **unremarkable except for an irregularly irregular pulse. She has no other medical problems and takes no medications**.A transthoracic echocardiogram (TTE) is normal. Which of the following is the most likely classification of this patient's AF according to guidelines from the **American College of Cardiology (ACC):**
a. Permanent
b. Persistent
c. Recurrent
d. Lone

115 An 81-year-old man with a history of **symptomatic permanent AF presents to your office** to discuss options for reestablishing sinus rhythm. He **hopes to decrease his symptoms of dyspnea. In addition to AF, the patient has congestive heart failure and echocardiographically documented significant mitral regurgitation**.Which of the following is not a risk factor for cardioversion failure in this patient?
a. Duration of AF of longer than 1 year
b. Older age
c. Left atrial enlargement
d. Normal-sized heart

116 A 45-year-old woman is **explored for a perforated duodenal ulcer 6 h after onset of symptoms.** She has a history of **chronic peptic ulcer** disease treated medically with **minimal symptoms**. The procedure of choice is:
a. Simple closure with omental patch
b. Truncal vagotomy and pyloroplasty
c. Antrectomy and truncal vagotomy
d. Highly selective vagotomy

117 A diagnosis of **bleeding esophageal varices** is made in this patient. Appropriate initial therapy would be:
a. Intravenous vasopressin
b. Endoscopic sclerotherapy
c. Emergency portacaval shunt
d. Emergency esophageal transection

118 **During an operation for carcinoma** of the hepatic flexure of the colon, an unexpected discontinuous 3-cm metastasis **is discovered in the edge of the right lobe of the liver. The** surgeon should:
a. Terminate the operation, screen the patient for evidence of other metastases, and plan further therapy after the reevaluation
b. Perform a right hemicolectomy and a right hepatic lobectomy
c. Perform a right hemicolectomy and a wedge resection of the metastasis
d. Perform a cecostomy and schedule reoperation after a course of systemic chemotherapy

119 A cardiac catheterization is **done in a healthy person. The blood sample withdrawn from the catheter shows 60% oxygen saturation, and the pressure recording shows oscillations from a maximum of 26 mm Hg to a minimum of 14 mm Hg**. The catheter tip was located in which of the following areas?
a. Ductus arteriosus
b. Foramen ovale
c. Left atrium
d. Pulmonary artery

120 An **inexpensive screening test** for a disease is available through analysis of venous blood. The distributions of blood **concentrations for persons with and without the disease** are depicted in the graph. The disease is irreversible and fatal if not **discovered and treated early**. Which of the following letters represents the most appropriate **cutoff point between normal and abnormal**?

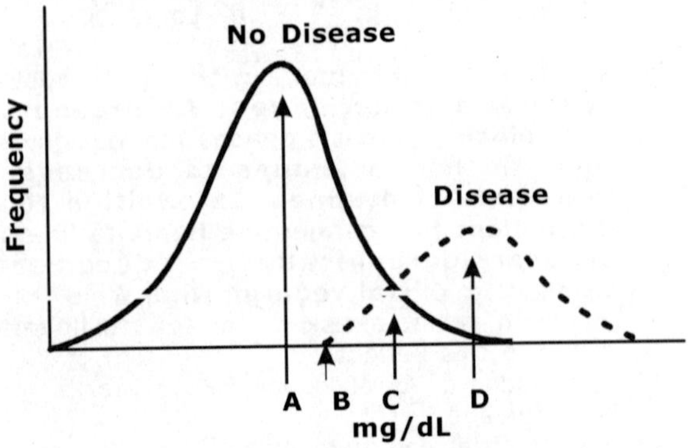

a. A b. B c. C d. D

121 A 40-year-old woman **has a 2-cm firm mass in the upper outer quadrant of her right breast. You order a mammogram.** The laboratory reports **"dense breasts with extensive fibrocystic changes, and no definite mass seen."** Which of the following strategies would be the most appropriate for this patient?
a. Reassure the patient because the mammogram did not identify any mass
b. Obtain a sonogram to correlate with the mammogram; if a mass is identified sonographically, perform biopsy
c. Repeat the breast examination and mammogram in 6 months
d. Since the mammogram showed only dense breasts and fibrocystic changes, recommend repeat mammography in 1 year

122 An 18-year-old female athlete **reports easy fatigability and weakness**. Physical examination shows **no abnormalities**. Laboratory **studies show:**

Serum

Na^+ 141 mEq/L
Cl^- 85 mEq/L
K^+ 2.1 mEq/L
HCO_3^- 35 mEq/L

Urine

Na+ 80 mEq/24 h
K+ 170 mEq/24 h

Which of the following is the **most likely diagnosis?**
a. Aldosterone deficiency
b. Anxiety reaction with hyperventilation
c. Diabetic ketoacidosis
d. Surreptitious use of diuretics

123 A 70-year-old man with a history of **chronic obstructive pulmonary disease, diabetes mellitus, and congestive heart failure presents to the emergency department with signs and symptoms of pneumonia. He was treated with levofloxacin 2 months ago for an acute exacerbation of chronic bronchitis. His vital signs are: respiratory rate, 33 breaths/min; BP, 90/60 mm Hg; pulse, 120 beats/min; temperature, 39°C.** What would be appropriate empiric antibiotic therapy?
a. Doxycycline 100 mg bid
b. Clarithromycin 500 mg bid
c. Ceftriaxone sodium, 1 g/day intravenously (IV), plus azithromycin, 500 mg/day IV
d. Levofloxacin, 500 mg/day

124 A 24-year-old man **presents with gonococcal infection of the urethra**. He says that he has just returned from California, and he **had a male sexual partner**. What would be the recommended treatment?
a. Levofloxacin,250 mg po, single dose, plus azithromycin, 1 g single dose
b. Ceftriaxone sodium,125 mg, single dose, intc. ramuscularly, plus azithromycin,1 g ,single dose
d. Ciprofloxacin 500 mg po, single dose Ciprofloxacin, 500 mg po, single dose, plus azithromycin, 1 g po, single dose

125 A 45-year-old man has a left **ventricular ejection fraction of 25% (N>55%) with diffuse hypokinesis.** He has a sedentary life-style. He eats red meat up to 6 times weekly and drinks 4 alcoholic beverages daily. **He is 185 cm (6 ft 1 in) tall and weighs 86 kg; BMI is 25 kg/m². His blood pressure is 90/60 mm Hg. Coronary arteriography** shows no evidence of atherosclerosis. To prevent further

heart damage,which of **the following is the most appropriate** recommendation?
a. Aerobic exercise program
b. Avoidance of alcohol
c. Ingestion of more vegetables and decrease in red meat intake
d. Isometric/weight-training exercise program

126 A patient being treated with **clindamycin for aspiration pneumonia develops diarrhea. The stool contains a toxin that kills cultured epithelial cells**. Stool culture grows an anaerobic grampositive rod. The same organism is **cultured from his bedpan**. Which of the following is most likely to sterilize the bedpan?
a. Boiling for 45 minutes
b. Exposure to benzalkonium chloride for 1 hour
c. Exposure to ethyl alcohol for 1 hour
d. Exposure to saturated steam (121°C) for 15 minutes

127 An 18-year-old woman has **gastroenteritis with nausea and vomiting and is able to ingest only small amounts of water.** After 3 days, she develops **light-headedness, especially when sitting or standing**. Arterial **blood gas analysis** is most likely to show which of the following sets of values?

pH	PCO_2 (mm Hg)	HCO_3 (mEq/L)
a. 7.30	28	15
b. 7.30	55	27
c. 7.40	40	24
d. 7.50	47	35

128 A 16-year-old male **presents after ingesting a battery**. Fig shows the upright abdominal radiograph of this patient. What is the **recommended treatment**?

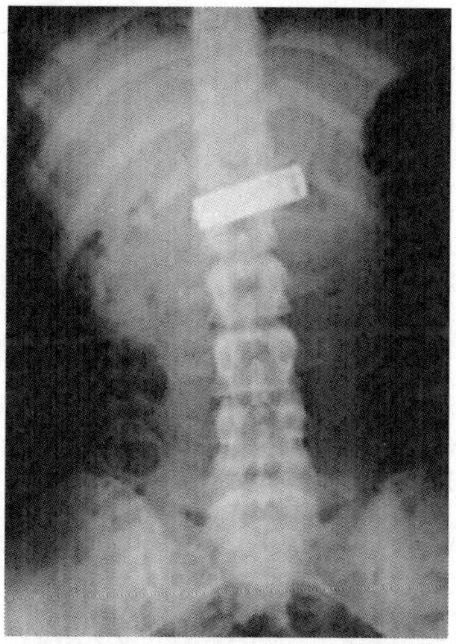

a. Prepare for emergent endoscopy
b. Induce vomiting with syrup of ipecac
c. No emergency intervention is required other than repeat abdominal x-rays
d. Insert a Foley catheter and remove the battery

129 Glycine is a diprotic amino **acid containing two ionizing groups available for titration. If the pKa values for** these groups are pK_1 = 2.4 and pK_2= 9.60**, what is the isoelectric point (pI) for glycine?**
a. 1.5 b. 6.0 c. 7.0 d. 9.0

130 A 10-yr-old boy **stubs his toe while walking barefoot**. The toe is tender,with bleeding **from the nail fold. This** child is at risk for:
a. Endocarditis
b. Osteomyelitis
c. Poor growth of the toe
d. Anemia

131 The study of **human relationships and of human behaviour for better understanding** of the pattern of human life, is **called**:
a. Anthropology
b. Social Psychology
c. Social epidemiology
d. Sociology

132 **Secular trend** is an example of :
a. Periodic fluctuation
b. Epidemic curve
c. Short term fluctuations
d. Long term fluctuations

133 **Assertion A**: Orthopnea and paroxysmal nocturnal dyspnea are rarely symptoms of isolated right heart failure.
Reason R: These symptoms usually reflect the decreased work of breathing
a. Both A and R are true and R is correct explanation of A
b. Both A and R are true and R is not correct explanation of A
c. A is true but R is false
d. A is false but R is true

134 **Assertion A**: Patients with large ventricular septal defects should be corrected surgically early in life
Reason R: Patients with large ventricular septal defects are those at greatest risk for developing pulmonary vascular obstruction
a. Both A and R are true and R is correct explanation of A
b. Both A and R are true and R is not correct explanation of A
c. A is true but R is false
d. A is false but R is true

135 **Assertion A**: **Obsessions** are defined as **persistent, intrusive ideas, images, or impulses**
Reason R: They bear relationship to **actual circumstances**
a. Both A and R are true and R is correct explanation of A
b. Both A and R are true and R is not correct explanation of A
c. A is true but R is false
d. A is false but R is true

136 A 36-year-old white female nurse **comes to the ER due to a sensation of fast heart rate, slight dizziness, and vague chest fullness. Blood pressure is 110/70.** The following rhythm strip is obtained, which shows:

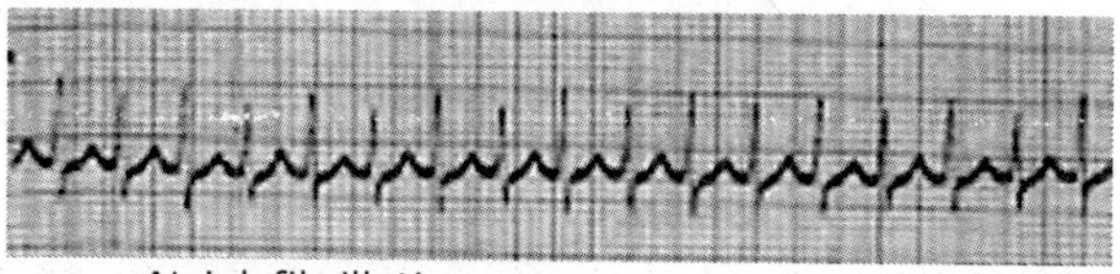

a. Atrial fibrillation
b. Atrial flutter

c. Supraventricular tachycardia
d. Ventricular tachycardia

137 You have been assigned to review the ECGs for the group this month. Many of the patients have renal problems and/or hypertension. For each electrolyte abnormality below, select the electrocardiographic finding with which it is most commonly associated.
No known electrocardiographic abnormalities.
a. Prolonged QT interval b. Short QT interval
c. Widened QRS complex d. Prominent U waves

1. Hypokalemia (SELECT 1 ECG FINDING)
2. Hyperkalemia (SELECT 1 ECG FINDING)
3. Hypocalcemia (SELECT 1 ECG FINDING)
4. Hyponatremia (SELECT 1 ECG FINDING)
Option:
a. 1-b; 2-e; 3-a; 4-d b. 1-c; 2-e; 3-a; 4-e
c. 1-c; 2-d; 3-e; 4-a d. 1-e; 2-d; 3-b; 4-a

138 The following data were obtained from a 70- kg female patient whose urine flow rate is 3 ml/min:

Plasma		Urine	
PAH concentration	0.04 mg/ml	PAH concentration	5.6 mg/ml
Urea concentration	0.50 mg/ml	Urea concentration	10 mg/ml
Inulin concentration	0.02 mg/ml	Inulin concentration	0.6 mg/ml

Renal plasma flow per minute in this woman is approximately:
a. 420 ml/min b. 90 ml/min
c. 350 ml/min d. 600 ml/min

139 Match these :-
1. Menstrual phase — a. High estrogen and progesterone; low FSH and LH
2. Follicular phase — b. Low estrogen and progesterone
3. Luteal phase — c. LH surge
4. Ovulation — d. Increasing estrogen; low LH and low progesterone

Options are :
a. (1-d) (2-a) (3-c) (4-b)
b. (1-b) (2-d) (3-a) (4-c)
c. (1-b) (2-c) (3-d) (4-a)
d. (1-c) (2-b) (3-a) (4-c)

140 The **dashed line** in the figure illustrates the effect of:

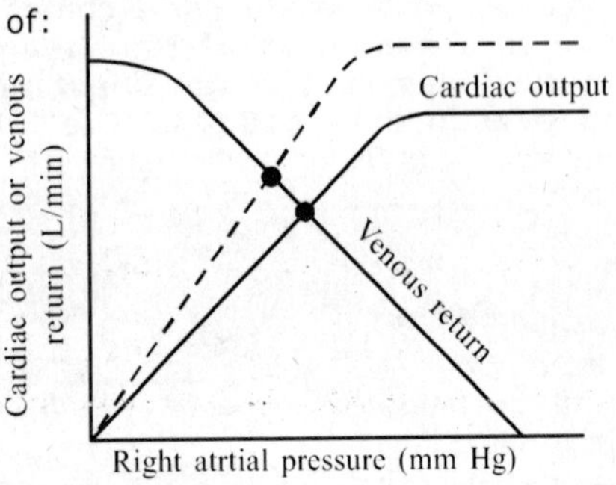

a. Increased total peripheral resistance (TPR)
b. Increased blood volume
c. Increased contractility
d. Increased mean systemic pressure

141 Which of the following features **defines toddler fractures**?
a. Subluxation of the radial head
b. Salter-Harris type 3 fracture of the distal fibular epiphysis
c. Fracture of the distal radius
d. Spiral fracture of the tibia

142 A 2-day-old boy manifests poor **feeding, vomiting, and lethargy leading to coma. Laboratory data reveal respiratory alkalosis and hyperammonemia.** The urine orotic acid level is also elevated. The most likely diagnosis is:
a. Methylmalonic acidemia
b. Carbamoylphosphate synthase deficiency
c. Ornithine transcarbamylase deficiency
d. Reye syndrome

143 A 15-year-old boy with tall stature **presents with decreased exercise tolerance over the past 2 months.** He states that he **used to play two games of basketball with no problem, but he now can play only one game.** On physical examination, his weight is at the 25th percentile, and his height higher **than the 95th percentile. He is thin and has a gangly body habitus. His fingers are long and thin**. There is pectus deformity in his chest. His joints are hyperextensible. An **ophthalmologic examination** reveals mild subluxation of the lens. Which of the following is the most **likely finding on an echocardiogram**?
a. Aortic root dilatation
b. Aortic stenosis
c. Bicuspid aortic valve
d. Dextrocardia

144 A newborn is **found to have congenital heart block**. Which of the following is the **most likely etiology**?
a. Group B streptococcal infection
b. Neonatal echovirus infection
c. Gestational diabetes
d. Maternal lupus

145 A 15-year-old white girl develops bloody diarrhea **on her sixth day of hospitalization for therapy of presumed bacterial pneumonia. She has been receiving intravenous ampicillin.** Her fever and tachypnea have resolved, and her oxygenation is now normal. In fact, she was scheduled for discharge. Which of the following **actions would be most appropriate**?
a. Switch the antibiotic to a third-generation cephalosporin
b. Discontinue ampicillin
c. Obtain ventilation-perfusion scan
d. Obtain CT scan of the abdomen

146 **If forbidden clones are** not deleted during T-cell development**, a person may develop:**
a. Hypogammaglobulinemia
b. A type I hypersensitivity reaction to exogenous antigens

c. An autoimmune disease
d. Tolerance to autoantigens

147 **Of the** following amino **acids, which one is released from skeletal muscle in amounts that exceed its** relative abundance in muscle **protein?**
a. Aspartate b. Alanine
c. Glutamate d. Leucine

148 **The left index finger from a febrile 28-year-old male** intravenous (IV) drug abuser reveals a painful, erythematous nodule on the finger pad and a linear hemorrhage beneath the fingernail. **Cardiac examination reveals a grade II high-pitched diastolic murmur heard best** along the second and third right intercostals space. **The lesions on the hand are most closely related to which of the following?**
a. Immunocomplex vasculitis
b. Thrombocytopenia
c. Coagulation factor deficiency
d. Disseminated intravascular coagulation (DIC)

149 **A 24-year-old woman,** gravida 0, para 0, complains of menstrual periods that are unpredictable in frequency and duration. **Her height is 152 cm (60 in) and she weighs 86 kg (190 Ib). Which of the** following statements is most likely true?
a. Mechanism is unopposed estrongen stimulation
b. Pelvic pathology is likely present
c. Treatment of choice is dilation and curettage
d. Regular **ovulation is common**

150 In the **initial psychiatric interview**, it is most **important to:**
a. Examine cognitive mental status
b. Recognize transference
c. Obtain a patient history
d. Assess motivation for change

151 Which of the following statements is **true** concerning **substance abuse**?
a. Tobacco is habituating, but does not cause addiction
b. Most cases of addiction to opioids are iatrogenic
c. Tolerance does not develop to cannabis use
d. If a narcotic analgesic is to be given to an opioid-dependent person, the dose should be significantly increased

152 A 68-year-old man has had low back **pain over the past 2 months. Laboratory studies show a normochromic, normocytic anemia and azotemia**. Serum and urine calcium concentrations are abnormally increased, and urinalysis **shows excessive protein (4+) and proteinaceous casts**. Bone marrow examination is most likely to show uncontrolled proliferation of which of the following cells?
a. Basophils b. Lymphocytes
c. Macrophages d. Plasma cells

153 **Norepinephrine stimulation of G proteins** results in an increased intracellular concentration of calcium. This increase is **not reversed by the extracellular calcium chelator EGTA**. Which of the following is the most likely source of the increased **intracellular calcium concentration**?
a. Endoplasmic reticulum b. Golgi complex
c. Mitochondria d. Nucleus

154 A 35-year-old man is admitted **to the hospital for an elective operation.** After 3 days in the hospital, during which various **examinations are performed, he receives general anesthesia for an abdominal operation.** Two days after the operation he becomes agitated and accusatory, is visibly tremulous, and seems to be hallucinating. **In relation to this man's agitation and possible hallucinations, a history of which of the following would have the most immediate relevance** in management plans?
a. Schizophrenia in the family
b. Alcoholism
c. LSD use
d. Traumatic early childhood

155 A 28-year-old woman complains of **several weeks' duration of pruritus and redness of the vaginal introitus.** She believes she **has a "yeast infection". She is nulliparous, and medical history is significant for type 2 diabetes mellitus of 4 years' duration, as well as severe sinusitis 8 weeks ago requiring a 2-week course of amoxicillin/ potassium clavulanate.**Over-the-counter topical yeast medications (eg, **fluconazole) have not been effective. Vaginal examination shows a thick, milky white discharge with reddened, swollen labia. A wet mount reveals small oval yeastlike organisms.** What is the next appropriate step in her care?
a. Prescribe oral metronidazole,500 mg, for 7 to 14 days
b. Obtain fungal culture for subtyping
c. Retreat with fluconazole cream for 7 days and prescribe one 150-mg tablet of fluconazole
d. Recommend vaginal douching with 1 tablespoon of white vinegar diluted in 1 quart of warm water

156 A 34-year-old man complains of **severe fatigue, which has become enough of a problem** that he has to go to bed shortly after arriving home from work. He has also developed a craving for ice. He denies any **abdominal pain or change in bowel habits but does describe persistent heartburn. His hemoglobin level is 114 g/L (normal, 140-170 g/L), mean corpuscular volume is 67 mm^3 (normal, 80-10 067 mm^3), and ferritin level is 8.4 μg/L (normal, 15-200 μg/L).** Despite treatment with a proton pump inhibitor, his heartburn persists, and he is referred for upper gastrointestinal (GI) endoscopy. **This does not reveal any abnormality or a bleeding site, although an esophageal biopsy is consistent with "mild esophagitis".** For "completeness", an air contrast barium enema is performed, which reveals a fullness and distention of the right cecum thought to be consistent with a leiomyoma. **What should the next step in management be?**
a. Reassure the patient that he has iron deficiency anemia and treat him with iron supplementation
b. Reassure him that he is not bleeding from his GI tract since his stool samples tested negative for blood
c. Refer him for colonoscopy with particular attention to the cecum

d. Perform a flexible sigmoid examination as his esophagogastroduodenoscopy and barium enema examinations should provide adequate visualization of the rest of the GI tract

157 T2-weighted-MRI head of an **AIDS** patient is shown below. What is the **most likely diagnosis**?

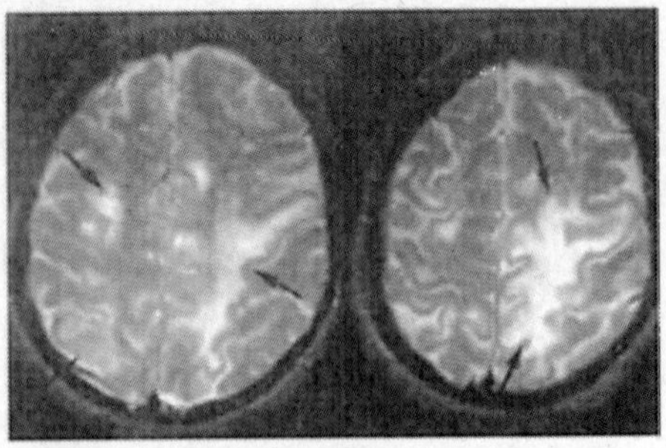

a. HIV encephalopathy
b. PML
c. HSV-I encephalitis
d. Primary CNS lymphoma

158 The following is **false** about **the picture given below** :

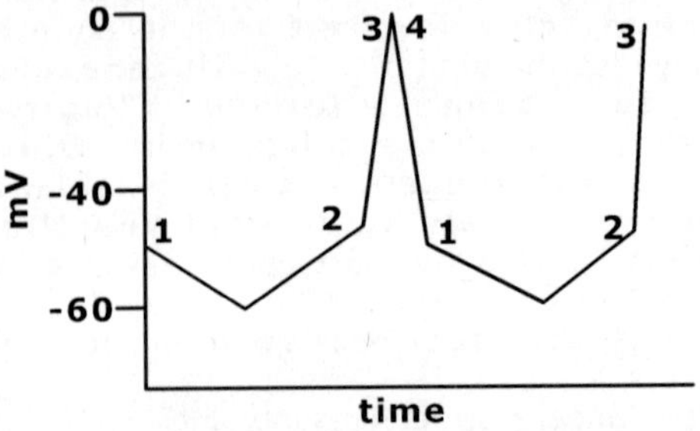

a. It denotes the membrane potential of pacemaker tissue
b. Segment 2 triggers the next impulse
c. Segment 3 is mainly due to Na+ influx
d. Segment 4 is due to K+ efflux

159 The acid fast staining **of biopsy obtained from a person having sensory loss of** skin shows following picture:

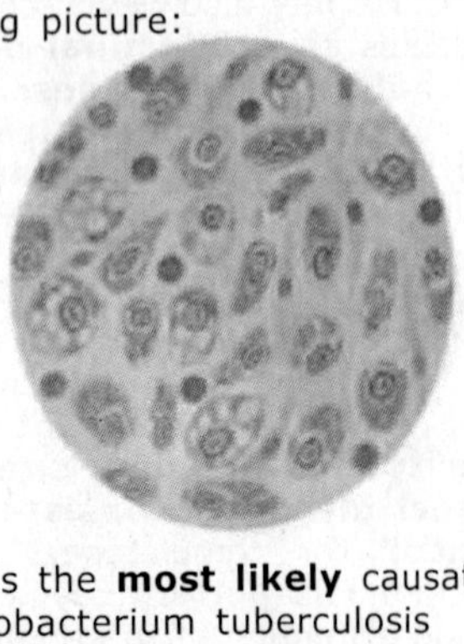

Which is the **most likely** causative organism?
a. Mycobacterium tuberculosis
b. Mycobacterium leprae
c. Anthrax bacillus
d. Clostridium

160 A patient with history of mild **diarrhoea since 11 months, presented with pain in right iliac fossa. On palpation a tender mass was palpable.** His small bowel enema showed this picture.

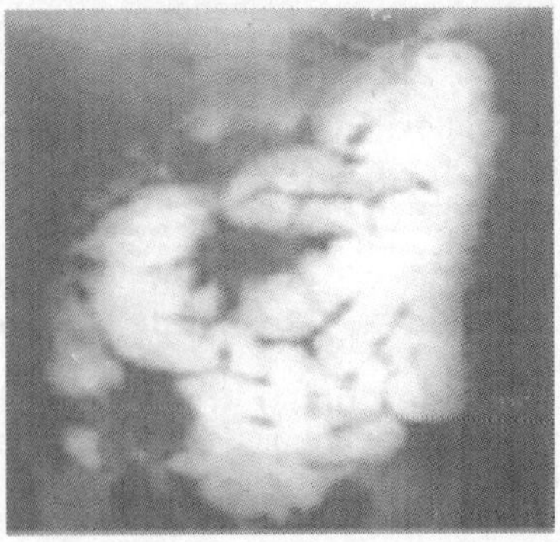

What is this radiological sign known as?
a. String sing of Kantor
b. Pincer deformity
c. Bird beak deformity
d. Coil spring sign

161 Following is the **endoscopic retrograde pancreatogram on the left and the operative pancreatogram and cholangiogram** on the right of a 25-year-old female with abdominal pain, nausea and vomiting for 20 years. The abdominal plain film was unremarkable. What is your **diagnosis**?

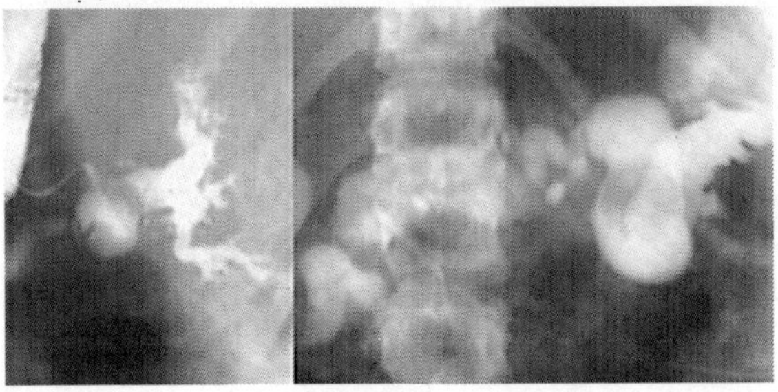

a. Hereditary pancreatitis
b. Chronic pancreatitis due to hyperparathyroidism
c. Chronic pancreatitis due to cystic fibrosis
d. Chronic pancreatitis due to cholelithiasis

162 Sangeeta a 40-year-old lady presented with **sudden onset breathlessness, right-sided chest pain and hemoptysis. She was taking oral contraceptives for last 5 years.** Laboratory tests revealed elevated levels of plasma D-dimer. Probable diagnosis of **pulmonary thrombo-embolism was made but lung scan was non-diagnostic of pulmonary embolism.** What should be the **next step (investigation)** in her evaluation?
a. Pulmonary angiogram (PAgram)
b. CT chest
c. Contrast phlebography of lower limbs
d. Ultrasonography (U/S) of lower limbs

163 A 60-year-old lady presents with right temporal **headache associated with fever, stiffness & pain in both shoulders and buttocks for last 6 months**. Last evening she developed loss of vision in right eye. On examination she has temporal **tender ness and fundus shows swollen optic disc in right eye. Laboratory investigations reveal; ESR = 150 mm in 1st hour, Hb = 8.5** gm %. The **treatment of choice** for this patient is :
a. Aspirin
b. Injection heparin
c. Corticosteroid
d. Clopidogrel

164 An adult Indian male (I.V. drug abuser) was **admitted to hospital with complain of dyspnoea.His chest X-ray reveals diffuse ground glass opacity**. **Bronchioalveolar lavage** shows thin walled trophozoites and thick walled spherical cysts containing **four or eight nuclei using methenamine** silver stain. Which of the following statement is not true :
a. Diagnosis is pneumocystis carinii pneumonia
b. Infecting organism is a fungus
c. Infecting organism specially destroy type II pneumocytes.
d. Lower lobe periphery of lung may be spared in this disease.

165 An adult male complaining of diffuse painful rash extending from mid thigh to his navel region. A skin scraping was sent to the laboratory for culture yielded a slow growing colony which produced numerous smooth walled macroconidia. Microconidia being absent. This is consistent with **isolation of a dermatophyte of genera** :
a. Trichophyton
b. Microsporum
c. Epidermophyton
d. Trichosporum

166 On 2nd day of life a new born **develops sepsis, respiratory distress and skin petechiae. On ultrasound examination he has multiple abscesses in liver and spleen. Lung and brain also shows similar lesions on CT scan.** The new born have history of preterm and prolong rupture of membrane during labour. **Diagnosis** is :
a. Granulomatosis infantisepticum
b. Staphylococcal sepsis
c. Toxic shock syndrome
d. Congenital tuberculosis

167 A 55-year-old smoker male presented with **high grade fever, cough and scanty sputum. Chest** X-ray revealed infiltrates. Patient is confused and **disoriented and reported watery diarrhoea. On laboratory examination leucocytosis, raised ESR and serum Na+ 126 mEq/L and K+ 4 mEq/L** have been found. Which test is useful for **early and specific diagnosis** of the condition :
a. Blood culture of the organism
b. Fluroscent antibody test in serum for legionella
c. ELISA in urine for detection of soluble antigen
d. A four fold or greater rise in antibody titre

168 A 20-year-old sexually active female college student presents with vaginal irritation, scant discharge, and fishy odour for 1 week. There is no dysuria. She denies any history of sexually transmitted diseases **most likely diagnosis** is:-
a. Trichomonas vaginitis
b. Candidal vaginitis
c. Gonococcal cervicitis
d. Bacterial vaginosis

169 There are two communities A and B. Both have **population of 1000 each. Prevalence of disease X in community A is 5% and in community B is 10%. same** screening test is applied for the disease in both the communities. In which of the communities more no of false positives **(People with positive test but no disease)** will be found :
a. Community A
b. Community B
c. Equal in both
d. None

170 A 40 years female presented with dysphagia **for solid food, regurgitation and weight loss. She also complains of fullness or gurgling in the chest.** These symptoms worsen whenever she eats parties and functions rapidly and exacerbates by **emotional stress. Since last 3 months she also complains of nocturnal choking or regurgitation.** X-ray chest shows widened mediastinum and air fluid level in chest. The **probable diagnosis** is :
a. GERD
b. Hiatus Hernia
c. Carcinoma Oesophagus
d. Achalasia Cardia

171 A 65-year-old male presented with **per rectal bleeding, mucous discharge and sensation of lump in anus since 3 months. Patient also complains of alteration in bowel habit. DRE revealed an ulcerated hard tender bleeding mass in anal canal**. Tissue biopsy was sent which was reported as well differentiated adenocarcinoma. **What will be the further plan of treatment**?
a. Radiotherapy
b. Chemotherapy
c. Abdominoperineal resection
d. Defuctioning colostomy alone

172 A 30-year-old woman presents with a 1.5 **cm mass below her right ear lobe. She has been aware of the mass for 4 years. Physical examination reveals a firm, non tender, movable mass and intact facial nerve function; cervical lymph nodes are not palpable**. The **most likely** diagnosis is :
a. Papillary cystadenoma lymphomatosum (Warthin's tumor)
b. Low-grade mucoepidermoid carcinoma
c. Benign mixed tumor (pleomorphic adenoma)
d. Malignant mixed tumor

173 A 35-year-old engineer presented with **bleeding from external meatus and perineal hematoma, after he fell astride on a scaffolding, half-an-hour back.** The patient had not passed urine since the accident. On physical examination there was **no evidence of extravasation of urine and the bladder was not distended.** What would be the **immediate management** ?
a. Encourage him to pass urine after adequate control of pain
b. Assess the urethral injury by ascending urethrography
c. Percutaneous suprapubic catheterisation of the bladder
d. Catheterization of the urethra

174 A 58-year-old woman with a history of **rheumatoid arthritis presents with severe pruritus,hepatomegaly, and marked elevation of her cholestasis enzymes** without elevation of bilirubin.Based on this history and her physical and laboratory abnormalities, you would expect that:

a. Mid-zonal liver cell necrosis with councilman bodies
b. Perivenular fibrosis of the terminal hepatic venules
c. "Pipe stem" cirrhosis
d. Granulomatous destruction of bile duct radicals

175 A 35-year-old-woman has been **admitted to hospital for investigation of progressive weakness in her legs, for the past 5 years.** The patient's mother **has similar difficulties with weakness and sensory problems. Examination revealed power of 3/5 distally in the upper and lower limbs with a glove and stocking pattern sensory loss to pain and touch.** The **diagnosis is** :
a. Hereditary neuropathy with liability to pressure palsies
b. Chronic inflammatory demyelinating poly-neuropathy
c. Multiple sclerosis
d. Hereditary sensory motor neuropathy

176 A 35-year-old-man is admitted with acute right **sided weakness and slurred speech. He** does not have a history of hypertension, diabetes or high **cholesterol. There is no family history of CVA. He does not smoke. He complains of headaches and generalised limb weakness infrequently. On examination, he has hypotonia and weakness** in the proximal muscles more than the distal muscles. His laboratory tests show a high lactate to pyruvate ratio. The **likely diagnosis** is :
a. Polymyositis
b. Inclusion body myositis
c. MELAS
d. Polymorphonuclear leukoencephalop

177 **Assertion A**: Omalizumab is a blocking antibody that neutralizes circulating IgM
Reason R: Omalizumab is usually given as a subcutaneous injection.
a. Both A and R are true and R is correct explanation of A
b. Both A and R are true and R is not correct explanation of A
c. A is true but R is false
d. A is false but R is true

178 **Assertion A**: **Sweat glands have** sympathetic innervation.
Reason R: Therefore **neurotransmitter is Acetylcholine.**
a. Both A and R are true and R is correct explanation of A
b. Both A and R are true and R is not correct explanation of A
c. A is true but R is false
d. A is false but R is true

179 **Assertion A**: Cockayne described syndrome as dwarfism with retinal atrophy and deafness.
Reason R: It differs from Xeroderma pigmentosa by the lack of dwarfism.
a. Both A and R are true and R is correct explanation of A
b. Both A and R are true and R is not correct explanation of A
c. A is true but R is false
d. A is false but R is true

180 **Assertion A**: **Herpes zoster** is generally limited to 1 dermatome or at most 2 or 3 adjacent dermatomes.
Reason R: The lumbar dermatomes are the most commonly involved sites.
a. Both A and R are true and R is correct explanation of A
b. Both A and R are true and R is not correct explanation of A
c. A is true but R is false
d. A is false but R is true

Ans. 1: (b) Discontinuation of oral contraceptives and a repeated CT scan of her abdomen in 3–6 months

Ref: Read the text below

Sol:

- The CT scan findings of this patient plus the history of prolonged use of oral contraceptives are **characteristic in hepatocellular adenoma.**
- Because the **tumor extensively involves both the right and left lobes of the** liver, oral contraceptive use must be discontinued, and the patient must be observed for 3–6 months. Significant reduction in size of the adenoma has been **noted in many cases after cessation of oral contraceptive use.**
- If there is no regression of lesions, then **liver transplantation should be recommended.**

Ans. 2: (b) Liver abscess

Ref: Read the text below

Sol:

- Fever, jaundice, **RUQ pain with tenderness, and leukocytosis are symptoms common** to both cholangitis and liver abscess.
- Elevation of the right diaphragm on chest x-ray favors a diagnosis of a liver abscess.
- Because of the popularity of treating **patients with cholangiocarcinoma with long-term** indwelling stents, the incidence of complications due to **pyogenic abscess has also increased.**

Ans. 3: (d) Administration of antibiotics and CT-guided percutaneous drainage

Ref: Read the text below

Sol:

- **Administration of antibiotics and CTguided percutaneous** drainage of a liver abscess (consequent to biliary stenting) can be **achieved with lower morbidity and mortality.**
- **Most pyogenic liver abscesses harbor multiple organisms (E. coli, Klebsiella, Proteus, Streptococcus, and anaerobes).**
- Broad-spectrum antibiotics should **be empirically started before the specific organism** has been identified and before sensitivities are known.
- Closed aspiration of a liver abscess without drainage is **inadequate in providing a more rapid resolution of the condition.**

Ans. 4: (d) Sigmoid diverticulitis

Ref: Read the text below

Sol:

- The most likely cause **of the finding depicted, which is** air in the bladder, is a colovesical fistula secondary to acute sigmoid **diverticulitis.**
- A renal stone, if visible at all, would be a calcific **density and would be in the dependent portion of the bladder. There is no motion visible.**
- **A bladder tumor would appear as a filling defect with the density** of soft tissue.

Ans. 5: (b) Both A and R are true and R is not correct explanation of A

Ref: Read the text below

Sol:

- Type 1 (autoimmune) diabetes mellitus is associated with MHC genes on more than one haplotype. The presence of both the DR3 and DR4 haplotypes in one individual confers a 20-fold increased risk for type 1 diabetes; the strongest single association is with DQB1*0302, and all haplotypes that carry a DQB1*0302 gene are associated with type 1 diabetes, whereas related haplotypes that carry a different DQB1 gene are not.
- However, the relative risk associated with inheritance of this gene can be modified, depending on other HLA genes present either on the same or a second haplotype.

Ans. 6: (b) Both A and R are true and R is correct explanation of A

Ref: Read the text below

Sol:

- **Because T cells are required for B cell responses to most antigens, any gene defect (or acquired disorder) that interferes with T cell development and cell-mediated immunity will also compromise antibody production and humoral immunity.**
- MHC class II deficiency results in one such immunodeficiency in that the TCRαβ? must see protein antigens as peptide fragments held within the α-helical grooves of class II and class I molecules encoded by the MHC.
- Antigen-presenting cells in individuals with this relatively rare disorder fail to express the class II molecules DP, DQ, and DR on their surface. Although some affected individuals produce CD4-bearing T lymphocytes in their thymus, these cannot recognize antigen properly to function as normal helper T cells.

Ans. 7: (b) Both A and R are true and R is not correct explanation of A

Ref: Read the text below

Sol:

- Rheumatoid nodules may develop in 20–30% of persons with RA. They are usually found on periarticular structures, extensor surfaces, or other areas subjected to mechanical pressure, but they can develop elsewhere, including the pleura and meninges. Common locations include the olecranon bursa, the proximal ulna, the Achilles tendon, and the occiput.
- Nodules vary in size and consistency and are rarely symptomatic, but on occasion they break down as a result of **trauma or become infected. They are found almost** invariably in individuals with circulating rheumatoid factor.
- Histologically, rheumatoid nodules consist of a central zone of necrotic material including collagen fibrils, **noncollagenous filaments, and cellular debris; a midzone of palisading macrophages**

that express HLA-DR antigens; and an outer zone of granulation tissue.

- Examination of early nodules has **suggested that the initial event may be a focal vasculitis. In some patients, treatment with m**ethotrexate can increase the number of nodules dramatically.

Ans. 8: (c) Oversewing the ulcer and performing a vagotomy and pyloroplasty

Ref: Read the text below

Sol:

- For the patient who is unstable and **has a pyloric or duodenal ulcer, oversewing** the ulcer and closing the pyloric incision **as a pyloroplasty and performing a vagotomy is the** procedure of choice because of its low operative mortality.
- However, this procedure carries a higher-recurrence rate.
- Major resections, such **as antrectomy and subtotal gastrectomy** are contraindicated in the unstable patient.
- At endoscopy biopsies for H. pylori should be taken and, if positive, treatment designed to eradicate H. pylori should be **started. Eradication of H. pylori reduces the recurrence rate of bleeding.**

Ans. 9: (c) It may spread rapidly through tissue planes

Ref: Read the text below

Sol:

- It is unclear **why patients develop overwhelming infection** at certain times.
- Asurgical wound must be **examined if a high fever occurs.**

Ans. 10: (a) Pseudomonas

Ref: Read the text below

Sol:

- **Ceftizoxime (Cefizox) is not effective** against many **strains of Pseudomonas.**
- If the drug is used, a higher **dosage may be indicated, and the antibiotic should** be changed if a quick response does not occur.
- Complications may occur in **patients who are allergic to penicillin.**

Ans. 11: (c) He has a history of biliary tract disease

Ref: Read the text below

Sol:

- **Pyogenic abscess** occurs after abdominal sepsis, biliary tract disease, and septicemia.
- Amebic liver **abscess should be considered, however**, if the patient has recently visited a tropical country or if **abdominal pain and diarrhea are present.**
- Metronidazole (Flagyl) is most effective in **treating amebic abscess, and laparotomy** should be avoided when possible unless complications specifically indicating intervention are present.

Ans. 12: (c) It can be partly prevented by ketoconazole

Ref: Read the text below

Sol:

- **Candida sepsis is an important** clinical problem in burn units and ICUs and in patients with immunosuppression.
- **Candida albicans is dimorphic, and both yeast and mycelial** forms are seen in infected tissues.
- Ketoconazole is given by **mouth; it cannot be given in liver disease or in a nonacid environment.**
- The main treatment of **Candida sepsis is administration of amphotericin B.**
- Actinomycin is an antibiotic that has antineoplastic action.

Ans. 13: (a) Claw hand involving the ring and little fingers

Ref: Read the text below

Sol:

- The **lumbrical muscles arise from the flexor digitorum profundus** tendons at a level distal to the small bones in the hand.
- The **hypothenar muscles are** on the ulnar side, and the thenar muscles are on the thumb side of the hand.
- The medial two **lumbrical muscles are paralyzed**, and this leads to the typical deformity.

Ans. 14: (d) The distal radial metaphysis is displaced dorsally

Ref: Read the text below

Sol:

- The distal **radial metaphysis is displaced dorsally**. This fracture was described by Colles over 150 years ago.
- The impact is caused by a fall on the **flexor surface of the wrist. The distal segment is displaced dorsally.**
- The reverse injury, involving a fall on **the extensor surface of the wrist and flexor deformity, is a Smith fracture.**
- Colles's fracture occurs more **commonly in older women. The styloid of the ulna—not the shaft of this bone—is fractured.**

Ans. 15: (d) Needle decompression

Ref: Read the text below

Sol:

- The X-ray shows a **tension pneumothorax.** Insertion of a needle in the second intercostals space, **midclavicular line can be a lifesaving procedure.**
- The diagnosis of tension pneumothorax should be made on the basis of clinical findings such as decreased **breath sounds and tympany to percussion on the affected** side. Neck veins may be destended if the patient is not phyovolemic.
- The patient will be short of **breath and hypotensive. The other answers are incorrect, especially A, which would** exacerbate the problem by introducing positive pressure into the airways.

Ans. 16: (a) 1-d; 2-c; 3-f
Ref: Read the text below
Sol:

- **WDHA, or VIPoma (vasoactive intestinal polypeptide) is characterized by voluminous** diarrhea, 5 L or more daily, rich in potassium, which looks like watery tea. The diarrhea is secretory and if refractory to antidiarrheal **agents. Patients are weak, with metabolic acidosis and hypokalemia.**
- Octreotide decreases diarrhea volume. The pancreatic tumor should be excised. Secretory diarrhea also occurs in some **patients with ZES, and is the only complaint in <10% of** ZES patients. More than 90% of ZES patients have peptic ulcer disease.
- **Unlike the diarrhea associated with ZES, the diarrhea of WDHA** continues with fasting and continuous nasogastric tub suctioning. 15% of patients with glucagonoma have diarrhea; glucagonoma is associated with migratory necrotizing dermatitis.
- **Gastrinoma, or ZES, should be suspected in patients with peptic ulcer disease refractory** to medical treatment, or in patients with multiple ulcers or ulcers in uncommon locations. **Gastrin secretion by the tumor**, most commonly found in the pancreas, results in hypersecretion of gastric acid. Common patient complaints are epigastric pain, melena, hematemesis, **diarrhea, and weight loss. ZES may occur as part of the MEN-1 syndrome; this patient presents with only atypical peptic ulcer disease. Omeprazole is the treatment of choice for control of peptic ulcers in ZES.**
- **MEN-1, or Werner's syndrome, and autosomal dominant disorder**, involves tumors or hyperplasia of two or more glands, most commonly parathyroid, pancreas, and pituitary glands.
- Hyperparathyroidism is most common, followed by various pancreatic isle cell tumors and pituitary adenomas. MEN-2A (Sipple's syndrome) consits of pheochromocytoma, medullary carcinoma of the thyroid, and often hyperparathyroidism. MEN-2B is characterized by medullary carcinoma of **the thyroid,pheochromocytoma, neuromas and marfinoid body habitus. MEN-2A and -2B are also autosomal dominant.**

Ans. 17: (b) Chronic pancreatitis
Ref: Read the text below
Sol:

- The **CT section through the upper abdomen** reveals **cal-cifications within the pancreas** and **inflammation of the peripancreatic mesenteric fat.**
- Pancreatitis classically pre-sents as **upper abdominal pain** that radiates through to the back; however, some patients **may describe it as chest pain.**

Ans. 18: (b) The steeple sign
Ref: Read the text below
Sol:

- The clinical presentation is of **croup** which is associated **with the steeple sign,** or a tapering of the **trachea on the frontal chest radiograph.**

Ans. 19: (b) T2-W images and STIR (short tau inversion recovery) sequences with fat suppression can identify tears in the supraspinatus tendon
Ref: Read the text below
Sol:

- **CT arthrography is of value** in the assessment of the glenoid labrum,the prone oblique position provides **more information about the posterior aspect of the glenoid labrum** and the capsular attachments, which are important in **patients with posterior dislocations.**
- The **supraspinatus tendon** is best seen in the coronal oblique plane.
- On **ultrasound, the supraspinatus tendinous** margin is echobright and central portion is echopoor.
- In **anterior dislocation of the shoulder**, cortical defects occur in the posterior aspect of the head of the humerus (**Hill–Sachs lesion**), which are best shown by a **Striker's view (patient** supine, **humerus 90° to the table with a cephald beam at 25°).**

Ans. 20: (b) Complete blood count (CBC)
Ref: Read the text below
Sol:

- **Bleeding occurs as a consequence of thrombocytopenia, deficiencies of coagulation factors,or both**. Thrombocytopenia usually presents as petechial bleeding that is first observed in the lower extremities.
- **Deficiencies in coagulation factor more often cause bleeding into the gastrointestinal tract or joints.** Intracranial bleeding, however, can occur with a **deficiency of platelets or coagulation factors and can be catastrophic.**
- **CBCs are routinely performed in most laboratories** through the use of an electronic particle counter,which **determines the total white blood cell and platelet counts and calculates the hematocrit and hemoglobin** from the erythrocyte count and the dimensions of the red cells.
- For this patient, a **CBC would likely disclose a decreased platelet count (thrombocytopenia).**Impaired hepatic synthetic function and vitamin K deficiency would result in prolongation of the **PT and INR. Coagulation factor deficiencies and coagulation factor inhibitors would result in prolongation of the PTT.**
- A mixing study is obtained to differentiate between a coagulation factor deficiency and a coagulation factor inhibitor by mixing patient **plasma with normal plasma in the laboratory.**

Ans. 21: (d) Extramedullary hematopoiesis

Ref: Read the text below

Sol:

- **Hematopoiesis begins in the fetal yolk sac and later occurs predominantly in the liver and the spleen.**
- Recent studies demonstrate that islands of **hematopoiesis develop in these tissues from hemangioblasts,** which are the common progenitors for both hematopoietic and endothelial cells.
- These islands then **involute as the marrow becomes the primary site for blood cell** formation by the seventh month of fetal development.
- **Barring serious damage**, such as that which occurs with myelofibrosis or radiation injury, the bone marrow remains the site of blood cell formation throughout the rest of life. In childhood, there is **active hematopoiesis in the marrow spaces of the central axial skeleton (i.e., the ribs, vertebrae, and pelvis) and the extremities, extending to the wrists, the ankles, and the calvaria.**
- With normal growth **and development, hematopoiesis gradually withdraws from the periphery. T**his change is reversible, however; distal marrow extension can result from intensive stimulation, as occurs with severe hemolytic anemias, long-term administration of hematopoietic growth factors, and hematologic malignancies.
- The term **medullary hematopoiesis refers to the production of blood cells in the bone marrow; the term extramedullary hematopoiesis indicates blood cell production outside the marrow in the spleen, liver, and** other locations.

Ans. 22: (d) Reticulocyte count

Ref: Read the text below

Sol:

- In many **renal diseases, the kidneys fail to produce sufficient amounts of erythropoietin**.
- **Replacement of endogenous erythropoietin** stimulates red cell precursors in the bone marrow to mature more quickly.
- If the patient has normal bone marrow, an **elevated reticulocyte count** should be seen several days after initiation of therapy.

Ans. 23: (c) 1-b; 2-a; 3-j

Ref: Read the text below

Sol:

- **Hereditary spherocytosis is the most common** symptomatic familial hemolytic anemia, and is transmitted as an autosomal dominant trait. A defect in the red cell membrane causes increased trapping in the **spleen and hemolysis. Anemia, jaundice, and splenomegaly are clinical findings.**
- **Splenectomy is the only treatment. Thalassemia is transmitted as a** dominant trait; anemia is the result of a defect in hemoglobin synthesis. Thalassemia major, or homozygous thalassemia, is associated with anemia, icterus, **splenomegaly, and early death. Transfusions are usually required.**
- **Splenectomy may reduce hemoloysis and transfusion requirements**. Sickle-cell anemia is hereditary hemolytic anemia. Serum bilirubin may be mildly elevated. Splenomegaly often precedes autoinfraction. Splenectomy may **be indicated for chronic hypersplenism or acute splenic sequestration.**
- In thalassemia, intracellular hemoglobin precipitates, or Heinz bodies, damage red cells and contribute to early **destruction. Cells are small, thin, misshapen, and resistant to osmotic lysis. Diagnosis is made by peripheral smear.Nucleated red cells, or target cells, are present.**
- **Distorted red cells, or target cells, are present**. Distorted red cells of different shapes and sizes are found. In sickle-cell disease, characteristic sickle cells are seen on peripheral smear. In hereditary spherocytosis, the peripheral smear shows small, thick, nearly spherical red cells. Cells have **increased osmotic fragility.**
- **The triad of rheumatoid arthritis, splenomegaly, and neutropenia** is known as Felty's syndrome. Gastic achlorhydria is common. Thrombocytopenia and mild anemia are sometimes seen. Splenectomy is sometimes used to **treat the neutopenia in patients with serious infections, anemia requiring transfusions, or severe thrombocytopenia.**

Ans. 24: (a) 1-h; 2-a

Ref: Read the text below

Sol:

- Breast cancer **commonly metastasizes to bone, lung, soft tissues, liver, and** brain. The patient should be worked up for local recurrence as well **as other distant metastasis.**
- **Benign liver cysts can be single or multiple.**
- Solitary nonparasitic **cysts usually contain clear, watery fluid. These cysts are more** common in the right lobe. They are most likely congenital and most are asymptomatic; many are found incidentally.
- An anechoic area on ultrasound is suggestive. **Hydatid cysts, caused by Echinococcus, are also more common in the right lobe. The colorless fluid** in the cyst is under high pressure, unlike parasitic cysts. Ultrasound will **show internal echoes.**
- **Hemangiomas can have a variable echogenic pattern on ultrasound; focal nodular hyperplasia is often hypodense.**
- Hepatocellular carcinoma and metastasis have a **characteristic sonographic appearance different from benign nonparasitic cysts.**

Ans. 25: (c) Tracheoesophageal fistula

Ref: Read the text below

Sol:
- It is also **commonly known as VATER association**. (vertebral, anorectal malformations, tracheoesophageal fistula, renal **and distal limb malformations).**
- The most common abnormalities are cardiac in origin and **involve ventriculoseptal defect (VSD) and atrial septal defect (ASD).**

Ans. 26: (b) Steinmann pin insertion and traction
Ref: Read the text below
Sol:
- The priorities in patient **care are to control hemorrhage in the abdomen and decompress the subdural hematoma.**
- The optional initial **surgical therapy of the supracondylar femur** fracture is the insertion of a Steinmann pin for traction.
- If traction fails to produce adequate alignment, **open reduction can be performed at a later date.**

Ans. 27: (a) Aspiration of the right chest cavity
Ref: Read the text below
Sol:
- In a patient presenting **with a chest wound in shock, the priorities are airway, breathing, and circulation.**
- **Thus, aspiration of the right chest to rule out a tension pneumothorax should be performed first.**
- Aspiration of the **pericardium does not definitively rule out cardiac injury**; a pericardial window provides both diagnosis and decompression.
- An echocardiogram is not indicated in **an unstable patient.**

Ans. 28: (d) Closure of the hole with sterile dressing
Ref: Read the text below
Sol:
- The immediate treatment is the **closure of the hole by any means available. Sucking** chest wounds allow shift of the **mediastinum to the opposite side.**
- Thoracotomy is not usually required. Laparotomy is indicated **for a gunshot wound below** the fourth intercostal space, but it should follow respiratory stabilization.
- A chest tube will be required, following closure of the **sucking wound, to prevent a tension pneumothorax.**

Ans. 29: (c) LeFort III fracture
Ref: Read the text below
Sol:
- The physical findings are characteristics of a Le Fort III fracture.
- In this injury,the fracture passes through maxilla and nasal bones and above the zygomatic bone.

Ans. 30: (b) Platelets
Ref: Read the text below
Sol:
- The **proliferation and maturation of platelets take longer than those of either red blood cells (7 to 10 days) or white blood cells (10 to 14 days)** and thus are the slowest to recover from an acute bone marrow injury, **such as occurs with chemotherapy**.

Ans. 31: (a) Serum folic acid levels more accurately reflect tissue stores than do red blood cell folic acid levels
Ref: Read the text below
Sol:
- Patients with **megaloblastic anemia who do not have glossitis**, a family history of pernicious anemia, or the neurologic features **described for cobalamin deficiency may have folic acid deficiency.**
- **Tests to determine folic acid deficiency vary in their accuracy**. Serum folic acid levels are less reliable than red blood cell folic acid levels.
- A serum folic acid level of **less than 2 ng/ml is consistent with folic acid deficiency, as is a red blood cell folic acid level of less than 150 ng/ml.** Because the combination of folic acid and iron deficiency is common, full **expression of megaloblastosis is often blocked**, and the patient will have a dimorphic anemia rather than the easily identifiable macro-ovalocytosis.
- **Hypersegmentation of PMNs persists**. The serum folic acid level decreases within 2 weeks after dietary folic acid ingestion completely ceases. Therefore, many hospitalized patients have low serum folic acid levels without real tissue folic acid deprivation.
- In **evaluating patients for folic acid deficiency, values for the levels of serum folic acid, serum cobalamin, and red blood cell folic acid** must be obtained. The red blood cell folic acid level reflects tissue stores.
- When it is difficult but necessary to distinguish the megaloblastosis of cobalamin deficiency from that of folic acid deficiency, **measurements of the serum methylmalonic acid and homocysteine levels are helpful.**

Ans. 32: (a) Ringed sideroblasts and ineffective erythropoiesis
Ref: Read the text below
Sol:
- **Sideroblastic anemias** are a heterogeneous group of disorders characterized by anemia and the presence **of ringed sideroblasts in the marrow.**
- There are **hereditary forms and acquired forms**, which are further subdivided into benign and malignant variants.
- **Abnormalities of heme synthesis** are the usual causes. Iron enters the RBC precursor but cannot be incorporated and accumulates to form ringed sideroblasts.

- The **diagnosis is established by the presence of reticulcytopenia and ringed sideroblasts** in the bone marrow. Cytogenetic studies of the bone marrow may reveal changes seen in myelodysplastic syndromes.
- **Alcohol abuse can cause a reversible form of sideroblastic anemia, and stopping alcohol is an important aspect of patient care.**

Ans. 33: (c) 8 years
Ref: Read the text below
Sol:
- The radiograph of the **wrist reveals a torus fracture of the radial metaphysis**.This is associated with a fall onto an out-stretched hand in a **child 5 to 10 years old.**
- A **two-month-old** would have a bowing type deformity after trauma.
- A 2-**year-ald would** most likely have a greenstick type frac ture.
- An adult would **likely have a Colle's type fracture.**

Ans. 34: (b) Tension pneumothorax
Ref: Read the text below
Sol:
- **Shift of the trachea** strongly **suggests a tension pneumothorax.**
- Subcutaneous emphysema is also more common with a **tension pneumothorax than with the other conditions listed.**
- Simple pneumothorax and chest wall laceration are **much less serious injuries than tension pneumothorax.**

Ans. 35: (c) CT scan with oral and intravenous contrast
Ref: Read the text below
Sol:
- **CT scan with oral and intravenous contrast** gives the best sensitivity and specificity in diagnosing blunt trauma to the pancreas.
- **ERCP could be useful in studying the integrity of the** pancreatic duct, but a CT scan is more accurate in revealing traumatic **pancreatitis without major ductal injury. An upper GI series may show widening of the duodenal C-loop.**
- **An isolated serum amylase elevation is not diagnostic** of pancreatic injury.
- Repeated testing of amylase levels, if amylase **levels increase with time, may be more diagnostic of traumatic pancreatitis than a single value.**

Ans. 36: (c) Exploratory laparotomy
Ref: Read the text below
Sol:
- The patient should prepared **and draped, with the nasogastric** tube and Foley catheter inserted, and then anesthetized **immediately prior to laparotomy.**
- Some surgeons initially control the aorta **through a thoracotomy incision through** the seventh intercostal space.
- Transfusion before control of **bleeding causes more bleeding.**

Ans. 37: (c) Apply direct pressure with sterile gauze
Ref: Read the text below
Sol:
- Apply direct pressure with **sterile gauze. Direct pressure is the best choice.**
- Attempting to clamp vessels can cause further vascular or **nerve injury. Tourniquet is used only if direct pressure fails.**
- As soon as direct pressure is attempted, a second **person should insert a large-bore peripheral intravenous line.**

Ans. 38: (b) ORIF of fracture plus three-compartment fasciotomy
Ref: Read the text below
Sol:
- A tense calf **with comminuted fractures (fractures exposed to exterior**) and pain on dorsiflexion necessitates a fasciotomy **because of the very high probability of a compartment syndrome.**
- Arterial injury is possible (but rare) in **lower leg injuries if the pulses are palpable.**

Ans. 39: (c) Displace the uterus to the left
Ref: Read the text below
Sol:
- Displace **the uterus to the left.**
- The first step in **restoring cardiac return in a patient** in the third trimester who has become hypovolemic is to displace the gravid **uterus off the vena cava by pushing it to the left**.
- The other choices (except for the use of the PASG) should be **considered following displacement of the uterus.**

Ans. 40: (c) Fat embolus
Ref: Read the text below
Sol:
- **Fat embolus** is usually associated with long bone or pelvic fractures and is associated with petechiae.
- Transfusion and **antibiotic reactions causing hypotension would occur relatively** quickly following administration.

Ans. 41: (c) Exsanguinating hemorrhage
Ref: Read the text below
Sol:
- **Exsanguinating hemorrhage is the predominant** risk, because bleeding may not be easily recognized, given that bleeding **into the pleural cavity and mediastinum can occur.**
- The abundant collateral blood supply generally protects against **upper extremities or cerebrovascular compromise.**

Ans. 42: (b) 1-c; 2-e; 3-a
Ref: Read the text below
Sol:

- The history is **typical of spontaneous pneumothorax**.Physical examination will reveal diminished breath sounds on the side of collapse and x-ray will confirm the diagnosis. A tension pneumothorax will cause hypotesios.
- **Lateral impact may cause fracture ribs causing** pain, difficulty in breathing, and may be associated with significant hemorrhage from intercostal vessels. The physical signs described are those of a massive hemothorax.
- **Precordial stab wound, distended jugular** veins, and hypotension should suggest a cardiac tamponade. It must be kept in mind that the same signs are those of a tension pneumothorax. Dyspnea and **deviation of trachea to the opposite side, absent breath sounds, and hyperresonant percussion note should** suggest the correct diagnosis.

Ans. 43: (c) 1-b; 2-f; 3-e
Ref: Read the text below
Sol:

- **Atemporal skull fracture crossing the** middle meningeal artery grove with lucid interval are pathognomonic of an **extradural hemorrhage.**
- **Head-on collision and bent steering** wheel should raise suspicion for head injuries, facial fractures, and **deceleration injuries.** The impact of knee against the dash-board forces the head of the femur posteriorly in **the acetabular socket and may** cause acetabular fracture.
- **Multiple rib fracture with often** multiple fractures in the same segment of a rib may cause flail chest and contribute to pain and hypoxia. It is the underlying pulmonary contusion that will determine the extent of **respiratory failure.**

Ans. 44: (b) Autoimmune hemolytic anemia may be idiopathic or secondary to disorders such as systemic lupus erythematosus, chronic lymphocytic leukemia (CLL), HIV infection, or hepatitis C infection
Ref: Read the text below
Sol:

- **Intravascular hemolysis** in autoimmune hemolytic anemia is rare and indicates that an extremely rapid rate of erythrocyte **destruction is occurring or that the extravascular removal mechanisms have been overwhelmed.**
- **Erythrocytes sensitized to IgG alone** are usually removed in the spleen, whereas RBCs sensitized to IgG plus complement or to complement alone are generally destroyed in the liver, because **hepatic Kupffer cells carry receptors specific for complement component C3b.**
- **Both an idiopathic variety of autoimmune hemolytic** anemia and a variety that occurs secondary to other disorders have been described. Such primary disorders include systemic lupus erythematosus, non-Hodgkin lymphoma (especially chronic lymphocytic leukemia), **Hodgkin disease, cancer, myeloma,dermoid cyst, HIV infection, angioimmunoblastic lymphadenopathy with dysproteinemia, hepatitis C infection, and chronic ulcerative colitis.**
- **Approximately 20% of patients remain well indefinitely after steroid therapy**, but the majority suffer from a chronic, treacherous disease that can produce sudden relapses with abrupt anemia.
- If the **corticosteroid dose required for long-term therapy produces significant morbidity, one can proceed empirically either to splenectomy** or to the use of immunosuppressive agents.
- **Splenectomy rarely results in extended remission but is valuable as a prednisone-sparing measure.**

Ans. 45: (b) Risk factors that predispose to painful crises include a hemoglobin level greater than 8.5 g/dl, pregnancy, cold weather, and a high reticulocyte count
Ref: Read the text below
Sol:

- **Sickle cell disease** develops in persons who are homozygous for the sickle gene (HbSS), in whom 70% to **98% of hemoglobin is of the S type**.
- **About 0.2% of African Americans** have sickle cell anemia. Risk factors that predispose to painful crises include **a hemoglobin level greater than 8.5 g/dl, pregnancy, cold weather, and a high reticulocyte count**.
- **Conversely, the low hematocrit** in sickle cell anemia reduces blood viscosity and is protective. The most definitive tests for sickle cell anemia are hemoglobin electrophoresis or high-performance liquid chromatography, which indicate the relative percentages of HbS and HbF.
- **Hydroxyurea produces an increase in F reticulocyte and HbF levels. In a phase III trial**, patients treated with hydroxyurea (starting dosage, 15 mg/kg/day) had fewer painful crises, fewer admissions for crisis, and fewer episodes of **acute chest syndrome and required fewer transfusions than patients given a placebo.**
- There was **no effect on stroke; however, after 8 years of follow-up, mortality was reduced by 40%.**

Ans. 46: (b) Phlebotomy and hydroxyurea
Ref: Read the text below
Sol:

- The **elevated hematocrit level**, reduced serum erythropoietin level, headache, fever, memory difficulties, and **weight loss seen in this patient are characteristic of polycythemia vera.**
- Although there is **not an overall consensus on treatment of polycythemia vera**, phlebotomy is frequently used as an initial treatment.

- Because this patient is **older than 70 years and has previously had a thrombotic event, a myelosuppressive agent such as hydroxyurea should be used in addition to phlebotomy**.
- This combination of hydroxyurea and phlebotomy has been demonstrated to be an effective therapeutic regimen in **controlling the hematocrit in most patients with polycythemia vera and in lowering the risk of thrombosis that occurs with use of phlebotomy alone.**
- When **hydroxyurea is used, complete blood counts should** be frequently monitored to avoid excessive myelosuppression.
- Patients may experience painful leg ulcers. Two reports have shown an increased risk of acute myeloid **leukemia in patients taking hydroxyurea, although it remains controversial whether the use of hydroxyurea increases the risk of acute myeloid leukemia.**

Ans. 47: (d) With serious bacterial infections, characteristic morphologic changes of the neutrophils include increased numbers of band forms and increased numbers of cells with Dohle bodies and toxic granulations
Ref: Read the text below
Sol:

- **Neutrophilia, or granulocytosis, is usually defined as a neutrophil count greater than 10,000/mm^3.**
- **Neutrophilia** most often occurs secondary to inflammation, stress, or corticosteroid therapy. **Neutrophilia is also associated with splenectomy.**
- Serious bacterial infections and chronic inflammation are usually associated with changes in both the number of **circulating neutrophils and their morphology.**
- Characteristic changes include increased numbers of young cells (bands), increased numbers of cells with residual endoplasmic **reticulum (Dohle bodies), and increased numbers of cells with more prominent primary granules (toxic granulation).**
- These changes are probably caused by the endogenous production of granulocyte colony-stimulating factor or **granulocyte-macrophage colony-stimulating factor and are also seen with the administration of these growth factors.**

Ans. 48: (c) Metastases
Ref: Read the text below
Sol:

- The **CT scan reveals multiple round, well-demarcated foci consistent with multiple metastases.**
- **Abscesses are not consistent with the history. Intracerebral hematomas** would not appear so focal and weil circumscribed.
- **Multiple sclerosis** does not usually have any findings on CT and can be seen only on MRI.
- **Glioblastoma multiforme is com-monly a large infiltrating lesion with surrounding edema.**

Ans. 49: (c) 1-c; 2-d; 3-e; 4-a
Ref: Read the text below
Sol:

- The 30-year-old-**female with mitral valve prolapse** has developed subacute bacterial endocarditis. The likely etiologic agent **is a viridans streptococci.**
- Viridans streptococci cause most cases of **subacute bacterial endocarditis. No other agent listed is likely to cause this infection.**
- The 80-year-old-male with a Foley catheter in place has developed a nosocomial infection likely secondary to **urosepsis. Providencia species frequently cause urinary tract infection in the hospitalized patient.**
- The young man with a fluctuant lesion and fistula over the mandible presents a classic picture of cervicofacial **actinomycosis.**
- **The sickle cell anemia patient who presents** with concomitant pneumonia and meningitis has overwhelming infection with S. **pneumoniae due to functional asplenia. S.** pneumoniae causes a particularly severe infection associated with sickle cell disease.

Ans. 50: (c) 1-c; 2-d; 3-e; 4-a; 5-b
Ref: Read the text below
Sol

- **Pneumonia due to P. carinii** was among the first recognized manifestations of AIDS. The chest radiograph typically shows **a diffuse bilateral interstitial pattern, but other patterns, including a normal radiograph, may occur.**
- **Pneumocystis infection may also occur at extrapulmonary** sites. Cytomegalovirus (CMV) is a frequent disseminated pathogen that causes retinitis that may lead to blindness. CMV may also cause pneumonitis, **adrenalitis, and hepatitis, as well as colitis with significant diarrhea.**
- The **protozoan Cryptosporidium may cause a chronic diarrhea that leads to malabsorption and wasting. It can be diagnosed** by direct examination of the stool with special concentration or staining **techniques or both. Salmonella infections have been recognized with increased frequency in patients with HIV**.
- These patients are typically bacteremic and develop bacteremic relapse; they do not usually present with a diarrheal **illness. Patients who present with seizures warrant evaluation for toxoplasmosis.**
- CNS lymphoma and certain **other infections may also cause seizures.** Patients with toxoplasmic encephalitis may also have toxoplasmic **chorioretinitis, although CMV remains the most common identified cause of retinitis in patients with AIDS.**

Ans. 51: (b) Bronchoscopy and transbronchial lung biopsy
Ref: Read the text below
Sol:
- **Sarcoidosis is a systemic illness** of unknown etiology. Many patients have respiratory symptoms, including cough and dyspnea.
- Hilar and peripheral **lymphadenopathy is common, and** 20 to 30% of patients have hepatomegaly. The chest x-ray shows symmetrical hilar lymphadenopathy.
- The diagnostic method of choice is **transbronchial biopsy, which will show a mononuclear cell granulomatous inflammatory** process.
- While liver and scalene node biopsies are often positive, noncaseating granulomas are so frequent in these sites that they are not **considered acceptable for primary diagnosis. ACE levels are elevated in twothirds of patients, but false**-positive values are common in other granulomatous disease processes.

Ans. 52: (a) Visual impairment
Ref: Read the text below
Sol:
- According to a study carried out by the **Voluntary Health Association of India, 88%** of the elderly reporting any ailment had **visual impairment, 40% had locomotor disorders, 13% had skin conditions and 8% had psychiatric problems**.

Ans. 53: (d) Negatively skewed
Ref: Read the text below
Sol:
- For a symmetric curve **such as gaussian - mean, median and mode coincide**. That is, they are the same value.
- A skewed distribution will have different mean, median and **mode. In fact, very different values of mean, median and mode is a clear indication of skewness.**

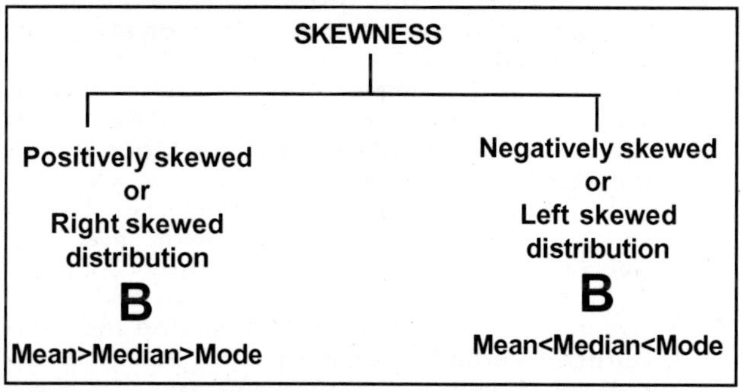

Ans. 54: (b) Radial nerve
Ref: Read the text below
Sol:
- The **radiograph demonstrates a transverse fracture of the distal half of the humeral shaft**. The radial nerve runs in a groove on the **posterior aspect of the humerus** as it courses into the forearm compartment and is **therefore at high risk of injury.**
- If the **nerve injury is apparent before any manipulation has been done**, the fracture should be reduced; the nerve injury should be observed since the nerve function will likely improve with time.
- If the **nerve injury is only present after reduction, immediate surgical exploration is warranted because the nerve might be trapped in the fracture site**. At this level of the arm, the ulnar and median nerves are well protected by muscle.
- The **posterior interosseous nerve** is a distal branch of the radial nerve and may be injured in fractures near the radial head, but it is in no danger from injuries at the level seen in this radiograph.**There is no "ascending circumflex brachial nerve".**

Ans. 55: (b) Manometry can be expected to show high resting pressures of the lower esophageal sphincter
Ref: Read the text below
Sol:
- **Patients with achalasia** typically present with distal esophageal obstruction, which leads to regurgitation **of saliva and undigested food.**
- The characteristic appearance of **the esophagram is the tapered "bird's beak" deformity at the level of the esophagogastric junction.**
- Chest pain may be seen in the early **stages of the disease. Manometry** yields high resting pressures of the lower esophageal sphincter, which fails to relax or only partially relaxes. The absence of peristaltic deglutitory contractions in the body of the esophagus is also noted during manometry.
- Although both **surgical intervention and forceful dilation** have been used to treat this disease, surgery results in improvement in over 90% of patients, compared with only 70% of patients treated by forceful dilation.
- Surgical treatment is an **esophagomyotomy. Patients with achalasia have seven times the risk of developing squamous cell carcinoma as compared with the general population.** This dreaded complication can occur even after successful treatment for the disease.

Ans. 56: (d) The chance for eventual continence is greater when the rectum has descended to below the levator ani muscles
Ref: Read the text below
Sol:
- Imperforate anus affects **males and females with equal frequency, occurring** in 1 of each 20,000 live births.
- It is due to failure of descent **of the urorectal septum. Imperforate anus may be broadly classified into "high" or "low",** depending on whether the rectum ends above or below the level of the levator ani complex. In 90% of females, but only 50% of males, the lesion is of the low variety.
- The rectal fistula may **end in the prostatic urethra or vagina in the high cases, while the low cases terminate in a perineal fistula.**

- For the low cases, only a **perineal operation** may be required and these children will be expected to be continent. A pull-through procedure will be required for the high imperforate anus and the likelihood of continence is smaller.
- If there is **doubt about the level or location of the termination of the rectum**, it is better to perform a temporary colostomy than to compromise **the ultimate chances of continence by an injudicious perineal approach.**

Ans. 57: (c) Parastomal hernia

Ref: Read the text below

Sol:

- The **most frequent serious complication of end colostomies is parastomal herniation**, which commonly occurs when the stoma is placed lateral to, rather than through, the rectus muscle.
- **Symptomatic herniation requires operative relocation of the stoma or mesh herniorrhaphy.** Minor problems are frequently encountered with colostomies.
- They include irregularity of function, irritation of the skin due to leakage of enteric contents, or **bleeding from the exposed mucosa following trauma.**
- **Prolapse occurs most frequently with transverse loop colostomies** and is likely due to the use of the transverse loop to decompress distal colon obstructions. As the intestine decompresses, it retracts from the edge of the surrounding fascia, which allows prolapse or herniation of the mobile transverse colon.
- **Optimal treatment of stomal prolapsed is restoration of intestinal continuity or conversion to an end colostomy**.Perforation of a stoma is usually due to careless instrumentation with an irrigation catheter.
- Perforations that cause minimal **peritoneal contamination may be treated with observation and antibiotics, while more extensive leaks require operative closure.**

Ans. 58: (b) Stage B

Ref: Read the text below

Sol:

- The **ACC/AHA classification** is a departure from the traditional New York Heart Association (**NYHA) classification, which characterizes patients by symptom severity**.
- The aim of the **new ACC/AHA guidelines** is to identify patients at risk for developing heart failure. Early recognition of contributing risk factors, as well as the identification and treatment of asymptomatic patients with ventricular dysfunction, can prevent pathologic progression to symptomatic heart failure.
- **Stage A** identifies patients who are at high risk for developing heart failure but who have no apparent structural abnormality of the heart.
- **Stage B denotes patients with a structural abnormality of the heart but in whom symptoms of heart failure have not yet developed.**
- **Stage C** refers to patients with a structural abnormality of the heart and symptoms of heart failure.
- **Stage D** includes the patient with end-stage heart failure that is refractory to standard treatment. This patient has stage B heart failure.
- **The goal of therapy is aimed at preventing progression to stage C or D**.

Ans. 59: (b) Implantable cardioverter defibrillator (ICD)

Ref: Read the text below

Sol:

- The **management of heart failure has** evolved from primarily noninvasive medical therapies to include invasive medical devices.
- In **addition to contributing to worsening heart** failure, ventricular arrhythmias are a likely direct cause of death in many of these **patients;the rate of sudden cardiac death in persons with heart failure is six to nine times that seen in the general population.**
- The **use of ICDs for the primary prevention of sudden death** in patients with left ventricular dysfunction has grown enormously in recent years.
- There is **increasing evidence that ICD placement** reduces mortality in patients with ischemic cardiomyopathy,regardless of whether they have **nonsustained ventricular arrhythmias**. The role of these devices in patients with heart failure of a nonischemic cause has yet to be elucidated and is the subject of several ongoing trials.
- **Biventricular pacing improves** prognosis in patients with severe CHF but has no role in the management of lethal arrhythmias.**Both IABP and VAD** are mechanical devices utilized as a bridge to cardiac transplantation for patients with very severe CHF.

Ans. 60: (d) Pulsus alternans

Ref: Read the text below

Sol:

- **Mitral regurgitation** resulting from annular dilatation is commonly audible in systolic heart failure. However, **the regurgitant murmur is generally** no louder than grade II to grade III in intensity and will wax and wane, depending on the extent of left ventricular dilatation.
- **Murmurs of greater intensity should suggest intrinsic rather than functional valve disease.Paradoxical splitting of S2 can occur** in systolic chronic heart failure as a result of either left bundle branch block or reversal **of A2 and P2 caused by prolonged ejection of blood by the impaired left ventricle.**
- Fixed splitting of S2 is associated with atrial septal defect or right ventricular failure. Orthopnea is not specific to CHF. Patients with COPD also find it easier to breathe with the head of the bed and thorax elevated. A **presystolic, or S4, gallop indicates reduced compliance of the left ventricle but not a failing left ventricle per se.**
- Pulsus **alternans, characterized by alternating** weaker and stronger pulsations in the peripheral arteries, indicates a diseased left ventricle with poor systolic function. Pulsus alternans will usually be accompanied by an S3 gallop.

Ans. 61: (c) Oral bioavailability of loop diuretics varies little from drug to drug

Ref: Read the text below

Sol:

- **Thiazides** may precipitate or exacerbate hyperglycemia, worsen hyperuricemia, and decrease sexual function.
- The blood level **of digoxin will plateau 7 days (four to five halflives)** after initiation of regular maintenance doses without loading, making this approach satisfactory for gradually increasing the digoxin levels of outpatients.
- The oral bioavailability **of furosemide varies widely (10% to 100%), but absorption of torsemide and bumetanide** is nearly complete, ranging from 80% to 100%. Of the potassium-sparing diuretics, spironolactone has been associated with gynecomastia; amiloride has been **associated with impotence; and triamterene has been associated with kidney stones.**
- Diuretic unresponsiveness may be caused by excessive sodium intake, use of agents that antagonize their effects (**NSAIDs), chronic renal dysfunction, or compromised renal blood flow.**

Ans. 62: (b) Furosemide
Ref: Read the text below
Sol:

- One important goal in **the management of CHF is to distinguish CHF caused by systolic** dysfunction from CHF caused by diastolic dysfunction, because therapies for the two differ distinctly.
- The goal of **treatment for CHF caused by diastolic dysfunction** is to reduce symptoms by lowering filling pressures without significantly compromising forward cardiac output.
- Symptom control is best achieved with **nitrates and mild diuresis**. Other goals of therapy are control of hypertension and tachycardia and alleviation of myocardial **ischemia. No pharmacologic agents have been shown to effectively improve diastolic distensibility or mortality.**

Ans. 63: (d) ACE inhibitor therapy can be started, provided it is accompanied by careful monitoring of his creatinine and potassium levels
Ref: Read the text below
Sol:

- All patients **with CHF should be on an ACE inhibitor** unless there is a very good reason not to use one.
- The only patients with **CHF in whom an ACE inhibitor cannot be used are those in whom an ACE inhibitor causes hypersensitivity,** hyperkalemia, or cough or those with bilateral renal artery stenosis. Neither this patient's age nor his creatinine level is a contraindication to **ACE inhibitor use (in fact, the improved forward flow may actually increase his glomerular filtration rate and improve his renal function).**
- His creatinine and potassium levels should be **checked 1 to 2 weeks** after starting the medication to ensure that the creatinine level has not increased by more **than 25% and that his potassium level is less than 5.0 mmol/L.**
- Preliminary data suggested that **angiotensin II receptor blockers** were preferred over ACE inhibitors in older patients, but a larger trial **failed to confirm these results.**

Ans. 64: (c) 0.45
Ref: Read the text below
Sol:

PROBABILITY AND IT'S RULES

Probability is the extent of belief in a phenomenon or a statement.

- **Addition rule :**
  - P(A or B) = P(A) + P(B) if A and B are mutually exclusive.
- **Multiplication rule :** P(A and B) = P(A) × P(B) if A and B are independent.
  - **e.g. Getting Rh +ve and being male both are independent factors so we apply rule of multiplication to get the probability.**

Ans. 65: (a) Ask the patient to keep a record for her physical discomfort and mood during the next 3 menstrual cycles
Ref: Read the text below
Sol:

- Before **treating premenstrual dysphoric disorder**, an accurate diagnosis must be established by asking the **patient to track her symptoms.**
- Several **tracking journals are available for accurate reporting**. If the suspected diagnosis is confirmed, **low-dose SSRI therapy** taken intermittently during the luteal phase of the menstrual cycle has been shown to be helpful.
- **Buspirone is not indicated for the treatment of premenstrual dysphoric disorder.**

Ans. 66: (c) Initiate a 6-week trial of fluoxetine and schedule follow-up visits
Ref: Read the text below
Sol:

- This patient's symptoms are **characteristic of binge-eating disorder, which is characterized by episodes of binge eating without bulimia**. The prevalence is 2% in the general population and 45% in obese persons.
- Although **cognitive behavioral therapy** may help reduce binge-eating, it does not seem to affect weight. Most studies have **focused on the use of SSRIs and d-fenfluramine.**
- **Fluoxetine reportedly reduces** both binging frequency and body weight.Preliminary studies suggest that **sibutramine is a possible adjunctive treatment for bingeeating** disorder, but serious adverse reactions have been reported.
- As a result, physicians must closely **supervise patients taking this drug.**

Ans. 67: (c) Early mobilization, air stirrup, strengthening, and proprioceptive exercise
Ref: Read the text below

Sol:

- The patient has **no signs that suggest the need for x-ray according to the Ottawa ankle rules.**
- There is **no evidence to suggest that surgical repair of a stable ankle** provides better outcomes.
- Early mobilization with strengthening and proprioceptive exercises would give this man the best chance of returning to play **at his former competitive level.**

Ans. 68: (c) Instruct the nurse to insert 2 large-bore IV lines, order type and crossmatch testing for administration of 2 units of packed red blood cells, and begin IV fluid resuscitation

Ref: Read the text below

Sol:

- This patient has **a postpartum hemorrhage and needs to be evaluated for the cause**. Initial management should always include fluid resuscitation.
- The most common **cause of postpartum hemorrhage is uterine atony.**
- Other causes include **tissue trauma, retained products of conception, and clotting disorders.**
- The patient **has already received oxytocin**, which is the drug of choice for treatment, so methylergonovine **would be appropriate once the source of the hemorrhage has been determined.**

Ans. 69: (d) Order laboratory evaluation of complete blood cell (CBC) count; liver function tests; uric acid, BUN, and creatinine levels; 24-hour urine collection for determination of total protein level

Ref: Read the text below

Sol:

- This patient probably has **gestational hypertension and needs an evaluation for preeclampsia.** Gestational hypertension is defined as a systolic BP of 140 mm Hg or a diastolic BP of 90 mm Hg on at least 2 measurements obtained at least 6 hours apart after 20 weeks' gestation in a **previously normotensive patient.**
- Preeclampsia is gestational hypertension **with proteinuria of 300 mg protein during a 24-hour urine collection.** Preeclampsia is a multisystem disease and laboratory evaluation is required. Fetal evaluation is also appropriate at this time.
- This patient does not need to be admitted unless the results of the laboratory testing and the **physical examination are abnormal or the antepartum fetal testing results are not reassuring.**

Ans. 70: (b) Start an IV bolus of normal saline at 100 cc/h and reevaluate after the initial bolus

Ref: Read the text below

Sol:

- This infant's history and clinical **assessment are consistent with hypovolemic shock**. The first step would be to give the infant a bolus of **isotonic normal saline or lactated Ringer's solution at 20 cc/kg.**
- The infant should then be **reassessed clinically for further treatment**. This is considered an emergency, and fluid resuscitation should not be **delayed for laboratory or radiologic evaluation.**

Ans. 71: (d) Test for high-risk subtypes of human papillomavirus (HPV) and, if positive, perform colposcopy

Ref: Read the text below

Sol:

- A **small but important minority of women** with atypical squamous cells of undetermined significance has high-**grade squamous intraepithelial lesions on colposcopy and biopsy.**
- **Testing for high-risk HPV subtypes** is an effective method of determining the need for colposcopy.
- An **accepted alternative is** repeat Pap smear testing, with colposcopy performed if the Pap smear reveals **atypical squamous cells of undetermined significance or a higher-grade lesion.**

Ans. 72: (b) Age related macular degeneration

Ref: Read the text below

Sol:

- **Indocyanine Green Chorioangiography (ICG) is a procedure** which images a layer of the posterior part of the eye. This **layer, the choroid**, is deeper than the retina and normally obscured by pigmentation. The choroid contains a unique network of blood vessels. These blood vessels flow very fast and probably help to control the temperature of the eyeball in addition to **carrying nutrients to the photoreceptors that convert light into vision. Unfortunately, these large, fast flowing vessels can be affected by disease and change as we age.**
- The **most practical clinical application of the procedure** has been in those patients with **age related macular degeneration (ARMD). This is the leading cause of new blindness in** patients over 55 years. ARMD has two forms. Most often, the loss of vision is due to slow, painless atrophy over the course of our life. The pigmentation breaks down and the visual receptors are slowly lost. This is called atrophic or dry ARMD. There is little in the way of positive treatment. About l5 - 20% of the time, patients' develop a new vessels which is growing from the rich choroidal vessels and up into and among the visual receptors. The vessels push the receptors away from their usual position and visual problems result. This condition is called exudative or wet ARMD. The specialist can use a special laser to close off these vessels and

prevent further damage. These vessels can grow very fast. They leak fluid and can hemorrhage. When that happens, the doctor can't see them clearly. They are called "occult" new vessels, meaning that they are obscured by fluid or blood.

- **A fluorescein angiogram might do a good job of showing where the laser should be pointed when there is nothing in the way. In occult situations, however, many ophthalmologists want to see an ICG study in addition, to confirm their suspicions or to provide a better idea of where the laser should be done. In wet ARMD patients, about 15 - 30% of the time, an ICG study might be helpful. This is a relatively small percentage of patients that have either form of ARMD.**

Ans. 73: (d) Choroid plexus
Ref: Read the text below
Sol:

- **Choroid plexus** is not a pain producing structure.
- **Much of the brain parenchyma, ventricular ependyma, pial veins and choroids plexus are not pain-producing structures.**
- **Few cranial structures are pain producing** - The scalp, middle meningeal artery,dural sinuses, falx cerebri and proximal segments of large pial arteries.
- The key structures involved in **primary headache** are few and the large intracranial vessels and **durameter innervated by the trigeminal nerve.**

Ans. 74: (a) Increased chest compliance
Ref: Read the text below
Sol:

- With **normal aging,** growth and development of the human lung continues to about age 20. Following the **variable period of stability**, many parameters of function decline steadily with advancing age.
- With **advancing age, loss of elastic recall causes closure of small airways** in the lower regions of the lung during normal respiration and decreases gas exchange, resulting in an increased residual volume and a **lower resting serum oxygen tension. Decreased lung elasticity is a result of changes in collagen.**
- **Respiratory muscle strength and endurance decreases with age.** There is decreased chest compliance with normal aging, not **increased chest compliance.**

Ans. 75: (c) Iodide oxidation and binding to tyrosine in the follicle lumen
Ref: Read the text below
Sol:

- **Thyroid peroxidase** is the enzyme responsible for iodide oxidation and binding to tyrosine in **the follicle lumen.**
- The other steps in thyroid synthesis including cleavage of iodine from iodinated **tyrosines, endocytosis of colloid, movement of iodide** from plasma into thyroid cells, and separation of thyroxine from thyroglobulin in lysosomes,do not require thyroid peroxidase and would therefore **not be inhibited in the transgenic animal.**

Ans. 76: (b) Cognitive behavioral therapy
Ref: Read the text below
Sol:

- The woman **experienced a panic attack, which can mimic heart attacks**. After the resolution of a panic attack, the **medical evaluation would be normal**, which distinguishes these attacks from multiple heart attacks.
- The **most appropriate nonpharmacologic therapy is cognitive behavioral therapy.** The goal of this therapy is to change the way a patient interprets the world in order to change the patient's response to problems. For patients who experience panic attacks, cognitive behavioral therapy can help them to increase **adaptive behavior and decrease emotional distress, thereby decreasing the amount of panic attacks. Assertiveness training is a subtype of cognitive behavioral therapy.**
- However, it is **not the most appropriate therapy since it only address one aspect of the woman's disorder.** Assertiveness training may help decrease social anxiety, but if that is not the only trigger for this woman's panic attacks, then it would not be sufficient for therapy.
- **Dynamic psychotherapy** is a form of talking and relational therapy that is best used for adjustment, personality, depressive, and eating disorders. It also takes several months to years for the therapy to be effective. Therefore, it would not be appropriate for helping the woman with her recurrent panic attacks.
- **Psychoanalysis is a specific type of treatment where the analyst, upon hearing the thoughts of the patient, formulates and then explains the unconscious basis for the patient's symptoms and character problems.** It can be used for panic attacks and anxiety disorders, but it would not be the most appropriate therapy since this woman would benefit more from relaxation training and systemic desensitization that are associated with cognitive behavioral therapy.
- **Psychodrama is a kind of group therapy** in which group members act out their problems in a way to better understand conflicts between people. This type of therapy would not be appropriate for the woman and may even provoke another panic attack.

Ans. 77: (c) Noncompetitive antagonism
Ref: Read the text below
Sol:

- A **noncompetitive antagonist** binds at a different site than the receptor, or irreversibly binds the receptor site. In either case, the system is not activated. Thus, response is lowered at a given dose of agonist, and this effect is not overcome with increased agonist dose. (The dose-response curve shifts downward.)

- A **competitive antagonist** reversibly binds to a receptor without activating the system, lowering the response at a given agonist dose. However, a response of maximum efficacy may be achieved with increased agonist dose. (The dose-response curve shifts to the right.). Further, it is not stated that the effect of drug W is overcome with increasing doses of drug V. A full agonist will produce a response of maximum efficacy if present in sufficient quantity. Drug W cannot be a full agonist, because it diminishes the physiologic effect of drug V. When administered alone, a partial agonist binds to the receptor site and elicits a less-than-100% response regardless of dose.
- When **administered with a full agonist, it acts like an antagonist because it competes for receptor binding sites. (The dose-response curve shifts downward, and may also shift left or right.) Drug W cannot be a partial agonist because it acts at a site other than the receptor for drug V.**

Ans. 78: (a) Granulocyte colony-stimulating factor
Ref: Read the text below
Sol:

- **Granulocyte colony-stimulating factor** increases neutrophil, eosinophil and basophil counts: the **patient's white blood cell differential shows an increase in the percentage of neutrophils from 9% to 90% after the growth factor was given.**
- The **percentage of eosinophils** did not change, but since the total number of cells increased, the **absolute eosinophil** amount also increased. The percentage of lymphocytes decreased.
- The **other growth factors** listed would not increase production of neutrophils.
- **Transforming growth factor-beta** is made by macrophages, endothelial cells, and T-cells and is involved in B-cell maturation.
- **IL-6** is an acute phase reactant made by macrophages, and **IL-8 is involved in neutrophil migration and chemotaxis.**

Ans. 79: (d) Common in personality disorders
Ref: Read the text below
Sol:

- **Delusions are fixed false beliefs of which a person** cannot be dissuaded by empathic or logical argument.
- They may be present whenever **reality testing is obstructed by a psychotic process**; thus, they may occur in association not only with schizophrenia but also with mania, depression, or organic disturbances.
- **Commonly encountered delusions include those of persecution, grandiosity, and physical disease.**

Ans. 80: (d) Sympathetic denervation
Ref: Read the text below
Sol:

- **Recall that that the sympathetic nervous system** causes **pupilary dilation** (mydriasis) via α-adrenergics, while the parasympathetic nervous system **constrics the pupil (miosis) via muscarinic cholinergics.**
- The diagram in this questions shows that the left pupil is smaller than the right pupil without treatment, **which points to either increased parasympathetic stimulation or decreased sympathetic stimulation in the left eye.**
- **Adding tyramine**, which is an **indirect sympathomimetic, has no effect on the left eye**, which is consistent with sympathetic denervation of the left eye.
- The **treatment with epinephrine** had a large effect on the left eye, however, which rules out blockade of alpha-adrenergic receptors since blocking the α-adrenergic receptors would have blocked any effect of epinephrine.
- **Blockade of β-adrenergic receptors** is incorrect since B-receptors are not involved in pupillary constriction and dilation.
- **Blockade of muscarinic receptors** is incorrect because the left eye is constricted without treatment, not dilated as it would be with unopposed sympathetic stimulation.

Ans. 81:(b) CCTAGG
GGATCC
Ref: Read the text below
Sol:

- **Restriction endonucleases** recognize specific base pair sequences usually of four to six base pairs **when they possess twofold rotational symmetry.**
- Such a symmetrical placement of base pairs leading to an **identical reading from 5.′ to 3.′ on one strand and from 3.′ to 5.′ on the other strand is called a palindrome**.
- Of the sequences shown in the question, only **CCTAGG GGATCC** contains a palindrome.
- The exact center of symmetry lies between **the complementary TA–AT base pairs.**

Ans. 82: (c) 60 g/d
Ref: Read the text below
Sol:
Recommended daily allowance
(***See*** table on the next page)

Ans. 83:(b) Can be used in management of alchohol withdrawl syndrome
Ref: Read the text below
Sol:

- Phenytoin is **an imidazolidine derivative**.
- It relates to **barbiturates in chemical structure**. Clinically effective seum level is in the range on **10-20 micrograms/ml.**
- A steady state blood **level is achieved by 7-10 days.**

Group	Energy(moderate work) kcal/d	Proteing/d	Fatg/d	CalciumMg/d	IronMg/d	Folic acidMicrog/d	RetinolMicrog/d
Man	2900	60	20	400	28	100	600
Woman Pregnant lactation 0-6 6-12 months	2200 +300 +550 +400	50 +15 +25 +18	20 30 45	400 1000 1000	30 38 30	100 400 150	600 600 950

Ans. 84: (d) Phosphorus
Ref: Park/19th ed./500
Sol:
Fish - Protein rich - (15-25%)
Rich in
- Unsaturated fatty acids.
- Vit A - also remember fish oil - richest natural source of Vit A (retinol).
- Vit D.

Ans. 85: (d) Inhibiting the activity of 3-hydroxy-3-methylglutaryl (HMG) CoA reductase
Ref: Read the text below
Sol:
- This patient is most likely taking a statin. Statins inhibit the activity of HMG CoA reductase.
- One of the major side effects reported from statin use is myalgia. This is an important presenting symptom because continued use can result in rhabdomyolysis and acute renal failure.
- Decreasing the production of LDL is an effect of statins, but not the direct action.
- Decreasing the binding of bile acids and decreasing the activity of lipoprotein lipase are not current methods for lowering serum cholesterol.

Ans. 86: (d) Small cell carcinoma of the lung
Ref: Read the text below
Sol:
- The first thing you **need to recognize to answer this question** is that this patient has hyponatremia **(110 mEq/L, normal is between 135-145**).
- Given the **clinical finding of a lung mass, the most likely explanation is that this patient has SIADH**, a **paraneoplastic complication** of small cell carcinoma of the lung.SIADH is syndrome of inappropriate **antidiuretic hormone (ADH) secretion**, in which the body, or in this case the lung tumor, secretes ADH that is not responsive to normal feedback mechanisms, resulting in inappropriate retention of water and dilution of the sodium concentration.
- The **other malignancies in the answer choices are not associated with SIADH. Adenocarcinoma of the lung is more common in non-smokers and is not associated with SIADH.**
- **Medullary carcinoma of the thyroid** could secrete excess calcitonin, but not ADH.
- **Renal cell carcinoma** can secrete excess erythropoietin, leading to polycythemia, or excess red blood cells, but this would have no effect on sodium concentration.

Ans. 87: (b) Technetium bone scan
Ref: Read the text below
Sol:
- **Osteomyelitis can be diagnosed** in its earliest stage by technetium bone scanning.
- **Plain roentgenographic films** typically take at least 10 days to reveal the early changes of osteomyelitis.
- **Gallium scans** are helpful in proving the effectiveness of therapy at the end of treatment.
- **Blood counts and sedimentation rates** are helpful in monitoring the progression and response to treatment of osteomyelitis.

Ans. 88: (c) Has had a recent hepatitis B infection
Ref: Read the text below
Sol:
- **Serologic markers** are extremely useful in the diagnosis of hepatitis B infections. In the typical case, titers of surface **antigen (HBsAg) and e antigen (HBeAg) rise** either before or simultaneously with clinical symptoms then fall to **unmeasurable levels.**
- Shortly thereafter, **antibodies to surface antigen (anti-HBsAg) appear**. The short interval between the disappearance of **HBsAg and the appearance of anti-HBsAg** is the so-called window period, when hepatitis is present despite negative serologic results.
- **Another antibody is present during this period—antibody to hepatitis B core antigen (anti-HBcAG)**.This antibody persists for years after the infection has resolved. In the case presented in the question, the serologic findings show either that the man is in the window period of acute hepatitis B infection, in which case anti- HBsAg will appear on retesting, or that anti- HBcAg is persisting from a previous hepatitis B infection and the current hepatitis is due to another agent (eg, hepatitis C) or a toxin.
- **Anti-HBcAg usually does not indicate either a chronic carrier state or immunity.**

Ans. 89: (d) Radial nerve
Ref: Read the text below
Sol:
- Fractures of the shaft of the humerus **involve the radial nerve, which winds around its posterior aspect, in the radial groove. As** a result, a wrist, a wrist drop may be present.
- **Dislocations of the shoulder or fractures involving the surgical neck of the humerus**

may be associated with trauma to the axillary nerve. In such an event, sensations over the lateral aspect of the shoulder will be impaired.

Ans. 90: (b) Small bowel obstruction
Ref: Read the text below
Sol:

- **The radiographs demonstrate a classic appearance of small bowel obstruction with dilated loops of small bowel on the supine film and air-fluid levels on the up-right film.**

Ans. 91: (c) Chlamydial pneumonia
Ref : Read the text below
Sol:

- Chlamydial pneumonia **in infants presents at 3 to 16 weeks of age. Typically, the infants appear quite well,** are afebrile, but have been ill with tachypnea and a repetitive staccato cough.
- Rales, and sometimes wheezing, **can be heard. Conjunctivitis is present in approximately 50% of patients.**
- Hyperinflation and patchy infiltrates **are seen on chest x-ray, and eosinophilia is apparent on complete blood count (CBC).**

Ans. 92: (d) A depressive episode
Ref: Read the text below
Sol:

- **A** depressive episode **is characterized by a depressed mood, coupled with rumination and** demoralization, trouble concerntrating, and changes in circadian rhythms.
- Hypersomnia and hyposomnia **are both fairly common.**
- Mania and anxiety **might both be associated with decreased sleep, but concurrent demoralization would be unusual.**

Ans. 93: (a) Streptococcus pneumoniae
Ref: Read the text below
Sol:

- Community-acquired pneumonia is most commonly caused by streptococcus pneumoniae.
- Other organisms, **such as** Haemophilus influenzae or Moraxella catarrhalis, **are commonly found in smokers or those with underlying lung disease, but S. pneumoniae remains the most common.**
- **There is now concern about the rising** percentage of S. pneumoniae strains that are resistant to penicillin.
- **The best way to protect elderly patients and those with underlying lung disease from pneumonia is by use of the pneumococcal vaccine, which is indicated in all people over age 65 and those** younger who have underlying lung disease or who are asplenic.

Ans. 94: (d) Cocaine
Ref. Read the text below
Sol:

- **A frequent adverse effect associated with** maternal prenatal use of many substances is intrauterine growth retardation and preterm delivery.
- **Although tobacco, alcohol, narcotics, and amphetamines all have an adverse impact on pregnancy outcome, only** cocaine has clearly defined vascular-disruption anomalies such as intestinal atresia, limb-reduction defects, and brain anomalies.

Ans. 95: (a) Carpal tunnel syndrome
Ref: Read the text below
Sol:

- Carpal tunnel syndrome **is caused by compression of the median nerve at the level of the wrist.**
- **The** median nerve supplies **sensation to the radial 3½ digits of the hand as well as** innervation of the thenar musculature.
- **Symptoms include numbness and tingling in the fingertips and pain that can awaken the** patient at night and that can travel proximally up the arm.
- **On physical examination,** Tinel's sign and Phalen's test **are usually positive, and there can be sensory loss in the median nerve distribution and muscle weakness.**

Ans. 96:(b) Flexor pollicis brevis
Ref: Harrison - 2404
Sol.

- The **flexor pollicis brevis has two heads and there is a sesamoid bone associated with each of the tendons of these heads.**
- **Sesamoid b**ones are isolated islands of bone that may occur in tendons passing over joints. The patella is the classic example.
- The **adductor pollicis also has two heads (transverse and oblique), but they are not associated with sesamoid** bones.

Ans. 97: (d) 90
Ref: Read the text below
Sol:

- From inspection of the **figure, the R-R interval** (time between heart beats) at rest is 0.83 seconds; 60 seconds/minute divided **by 0.83 yields a resting heart rate of 72 beats/minute.**
- Since activation of b1 receptors in the sinoatrial node will result in increased heart rate, the only alternative larger than **72 beats/minute is 90 beats/minute.**

Ans. 98: (b) Dehydration
Ref: Read the text below
Sol:

- The increased pulse and decreased blood **pressure indicate a loss of fluid** (volume contraction).
- The **patient's hemoglobin**, urea nitrogen, and sodium all rise to above the normal values by **Day 3, whereas his glucose and creatinine remain normal.**

- These changes are consistent **with an hyperosmotic volume contraction, a loss of water without losing solute.** This typically occurs due to dehydration.
- **Choice A** is incorrect because renal failure would decrease creatinine clearance.
- **Choice C** is incorrect because diabetic ketoacidosis would cause increased blood glucose levels.
- **Choice D** is incorrect because gastrointestinal hemorrhage would present with additional symptoms and hemoglobin would decrease.

Ans. 99: (d) Increased chylomicrons
Ref: Read the text below
Sol:

- **Lipoprotein lipase deficiency is autosomal recessive** and associated with increased chylomicrons and **marked hypertriglyceridaemia.**

Ans. 100: (c) RNA
Ref: Read the text below
Sol:

- **Reverse transcriptase PCR** is a means of **amplifying RNA.**
- The RNA is **transcribed into complimentary DNA (cDNA)** using the enzyme reverse transcriptase, the cDNA is then **amplified by conventional PCR.**

Ans. 101:(b) Acromegaly
Ref: Read the text below
Sol:

- **Acidophilic cells of the anterior pituitary are** those cells that stain with acidic dyes. The major peptide hormones found in cells of this type are growth hormones and prolactin.
- **Tumors of acidophilic** cells may lead to excessive secretion of growth hormone, causing gigantism in children and acromegaly in adults. Acromegaly is associated with changes in facial features and enlargement of the hands and feet.
- **Dwarfism may be the result of deficiencies** in growth hormone or of growth factors. Cushing's syndrome is caused by excess secretion of glucocorticoids and may result from tumors of ACTH-containing cells in the pituitary. In contrast to the growth-hormone–containing cells, the cells that synthesize ACTH may be chromophobic or basophilic.
- **Adrenogenital syndrome results from excessive adrenal secretion of androgens.**

Ans. 102: (c) Triiodothyronine
Ref: Read the text below
Sol:

- The **thyroid gland synthesizes and secretes thyroxine** (3,5,3′ ,5′ ,-tetraiodothyronine, T4) and 3,5,3′-triiodothyronine (T3) as well as lesser amounts of reverse triiodothyronine (3,3′ ,5′ -triiodothyronine, RT3) and monoiodotyrosine.
- Of these, **T3 is most active in stimulating oxygen** consumption in the body, being three to five times as potent as **T4, although it is secreted in smaller amounts. RT3 and monoiodotyrosine are not active.**
- **Thyroglobulin is a glycoprotein of the thyroid gland** that plays a major role in the syn thesis of thyroid hormones. It is not, however, believed to play a role in the actions of the thyroid hormones.

Ans. 103:(c) Fatty acids
Ref: Read the text below
Sol:

- Although the **heart is versatile in its use of substrates**, more than 60% of myocardial oxygen consumption is **derived from free fatty acids.**
- **Glucose and lactate are the major carbohydrate** sources but make up only 30% to 35% of the total sources for myocardial energy.
- In the normal heart, **pyruvate uptake is very low and oxidation of amino acids** provides little input to myocardial energy expenditure. In general, the heart uses the substrate in greatest supply—for example, ketone bodies may be used during diabetic acidosis.
- **However, under normal conditions free fatty acids are the major substrate.**

Ans. 104:(d) Increased glucagon secretion
Ref: Read the text below
Sol:

- **One of the effects of insulin is to inhibit the secretion of glucagon** from the α cells in pancreatic islets.
- Thus, a **deficiency of insulin, such as occurs in diabetes mellitus**, is associated with increased secretion of glucagon, which contributes to the observed hyperglycemia.
- The **increased levels of glucagon** are also apparently due to increased glucagon release by cells in the gastrointestinal tract. Although insulin deficiency may cause coma from a variety of **causes, insulin does not control glucose uptake in the brain.**
- In insulin deficiency, an increase in the rate of uptake of glucose into skeletal muscle may still be **observed with exercise, and the rate of catabolism of proteins is increased. The latter effect contributes to increased gluconeogenesis in the liver.**

Ans. 105:(c) Before the onset of slow movements
Ref: Read the text below
Sol:

- The **basal ganglia constitute part of the extrapyramidal system concerned with the control of movement.**
- **Many neurobiologists** believe that the basal ganglia play an important role in the initiation **of voluntary movement.**

- **Consistent with such a notion is the experimental observation** that unit activity in the basal ganglia is associated with movements and that many units start to fire before the onset of slow, sustained movements.
- **Basal ganglia units are less likely to discharge during rapid movements.**
- The discharge of units in basal ganglia has not been **linked to somatosensory stimulation, acoustic stimulation, or visual accommodation.**

Ans. 106: (d) 0.75
Ref: Read the text below
Sol:

- Sensitivity, as defined in biostatistics, is the number of true positive results divided by the total positive test results (true positive plus false negative). Sensitivity = 60/(60+20) = 0.75

Ans. 107: (a) 2nd quartile
Ref: Read the text below
Sol:
Quartiles: Three cutpoints for values of a measurement that divide a group in four equal parts with regard to number of subjects, after the values are arranged in ascending order. eg. If we want to find central value of a set of 240 values, these have to be first arranged in a ascending order, then quartile will divide in four equal parts.

- **1st quartile** : Divide in a ratio of 1 : 3
- **2nd quartile** : Divide in a ratio of 1 : 1
- **3rd quartile** : Divide in a ratio of 3 : 1

So Central value of a set of 240 values can be obtained by 2nd quartile.

Ans. 108: (c) Mean is one
Ref: Read the text below
Sol:
Standard normal curve
Standard normal curve is a **smooth**, **bell shaped** perfectly symmetrical curve, based on an infinitely large numbers of observations.

- The total area of curve is **1**.
- Its mean is **zero**.
- Its standard deviation is **1**.
- The mean, median and mode all coincide.

Ans. 109: (b) Mid-day meal scheme
Ref: Read the text below
Sol:
Co-operative for assistance and relief every where (Care)

- Was founded in **North America in the wake of the second world war in the year 1945.**
- **CARE provides emergency** aid and long term development assistance.
- **CARE began its operation in India in 1950.**
- Till the end of 1980s, the promary objective of **CARE – India was to provide food for children in** the age group of 6-11 years.
- From mid 1980s, CARE-**India focused its food support in the ICDs programme an**d in development of programmes in the areas of health and income supplementation.

Ans. 110: (b) 3 out of 100,000
Ref: Read the text below
Sol:
Estimation of probability
Z also follows a normal distribution.
The relative deviate (Z)

$$= \frac{|x - \bar{x}|}{\text{Standard deviation}} = \frac{80 - 72}{2} = 4$$

The area of the normal curve correspnding to a deviate 4 = 0.4997. Since we are dealing with only half the total area (0.5) the area beyond 0.4997 is equal to 0.5 - 4997 or 0.0003. Therefore, the probability is that only 3 out of 100,000 individuals would likely have a pulse rate of 80, or higher.

Ans. 111: (a) A **retinal examination should now be performed on this patient**
Ref: Read the text below
Sol:

- **Secondary hypertension may be suspected on finding features that are not consistent with essential hypertension.**
- Such features include age at onset younger than **30 years or older than 50 years; blood pressure higher than 180/110 mm Hg at diagnosis;** significant targetorgan injury at diagnosis; hemorrhages and exudates on **fundus examination; renal insufficiency;LVH;** poor response to appropriate three-drug therapy; and accelerated or malignant hypertension.
- The clinician should inquire about a **family history of hypertension**, premature CV disease, and disorders that would increase the possibility of secondary hypertension. The examination should **include at least two standardized measurements of blood pressure with the patient in the seated position.**
- Initially, blood **pressure should also be measured in the opposite arm (to** identify arterial narrowing, which can cause an inaccurately low reading in one arm) and in the standing position, especially in diabetic patients and older patients (to identify orthostatic declines).
- **Retinal examination should be performed, primarily to identify retinal changes of diabetes or severe hypertension (i.e., hemorrhages, exudates, or papilledema).**

Ans. 112: (b) Stenosing lesions of the renal circulation cause hypertension through ischemia-mediated activation of the renin-angiotensin-aldosterone system
Ref: Read the text below
Sol:

- **Renovascular hypertension** is the most common form of potentially curable secondary hypertension.
- It probably **occurs in 1% to 2% of the overall hypertensive population**. The prevalence may be as high as 10% in patients with **resistant hypertension**, and it may be even higher in patients with accelerated or malignant hypertension. Stenosing lesions of the renal circulation cause hypertension through ischemia-mediated stimulation of the rennin angiotensin-aldosterone axis.
- **Fibromuscular disease** is the most common cause of renovascular hypertension in younger patients, especially women between 15 and 50 years of age; it accounts for approximately 10% **of cases of renovascular hypertension.**
- **Atheromatous disease** is the most common cause of renovascular hypertension in middle-aged and older patients and accounts for **approximately 90% of cases of renovascular hypertension.**
- The prevalence **of atheromatous renal artery disease** increases with age and is common in older hypertensive patients, especially in those with diabetes or with atherosclerosis in other vascular beds. Most patients with atheromatous renal vascular disease and hypertension have essential hypertension.

Ans. 113: (c) < 130/85 mm Hg
Ref: Read the text below
Sol:

- This patient has **stage 2 (moderate) hypertension** and is in risk group C because of her history of myocardial infarction and **diabetes (either one alone would suffice to put her in this risk group).**
- **As such, her target blood pressure is less than 130/85** mm Hg. Note that there is some evidence that lowering patients' **diastolic blood pressure to less than 70 mm Hg is associated with increased mortality.**

Ans. 114: (d) Lone
Ref: Read the text below
Sol:

- The **ACC/AHA/ESC guidelines** include the following categories: **recurrent**—more than one episode of AF has occurred; **lone**—AF occurring in a patient younger than 60 years who has no clinical or echocardiographic evidence of cardiopulmonary disease; **valvular**—AF occurring in a patient with evidence or history of rheumatic mitral valve disease or prosthetic heart valves is defined as valvular; **paroxysmal**—AF that typically lasts 7 days or less, with spontaneous conversion to sinus rhythm; persistent—AF that typically lasts longer than 7 days or requires pharmacologic or direct current (DC) cardioversion; **permanent**—AF that is refractory to cardioversion or that has persisted for longer than 1 year.
- **Paroxysmal, persistent, and permanent AF categories do not apply to episodes of AF lasting 30 seconds or less or to episodes precipitated by a reversible medical condition.**
- Reversible conditions include acute myocardial infarction, cardiac surgery, pericarditis, myocarditis, hyperthyroidism, pulmonary embolism, and **acute pulmonary disease.**

Ans. 115: (d) Normal-sized heart
Ref: Read the text below
Sol:

- Although success rates are high with **DC cardioversion, a number of risk factors for cardioversion failure have been identified.**
- These include **longer duration of AF (notably, longer than 1 year), older age, left atrial enlargement, cardiomegaly,** rheumatic heart disease, and transthoracic impedance.
- Pretreatment with **amiodarone, ibutilide, sotalol, flecainide, propafenone, disopyramide, and quinidine** have been shown to increase DC cardioversion success rates.

Ans. 116: (c) Antrectomy and truncal vagotomy
Ref: Read the text below
Sol:

- **Perforation of a duodenal ulcer is an indication for emergency celiotomy and closure of the perforation.**
- In patients with **no prior history of peptic ulcer disease, simple closure with an omental patch is recommended**. Seventy-two percent of patients who are asymptomatic preoperatively will remain so postoperatively.
- **Patients with long-standing ulcer disease require a definitive acidreducing procedure**, except in high-risk situations. The choice of procedure is made by weighing the risk of recurrence against the incidence of undesirable side effects of the procedure, and considerable controversy persists about this issue.
- **Antrectomy and truncal vagotomy offers a recurrence rate of 1%**, but carries a 15–25% incidence of sequelae such as diarrhea, dumping syndrome, bloating, and gastric stasis.
- **Highly selective vagotomy**, if technically feasible, offers a 1–5% incidence of side effects but carries a recurrence rate of 10–13% in some series, although results are better when gastric and prepyloric ulcers are excluded. In general, definitive acid-reducing procedures should be postponed if the perforation is more than 12 h old or if there is extensive peritoneal soilage.
- **Pyloroplasty and truncal vagotomy** carries intermediate rates of recurrence and side effects, but has the advantage of speed in the setting of very ill patients with acute perforation.

Ans. 117: (b) Endoscopic sclerotherapy
Ref: Read the text below
Sol:

- The diagnosis of **bleeding esophageal varices** is aided in the adult by stigmata of portal hypertension.
- Upper gastrointestinal **hemorrhage in cirrhotics is due to esophageal varices in less than half of patients.** Gastritis and peptic ulcer disease

account for the majority of cases. Esophagoscopy is the single most reliable means of establishing the source of bleeding, though variations in transvariceal blood flow may result in nonvisualization of the varices.

- In addition, **endoscopic sclerotherapy is reported to control acute variceal hemorrhage in 80–90% of cases and carries** an acute mortality lower than that of other procedures. Barium swallow has a high false negative rate and offers no therapeutic advantage. Celiac angiography will rule out **arterial hemorrhage and will demonstrate venous collateral circulation, but will not demonstrate variceal bleeding.**
- **Parenteral vasopressin controls variceal hemorrhage** by constriction of the splanchnic arteriolar bed and a resultant drop in portal pressure. Intraarterial vasopressin offers no advantage over intravenous administration and requires a mesenteric catheter. The reported control rate is 50–70%.
- **Esophageal balloon tamponade controls variceal hemorrhage** in two-thirds of patients, but may also control bleeding ulcers and thereby obscure the diagnosis. Although balloon tamponade has reduced the mortality and morbidity from variceal hemorrhage in good-risk patients, an increased awareness of associated complications (aspiration, asphyxiation, and ulceration at the tamponade site), as well as a rebleeding rate of 40%, has reduced its use. It is indicated as a temporary measure when vasopressin and sclerotherapy fail.
- **Emergency portacaval shunt is advised in good-risk cirrhotic patients whose bleeding is not controlled with vasopressin or sclerosis.**
- The **mortality for patients with bleeding varices not subjected to shunting is between 66 and 73%, whereas operative mortality** of emergency shunts ranges from 20 to 50%. Esophageal transection with the autostapler carries the same mortality as shunt procedures and the rebleeding **rate is estimated to be 50% at 1 year.**

Ans. 118: (c) Perform a right hemicolectomy and a wedge resection of the metastasis
Ref: Read the text below
Sol:

- Because **approximately 5% of colorectal** cancers are associated with resectable hepatic metastases, appropriate preoperative discussion should include obtaining permission for removal of synchronous **peripheral hepatic lesions if they are found.**
- If gross tumor is removed, **a 25% "cure" rate can be anticipated.Adequate local resection, either by wedge or by limited partial hepatectomy**, may be carried out whenever no extrahepatic disease is found and the hepatic lesion is technically removable.
- Any option that leaves the potentially obstructing primary cancer unremoved would be unacceptable.**Radiation therapy has little to offer in colon cancer or its hepatic metastases.**
- Local **infusion of floxuridine (FUDR) via an implantable Infusaid pump for 14 days at** 0.3 mg/kg/day has been reported to provide some acceptable palliation in selected patients with unresectable hepatic lesions.

Ans. 119: (d) Pulmonary artery
Ref: Read the text below
Sol:

- **Blood pressures in the pulmonary artery** are in the range of 15-**30mmHg systolic and 4-12mmHg diastolic,** which are pressures that most closely match those found in this patient's catheterization.
- **Left atrial pressures range from 1-10mmHg**, and right atrial pressures range from **0-8mmHg.**
- Prior to birth, the **ductus arteriosus** diverts blood from the pulmonary artery to the aorta, and the foramen **ovale provides a communication** between the two atria, equalizing their pressures, and shunting blood from the pulmonary circulation to the systemic circulation.

Ans. 120: (b) B
Ref: Read the text below
Sol:

- This question involves the relation of **predictive value to disease diagnosis.**
- **Choosing Point B as the cutoff** will cause the test to have a relatively high false-positive rate: some people with concentrations within the normal range will test positive for the disease. However, because this disease is irreversible and fatal unless treated early, it is appropriate in this case to set a cutoff point that will not generate any false-negative results. Thus, setting the cutoff point at B will ensure that the negative predictive value of the test is 100%, at the expense of having a somewhat lower positive predictive value.
- **Choice A is incorrect because the false-positive rate would be so high that the test would not be clinically useful (the positive predictive value will be too low).**
- **Choices C-D are incorrect** because all these choices would give some false-negative results (the **negative predictive value will not be 100%).**

Ans. 121: (b) Obtain a sonogram to correlate with the mammogram; if a mass is identified sonographically, perform biopsy
Ref: Read the text below
Sol:

- **A dominant breast mass on physical examination requires further evaluation even if the mammogram is negative.**
- **Mammographic interpretation** is frequently

difficult in younger patients because of the presence of dense breast tissue.

- **A sonogram is frequently required.**
- **Mammograms become easier** to interpret in older patients as the breast tissue becomes **increasingly replaced by fat.**

Ans. 122: (d) Surreptitious use of diuretics
Ref: Read the text below
Sol:

- This patient's serum bicarbonate is high, while her potassium is low. The potassium level in her urine is high. (**Typical range is 50-150mEq per day).**
- This **indicates the use of a diuretic which blocks the reuptake of potassium.**
- **Choice A** is incorrect because aldosterone increases potassium secretion, therefore aldosterone deficiency would cause decreased potassium secretion.
- **Choice B** is incorrect because hyperventilation causes respiratory alkalosis, resulting in decreased bicarbonate in the serum.
- **Choice C** is incorrect because acidosis causes decreased potassium secretion. Also, diabetic ketoacidosis would cause additional symptoms and abnormally high blood glucose levels.

Ans. 123: (c) Ceftriaxone sodium, 1 g/day intravenously (IV), plus azithromycin,500 mg/day IV
Ref: Read the text below
Sol:

- Current guidelines for the management of **community-acquired pneumonia advocate the use of the Pneumonia Severity Index** as an objective measure of risk stratification to help determine the initial site of treatment.
- **Based on age, comorbidities, and clinical findings, this patient is assigned to class IV (moderate risk).** He should be hospitalized (not in the intensive care unit) and treated with **IV therapy until clinically improved.**
- Since he was given a course **of antibiotics within the past 3 months, he is at risk for drug-resistant S pneumonia**e. In this case, a beta-lactam (ie, cefuroxime, cefotaxime sodium, ceftriaxone sodium, **ampicillin sodium/ sulbactam sodium and an advanced macrolide (ie, azithromycin, clarithromycin) or respiratory fluoroquinolone (ie, moxifloxacin HCl, gatifloxacin, levofloxacin, gemifloxacin mesylate would be appropriate.**
- Depending on the class of antibiotics recently given, one or another of the suggested options may be selected. **Recent use of a fluoroquinolone should dictate selection of a nonfluoroquinolone regimen.**

Ans. 124: (b) Ceftriaxone sodium,125 mg, single dose, intramuscularly, plus azithromycin,1g, single dose
Ref: Read the text below
Sol:

- **Recommended antibiotics for gonococcal infections are a single dose of cefixime,400 mg; ceftriaxone sodium, 125 mg; ciprofloxacin, 500 mg; ofloxacin, 400 mg; or levofloxacin, 250 mg.**
- Recent data from **the CDC-sponsored sentinel surveillance system indicate an increase in the prevalence of quinolone-resistant Neisseria gonorrhoeae** among men who have sex with men (MSM).
- Patients infected with N gonorrhoeae **are often coinfected with Chlamydia trachomatis.** Hence, patients treated for gonococcal infection should also be treated with an agent effective against uncomplicated **genital C trachomatis infection, unless chlamydial infection is ruled out.**
- Recommended antibiotic **regimens for chlamydial infection are azithromycin, 1 g, in a single dose, or doxycycline 100 mg bid, for 7 days. Oral azithromycin, 2 g, in a single dose is not recommended for the treatment of gonorrhea** because of a high rate of gastrointestinal (GI) side effects and high cost.

Ans. 125: (b) Avoidance of alcohol
Ref: Read the text below
Sol:

- This patient has heart **failure, hypotension, and no signs of atherosclerosis** in the setting of alcohol abuse, **sedentary lifestyle, and poor dieting.**
- The **most likely diagnosis is dilated cardiomyopathy** secondary to alcohol abuse. Dilated cardiomyopathy is the **most common cardiomyopathy** and etiologies include alcohol abuse, thiamine **deficiency, coxsackie viral infection, cocaine abuse, doxorubicin toxicity, and idiopathic.**
- **Ultimately, patients suffer from** systolic dysfunction with eventual cardiac arrest. The most appropriate **recommendation for this patient is to remove the source of his cardiomyopathy—alcohol.**
- **Diet, exercise and weight loss** will definitely have cardio-protective effects; however, removing the etiology of the patient's heart failure **needs to have highest priority in the management of this patient.**

Ans. 126: (d) Exposure to saturated steam (121°C) for 15 minutes
Ref: Read the text below
Sol:

- The bacteria in **question is Clostridium difficile** (the most common cause of antibiotic-associated diarrhea).
- **C. difficile is a anaerobic gram positive rod that forms spores.** These spores are only destroyed by autoclaving (**exposure to saturated steam for 15 minutes**), because the spore shell is resistant to other forms of sterilization.

- As a side note, using **alcohol based cleaners** (like Purell) will not sterilize your hands after you see a patient with C. **difficile infection.** Therefore, it is important to physically wash your hands with soap and water, in order to mechanically **wash the spores off your hands.**

Ans. 127: (d)7. 50 47 35
Ref: Read the text below
Sol:

- Due to the vomiting, this **woman is losing HCl** (the main stomach acid). Since she is unable to control the vomiting and is not eating she cannot adequately compensate for the acid loss. Therefore, she is **in a state of metabolic alkalosis (pH>7.40).**
- Although her kidneys will eventually compensate by **excreting HCO_3,** this process takes about a week to **compensate, and therefore HCO_3 will be increased (>24).**
- In order to compensate, the respiratory drive decreases so that the body retains more CO_2, and **therefore pCO2 is increased (>40). Only option D has increased pH, pCO_2 and HCO_3.**

Ans. 128:(c) No emergency intervention is required other than repeat abdominal x-rays.
Ref: Read the text below
Sol:

- **Fig shows a battery (size AA) in the region of the stomach** ingested by the 16-year-old patient.
- The **majority of ingested objects pass** through the gastrointestinal tract spontaneously without **the need for any intervention.**
- **Special cases** that require specific intervention include ingestion of sharp objects, such as razor blades or pins, or especially long or wide objects that are not **likely to pass (>5 cm long or 2 cm wide).**
- **Button battery and lithium battery** ingestions also require specialized care due to concerns of esophageal erosion.
- **Induced vomiting or attempted removal by gastric lavage** is not recommended for any ingested foreign body.

Ans. 129: (b) 6.0
Ref: Read the text below
Sol:

- Titration of the diprotic form of glycine **involves the net removal of one proton from one** molecule of glycine.
- **When observing a titration curve for glycine, the addition of base results in two stages on the curve with** two pK_a values (pK_a represents the negative logarithm of the acid ionization constant).
- **At very low pH values, the** fully protonated form of glycine predominates **($+H_3N - CH_2 - COOH$).**
- **The midpoint of the first stage of the curve, the pH = pK_1 of the ionizing group (COOH), is equal to 2.4 At** very high pH values, a proton is removed from the ionizable group $^+NH_3$ so that the predominate form of glycine is $H_2N - CH_2$ _COO^-.
- **The midpoint of this section of the curve is 9.6 where the pH = pK_2. The isoelectric point (pI) is the** midpoint between the two stages in the titration curve and represents the fully ionized, dipolar form of glycine with no net electric charge.
- **Because glycine has no ionizable** group in its side chain, pI is determined by the equation pI = ½(pK_1 + pK_2).

Ans. 130: (b) Osteomyelitis
Ref: Read the text below
Sol:

- **Bleeding from the nail bed suggests an open fracture** (Salter-Harris type 1) and places the patient at risk for **osteomyelitis.**
- In the **absence of infection**, the toe should heal quite well without deformity or limitation of growth.

Ans. 131: (d) Sociology
Ref: Read the text below
Sol:
SOCIOLOGY

- **Sociology** can be viewed from two angles :

(a) First, it can be seen as the study of relationships between human beings, and how these relationships change or vary in different parts of the world and at different times. The unit of study can be a small group (e.g., family) consisting of parents and children, or the study can extend beyond the family or small groups into the complex society where a greater number of people interact and interdepend in terms of economics, political power, general organisation and ways of living.

(b) The other part of sociology is concerned with the study of human behaviour. Human behaviour is determined not merely by biological and physical environmental factors but also by social factors. **Every form of human behavior has a social component. Sociologists are interested in the study of the social determinants of human behaviour. In the final analysis it may be stated that the aim of sociology is to search for the pattern of relationships between people in order to pave the way for the betterment of individuals in relation to society.**

Ans. 132: (a) Congenital
Ref: Read the text below
Sol:
Long-term or secular trends

- The term **"secular trend"** implies changes in the occurrence of disease (i.e., a progressive increase or **decrease) over a long period of time, generally several years or decades.**
- Although it may have short-term fluctuations imposed on it, a secular trend implies a consistent tendency to change in a **particular direction or a definite movement in one direction.**

- Examples include coronary **heart disease, lung cancer and diabetes which have** shown a consistent upward trend in the developed countries during the past 50 **years or so, followed by a decline of such diseases as tuberculosis, typhoid fever, diphtheria and polio.**

Ans. 133: (c) A is true but R is false
Ref: Read the text below
Sol:

- Orthopnea and paroxysmal nocturnal dyspnea are rarely symptoms of isolated right HF. However, when present, these symptoms usually reflect the increased work of breathing in the supine position that results from compromised excursion of the diaphragm.
- Tussive or effort-related **syncope may occur in patients with cor pulmonale with severe pulmonary hypertension because of the inability of the RV to deliver** blood adequately to the left side of the heart.
- The abdominal pain and ascites that occur with cor pulmonale are similar to the right heart failure that ensues in chronic HF. Lower-**extremity edema may occur secondary to neurohormonal activation, elevated RV filling pressures,** or increased levels of carbon dioxide and hypoxia, which can lead to peripheral vasodilation and edema formation.

Ans. 134: (a) Both A and R are true and R is correct explanation of A
Ref: Read the text below
Sol:

- Patients with large ventricular septal defects and pulmonary hypertension are those at greatest risk for developing pulmonary vascular obstruction.
- Thus, large defects should be corrected surgically early in life when pulmonary vascular disease is still reversible or not yet developed.
- In patients with **severe pulmonary vascular obstruction (Eisenmenger** syndrome), symptoms in adult life consist of exertional dyspnea, chest pain, syncope, and hemoptysis.
- **The right-to-left shunt leads to cyanosis, clubbing, and erythrocytosis. In all patients, the degree to which pulmonary vascular resistance is elevated before operationis a critical factor determining prognosis.**
- **If the pulmonary vascular resistance is one-third or less of the systemic value, progression of pulmonary vascular disease after** operation is unusual. However, if a moderate to severe increase in pulmonary **vascular resistance exists preoperatively, either no change or a progression of pulmonary vascular disease is common postoperatively.**

Ans. 135: (c) A is true but R is false
Ref: Read the text below
Sol:

- **Obsessions** are defined as **persistent, intrusive ideas, images, or impulses** that are recognized as absurd but cannot **be forced out of consciousness.**
- Although they **create anxiety**, obsessions differ from typical anxious thoughts in that they bear no relationship to **actual circumstances and are extremely unlikely to actually occur.**
- Older theories held that obsessions represented the emergence into consciousness of **unconscious desires or impulses, but treatment based on this assumption is ineffective.**
- **Obsessive impulses to jump from heights** may occur but fear of heights is called acrophobia. By definition, obsessions are not psychotic symptoms because the patient is aware that they are unrealistic.
- Obsessions that a **patient becomes convinced are true are called delusions.**

Ans. 136: (c) Supraventricular tachycardia
Ref: Read the text below
Sol:

- **Paroxysmal supraventricular tachycardia due to AV nodal reentry** typically displays a narrow QRS complex without clearly discernable P **waves, with a rate in the 160 to 190 range.**
- The atrial rate is faster in atrial flutter, typically with a classic sawtooth pattern of P waves, with AV conduction ratios most **commonly 2:1 or 4:1, leading to ventricular rates of 150 or 75/min.**
- Atrial fibrillation would show an irregularly **irregular rhythm. Wide QRS complexes would be expected in ventricular tachycardia.**

Ans. 137: (d) 1-e; 2-d ; 3-b; 4-a
Ref: Read the text below
Sol

- **Hypokalemia typically increases automaticity** of myocardial fibers, which results in ectopic beats or arrhythmias.
- Electrocardiography in **hypokalemia reveals flattening of the T wave and prominent U waves. Hyperkalemia decreases the rate** of spontaneous diastolic depolarization in all pacemaker cells.
- It also results in slowing of **conduction. One of the earliest electrocardiographic signs of hyperkalemia is the appearance of tall**, peaked T waves. More severe elevations of the serum potassium result in widening **of the QRS complex. Hypocalcemia results in prolongation of the QT interval.**
- Low serum calcium levels may also be associated with a decrease in myocardial contractility. At serum sodium levels **compatible with life, neither hyponatremia nor** hypernatremia results in any characteristic **electrocardiographic abnormalities.**

Ans. 138: (a) 420 ml/min
Ref: Read the text below
Sol:

To determine renal plasma flow (RPF) calculate the clearance of PAH as follows :

$$RPF = C_{PAH} = \frac{U_{PAH} \times V}{P_{PAH}}$$

where :

U_{PAH} is the urine concentration of PAH (mg/ml)

V is urine flow rate (ml/min)

P_{PAH} is the plasma concentration of PAH (mg/ml)

$$RPF = \frac{5.6 mg/ml \times 3 ml/min}{0.04 mg/ml}$$

RPF = 420 ml/min

Ans. 139: (b) (1–b) (2–d) (3–a) (4–c)
Ref: Read the text below
Sol:
(*See* figure on the bottom)

Ans. 140: (c) Increased contractility
Ref: Read the text below
Sol:

- An **upward shift** of the cardiac output curve is consistent with an increase in myocardial contractility; **for any right atrial pressure (sarcomere length)**, the force of contraction is increased. Such a change causes an **increase in stroke volume and cardiac output.**
- Increased blood volume and increased mean systemic pressure are related and would cause a rightward shift in the venous return curve.
- A negative inotropic **agent would cause decrease in contractility and a downward shift of the cardiac output curve.**

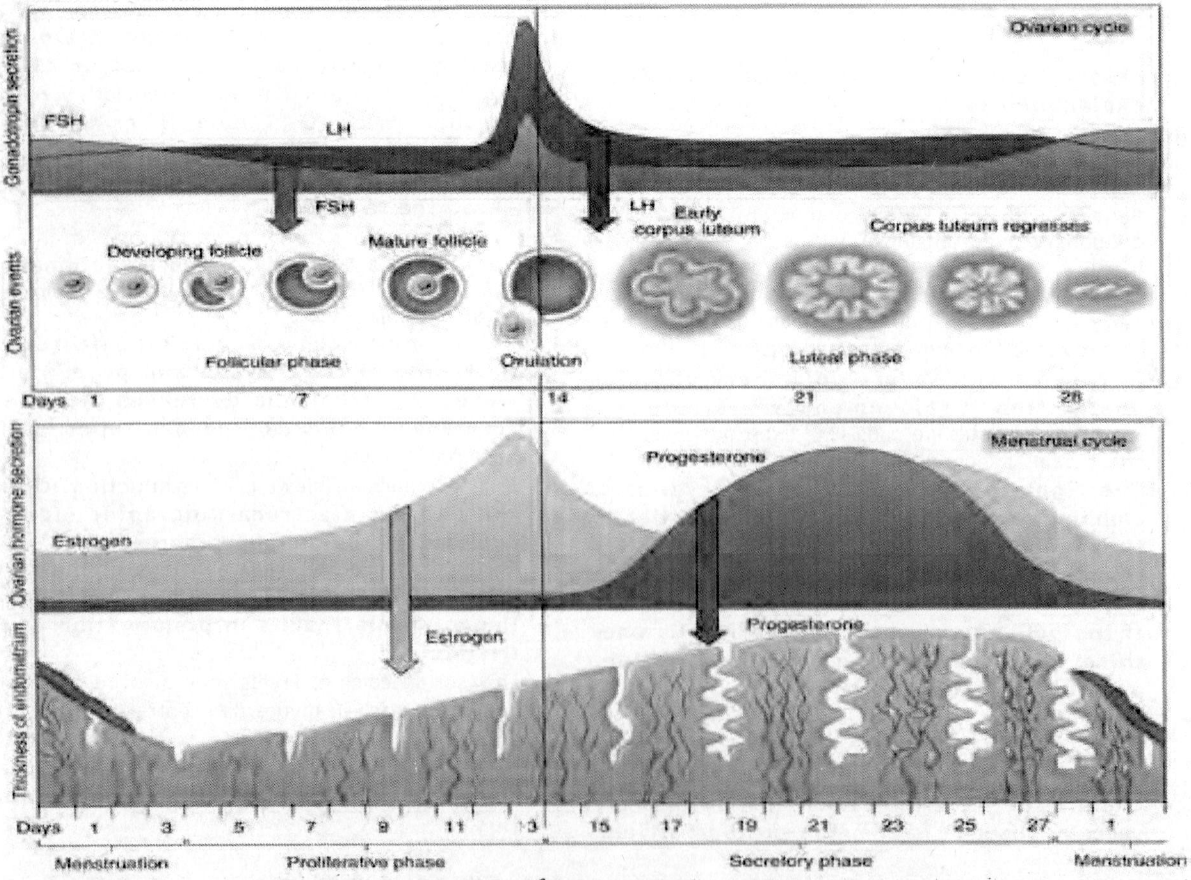

THE CYCLE OF OVULATION AND MENSTRUATION.

The downward arrows indicate the effects of the hormones.

Ans. 141: (d) Spiral fracture of the tibia
Ref: Read the text below
Sol:
- **Toddler fractures** represent a spiral fracture of the distal third of the tibia.
- They are usually the result of simple falls during running or playing.These fractures occur in **children 2-4 yr of age and occasionally up to 6 yr of age.**
- Clinical features **include pain, refusal to walk, minimal soft tissue swelling, a slight increase in warmth to palpation** over the fracture, and pain with palpation.

Ans. 142: (c) Ornithine transcarbamylase deficiency
Ref: Read the text below
Sol:
- **Ornithine transcarbamylase (OTC) deficiency** is an X-linked disorder and is most severe in males.
- Superficially it looks like **Reye syndrome**, and in older children, OTC deficiency may mimic **Reye syndrome.**
- Unfortunately, infants with a severe **neonatal onset have a very poor prognosis.**

Ans. 143: (a) Aortic root dilatation
Ref: Read the text below
Sol:
- The boy is this **clinical condition most likely has Marfan syndrome**, which is an autosomal-dominant **disorder of the connective tissues.**
- The genetic defect results in abnormal **synthesis and secretion of fibrillin, which is an essential component in connective tissues.**
- Patients with **Marfan syndrome** often have involvement in the skeletal, ocular, and cardiovascular systems. Most of the morbidity and mortality with this disease are related to the **cardiovascular manifestations; patients develop aortic root dilatation.**
- This may be associated with aortic insufficiency and aortic arch dissection. They may also have **mitral valve prolapse with significant hemodynamic consequences. Aortic root, aortic valve, and mitral valve replacement may be needed during the lifetime of the patient.**
- Patients with **Marfan syndrome** may frequently complain of chest pain; these patients must be viewed as having aortic dissection until proven otherwise. In this population, a **spontaneous pneumothorax is another potential cause of chest pain.**
- No data exist for recommending beta-blockers to all patients **with Marfan syndrome, however, beta-blockers clearly slow the progression of aortic root** dilatation in those with mild aortic root dilatation.
- **Exercise should be limited to aerobic activities.** Patients must avoid contact sports that cause acceleration-deceleration **injury and isometric maneuvers that tend to increase central blood pressure.** Aerobic activity is encouraged, but those with established aortic root dilatation should have adequate heart rate control with beta-blockers.
- **Aortic stenosis is not associated with Marfan** syndrome. Marfan syndrome can cause aortic regurgitation instead. **Aortic stenosis, in the context of genetic diseases, is associated with William's syndrome**, which also manifests as mental retardation and characteristic facies, as well as pulmonary artery stenosis.
- **Bicuspid aortic valve is not associated with Marfan syndrome. Bicuspid aortic valve can lead to aortic valvular stenosis.**
- **Dextrocardia refers** to the apex of the heart pointing toward the right. It is associated with **Kartagener syndrome.**

Ans. 144: (d) Maternal lupus
Ref: Read the text below
Sol:
- **Congenital heart block** is a prominent feature of neonatal lupus, which results from **maternal transfer of IgG autoantibodies**, usually anti-Ro, between the **12th and 16th wk of gestation.**
- The **heart block** is permanent and often requires cardiac pacing.

Ans. 145: (b) Discontinue ampicillin
Ref: Read the text below
Sol:
- The **first and essential step in treatment of Clostridium difficile-associated diarrhea** is the discontinuation of the current antibiotics, if at all possible.
- In most instances this course combined **with appropriate fluid and electrolyte replacement** is sufficient.

Ans. 146: (c) An autoimmune disease
Ref: Read the text below
Sol:
- **Forbidden clones provide a supply of cells that can recognize self - antigens and will serve as cells to** stimulate both humoral and cell-mediated immune responses, leading to autoimmunity.
- **B-**cell deficiency - primarily a lack of circulating B cells**–is a major cause of hypogammaglobulinemia.**
- Type I hypersensitivity **(anaphylactic hypersensitivity) is mediated by humoral antibodies, which result from a normal immune response to exogenous antigens.**
- **The** deletion of forbidden clones **leads to tolerance to autoantigens - the opposite of autoimmunity.**

Ans. 147: (c) Glutamate
Ref: Read the text below
Sol:

- **The** amount of alanine released from skeletal muscle **is greater than the amount that can be accounted for in muscle protein.**
- **The** catabolism of many amino acids in muscle **involves the transamination of α-amino group from amino acids to** pyruvate, producing alanine.
- **Thus, the carbon skeleton of much of the alanine released from muscle is derived from** glucose via the glycolytic pathway.

Ans. 148: (a) Immunocomplex vasculitis
Ref: Read the text below
Sol:

- **The** patient has acute infective endocarditis **due to staphylococcus aureus involving the aortic valve.**
- **The high-**pitched diastolic murmur between **the right second and third intercostals space is aortic regurgitation. It is heard best with the patient exhaling while sitting up and leaning forward.**
- **The** nail-bed finding is a splinter hemorrhage. **Painful, erythematous, nodular lesions on the finger pad are called Osler's nodes.**
- **Both lesions are examples of immunocomplex vasculitis, although some cases of Osler's nodes are embolic in origin.**
- **Immunocomplexes are also operative in acute glomerulonephritis and Roth's spots in the retina, which** are hemorrhages in the retinal vessels.

Ans. 149: (a) Mechanism is unopposed estrongen stimulation
Ref: Read the text below
Sol:

- **The** case scenario **is characteristic of dysfunctional uterine bleeding, a disorder resulting from** unopposed estrogen stimulation.
- **The usual findings are normal pelvic examination without pelvic pathology, anovulatory** cycles (not regular vovulation and extremes of reproductive age (adolescent and perimenopausal).
- **Serum prolactin levels may be elevated in some anovulatory conditions.**
- **Progestin cycling (not** surgical dilation and curettage is the treatment of choice.

Ans. 150: (c) Obtain a patient history
Ref: Read the text below
Sol:

- **Regardless of the clinical setting or the type of treatment** being contemplated, it is of primary importance in the initial **psychiatric interview** to obtain a careful patient history.
- **Evaluation of mental status is next in importance**, because it sheds light on the patient's orientation, cognition, and reality testing and may disclose the presence of organic disturbances.
- **Establishing a working alliance is critical but should occur as a concomitant of careful and empathic introductory interviews.**

Ans. 151: (d) If a narcotic analgesic is to be given to an opioid-dependent person, the dose should be significantly increased
Ref: Read the text below
Sol:

- **Cocaine abuse and withdrawal** is often associated with depression, protracted dysphoria and anhedonia.
- **Tobacco addiction is the most common type of drug dependency in the developed countries.**
- **Opioids administered** to treat pain seldom results in addiction. Repeated use of cannabis results in tolerance.
- If **indicated for pain, narcotic analgesics should be increased by 25 to 50% in an opioid-**dependent individual because of tolerance to the analgesic action.

Ans. 152: (d) Plasma cells
Ref: Read the text below
Sol:

- The patient described has **multiple myeloma,** which is characterized by proliferation of plasma cells and hyperproduction **of monoclonal light chains (Bence-Jones proteins). Accumulation at the renal tubules causes renal insufficiency.**
- **MM** also causes bone destruction, both from marrow expansion and stimulation of osteoclasts.
- This causes **hypercalcemia, which also contributes to renal dysfunction**. As with any leukemia, other cell lines are suppressed,causing anemia and thrombocytopenia.

Ans. 153: (a) Endoplasmic reticulum
Ref: Read the text below
Sol:

- **To answer this question**, you must know which organelles are sources of calcium available for use within the cell. The main sources of calcium in eukaryotic cells are the Smooth **Endoplasmic Reticulum (SER) and the mitochondria.**
- **Release of intracellular calcium** stores upon G protein activation follows a well established pathway: **the beta-gamma subunit of a G-protein** is cleaved and proceeds to **activate Phospholipase C (PLC).**
- **PLC, in turn, cleaves the membrane bound phospholipid [phosphatidylinositol** 4,5-bisphosphate] (PIP2) molecule into 2 components: Diacylglycerol (DAG) and Inositoltriphosphate (IP3). IP3 then binds to IP3 receptors present on the surface of the SER, which opens calcium channels and releases Ca^{2++} into the cytosol.
- **Calcium release by the mitochondria is not the direct target of the G-protein mediated calcium release.**

Ans. 154: (b) Alcoholism

Ref: Read the text below

Sol:

- **Agitation, tremulousness, and hallucinations** indicate the likely presence of delirium tremens.
- If the **hallucinations are primarily visual and frightening**, and if there is other evidence of sympathetic activation, the diagnosis would be more likely.
- Physicians should be **aware that alcoholic patients** often drink in the hospital and fail to disclose the extent of their alcohol use.
- Following an operation, **patients may develop an alcoholic withdrawal** state as a result of their restricted oral intake.

Ans. 155: (b) Obtain fungal culture for subtyping

Ref: Read the text below

Sol:

- The patient probably **has vaginitis caused by Candida glabrata** (which is responsible for about 14% of vulvovaginal candidiasis cases).
- This is more probable after antibiotic use in **patients with diabetes. C glabrata**, which is identified by germ tube testing, is resistant to **conventional treatments.**

Ans. 156: (c) Refer him for colonoscopy with particular attention to the cecum

Ref: Read the text below

Sol:

- **Even though this patient is young, this case has disturbing features. A young man should not have iron deficiency anemia.**
- **Esophagogastroduodenoscopy** does not identify a bleeding site or provide an adequate explanation for his anemia. Colon cancer, especially cecal cancer, can be associated with intermittent bleeding, so **even 3 consecutive stool samples** that are negative for blood are not proof that he is not bleeding.
- **Cecal cancer can mimic leiomyoma** on air contrast barium enema. On colonoscopy, the patient was found to have invasive cecal cancer.

Ans. 157: (b) PML

Ref: Read the text below

Sol:

(Progressive multifocal leukoence-phalopathy) is the correct diagnosis because;

- The **subcortical white matter (arrows) is primarily involved** in this patient.
- The **sharply defined margins, multiple areas, and lack of symmetry** on this MR examination distinguish PML from HIV encephalopathy.
- Unlike in HIV encephalopathy this process is **typically multifocal and lesions may coalesce** and have a **predilection for the occipital and parietal lobes.**
- The involved areas usually **begin in the subcortical white matter** and on the **T2-weighted images exhibit nonspecific areas of high signal.**

HIV encephalopathy

- On MR, the **white matter tracts such as corona radiata, the cerebral peduncles, and the brain stem** exhibit poorly defined symmetric areas of **abnormal high signal images on T2-weighted images.**

Generalized cortical atrophy also occurs.

- The **symmetry, diffuse nature, and poorly defined margins are typical features** of HIV encephalopathy.

HSV-I encephalitis

- The high signal edema representing encephalitis is best seen on T2-weighted images and has a **propensity to involve frontal and temporal lobes.**

Primary CNS lymphoma

- **MRI or CT** generally reveals a **limited number (one to three) of 3- to 5-cm lesions.** The lesions often show **ring enhancement on contrast administration and may occur in any location.**
- Locations that are **most commonly** involved with **CNS lymphoma** are deep in the white matter.

Ans. 158: (c) Segment 3 is mainly due to Na+ influx

Ref: Read the text below

Sol:

- The picture above is the graphical representation of **ionic activity of the pacemaker tissue.**

Ans. 159: (b) Mycobacterium leprae

Ref: Read the text below

Sol:

- The picture shows lepra **cells and characteristic arrangement of acid fast lepra** bacilli.
- Sensory loss is **also a feature of leprosy.**

Ans. 160: (a) String sing of Kantor

Ref: Read the text below

Sol:

This small bowel enema is showing a narrowed terminal ileum involved with crohn's disease- the 'string' sign of Kantor.

- Bird beak deformity - Caecal volvulus.
- Pincer shaped deformity- Intussusception.
- Coil spring sign - Intussusception.

Ans. 161: (a) Hereditary pancreatitis

Ref: Read the text below

Sol:

Hereditary pancreatitis.

Endoscopic Retrograde Cholangiopancreato-gram (ERCP)

- The **endoscopic retrograde pancreatogram** on the left shows a ventral pancreatic ductal system with many non-calcified **intraductal filling defects (arrows). The operative pancreato-gram and cholangiogram on the right demonstrates the dorsal duct with dilatation and large intraductal filling defects (arrows).**
- **The presence of large, peripherally dense, round** or oval calculi of the pancreatic ducts in a

patient with typical clinical characteristics is strong confirmatory evidence of hereditary pancreatitis. The calculi are calcified in **about 60 to 75% of cases of hereditary pancreatitis. In other cases, ERCP may be necessary to make the diagnosis.**

- **Chronic pancreatitis is found with familial occurrence** in kindreds with hyperlipidemia, hyperparathyroidism, cystic fibrosis, and cholelithiasis. In addition, there is a distinct group of patients in whom precipitating factors are not identified. This is generally termed hereditary pancreatitis, and it is thought to be inherited as an autosomal dominant with variable penetrance. The typical **clinical features include an early age of onset with varying degrees of abdominal pain and disability. There may be complications of endocrine and exocrine pancreatic insufficiency**, pseudocyst formation, and adenocarcinoma of the pancreas.
- The clinical **features of this entity are often not distinctive. This** is emphasized by an average 20 year delay from onset of symptoms to **diagnosis. Appreciation of characteristic pancreatographic findings of this disease should assist in making earlier diagnosis and direct appropriate treatment.**
- The etiology of hereditary pancreatitis remains undetermined. A defect in protein metabolism may be the cause in **that 50% of patients and their family members have associated amino-acidurias.**
- **Other reports suggest an anatomic etiology** with obstructing stenosis of the main pancreatic duct at one or both papillae. An anatomic etiology such as this could be related to defects in duodenal vacuolization as described in the embryogenesis of other duodenal anomalies such as congenital diaphragms, stenoses and duplications.

Ans. 162: (d) Ultrasonography (U/S) of lower limbs

Ref: Read the text below

Sol:

PTE DIAGNOSTIC STRATEGY

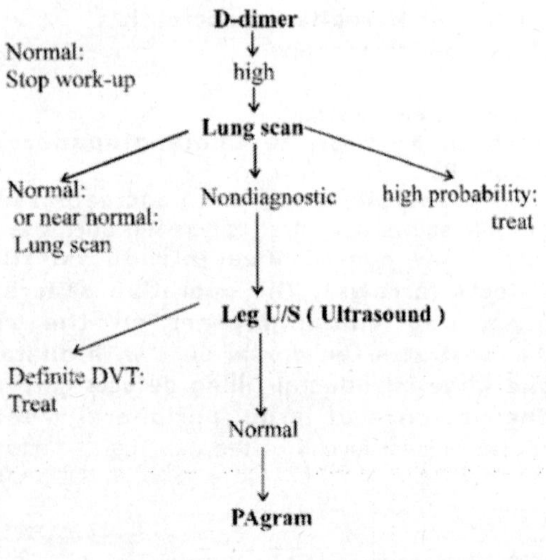

Ans. 163: (c) Corticosteroid

Ref: Read the text below

Sol:

TEMPORAL ARTERITIS

1. The clinical picture is highly **suggestive of temporal arteritis. The disease** is characterized clinically by the classic complex of fever, anemia, high ESR, and headaches in an elderly patient.
2. The disease is closely **associated with polymyalgia rheumatica, which is more common than giant cell arteritis.**
3. Characteristic lab finding in addition **to elevated ESR include normochromic** or slightly hypochromic anaemia.
   Alkaline phosphatase is increased **but creatine kinase is not elevated.**

Ans. 164: (c) Infecting organism specially destroy type II pneumocytes

Ref: Read the text below

Sol:

- This is a case of **Pneumocystis carinii pneumonia in an immunocompromised** (i.v. drug abuser) patients once considered a protozoan, **now proved to be a fungus on ribotyping.**
- Pneumocystis attaches to and kills type I pneumocytes, causing excess replication of type II pneumocytes. Alveoli gives honey combing appearance on **H and E stain.**
- **On X-ray - Patchy infiltration (ground glass appearance) is seen. The lower** lobe periphery may be spared.

Ans. 165: (c) Epidermophyton

Ref: Read the text below

Sol:

Numerous smooth walled macroconidia and absent microconidia	– Epidermophyton
Rough wall macroconidia few microconidias	– Microsporum
Absent macroconidia abundant microconidias	– Trichophyton

Ans. 166: (a) Granulomatosis infantisepticum

Ref: Read the text below

Sol:

- This is classical presentation of **neonatal listeriosis** specially with history of preterm labour and prolonged rupture of membrane.
- **Early onset infection** generally present on 2nd day of infection. Disseminated infection by listeriosis is called **Granulomatosis infantisepticum**. In this infection multiple abscess formation occur throughout the body.
- **Mortality** is very high. **No treatment** has been found effective.

Ans. 167: (c) ELISA in urine for detection of soluble antigen.

Ref: Read the text below

Sol:

- Antibodies takes at least 8 days to develop. It may cross react with **campylobactor infection** induced antibodies.
- Culture also takes 3 to 5 days. The examination of urine for legionella antigen by **enzyme linked immunosorbant assay (ELISA)** is a rapid and specific method of identifying **L. Pneumophila** as the likely cause of pneumonia.

Ans. 168: (d) Bacterial vaginosis
Ref: Read the text below
Sol:

- History consistent with vaginitis and description of foul odour and vaginal irritation are characteristic of **bacterial vaginosis**.

Ans. 169: (a) Community A
Ref: Read the text below
Sol:

- **Greater the prevalence of a disease in a community**, greater the positive predictive value of a screening test **in that community.**
- So if same screening test is used in **both the communities with dissimilar prevalences of** disease, positive predictive value will be more in the community with more **prevalence, i.e. community B in this question.**
- Positive predictive value will be less in community A thus more **number of false positives.**

Ans. 170: (d) Achalasia cardia
Ref: Read the text below
Sol:

- The disease is most **common in middle life but can occur at any age**. It typically presents with dysphagia.
- In patients who have remained untreated for many **years, regurgitation is frequent and there may be overspill into trachea especially at night.**

Ans. 171: (c) Abdominoperineal resection
Ref: Read the text below
Sol:

- **Adenocarcinoma of anal canal are considered to be started** from lower rectum and these tumors are **comparatively radioresistant.**

Ans. 172: (c) Benign mixed tumor (pleomorphic adenoma)
Ref: Read the text below
Sol:

- **Benign mixed tumors** (pleomophic adenomas) are the most common tumors glands; they account for 50 percent of all tumors and over 80 percent of all benign tumors in this location.
- In the parotid gland**, 65 to 75 percent of tumors are pleomorphic adenomas**. The female to male ratio is 4:3 and the peak incidence occurs **between 30 and 40 years of age.**
- The tumor is slow growing firm, Recurrence of the tumor **is the result of incomplete removal.**
- Facial nerve weakness in a patient who has a parotid **tumor almost indicates the presence of a malignant lesion.**

Ans. 173: (b) Assess the urethral injury by ascending urethrography
Ref: Read the text below
Sol:

- The **bulbous urethra may be injured as a result falling astride** an object. Urethral contusion may cause a perineal hematoma **without urethral disruption. Perineal hematoma usually resolves without complications.**
- Laceration will **lead to urinary extravasation.**
- The patient usually has a desire to void, but voiding should not be allowed until assessment of the urethra is **complete. No attempt should be made to pass a urethral** catheter, but if the patient's bladder is overdistended, **percutaneous suprapubic cystostomy can be done as a temporary procedure.**
- A urethrogram with instillation of 15-20 ml of **contrast material, will demonstrate extravasation and the location of injury**. The contused urethra will show no evidence of extravasation. If there is no evidence of extravasation on the urethrogram, a urethral catheter may be passed into the bladder**. Extravasation is a contraindication to further instrumentation at this time.**
- After the urethrography, the patient with urethral contusion is allowed to void; and if the voiding occurs normally, without pain or **bleeding no additional treatment is necessary. If bleeding persists urethral catheter drainage can be done.**
- **If urethral laceration is detected on urethrography** instrumentation of the urethra should be avoided. A suprapubic cystostomy tube should be inserted (through a small incision in the suprapubic area to expose the dome of the **bladder) to allow complete urinary diversion while the urethral laceration heals.**

Ans. 174: (d) Granulomatous destruction of bile duct radicals
Ref: Read the text below
Sol:

- With a history of **rheumatoid arthritis (autoimmune disease), pruritus (bile salt deposition** in the skin), normal bilirubin levels, and elevation of the cholestasis enzymes in a middle-aged woman, **primary biliary cirrhosis** is the most likely diagnosis. It is characterized by the development of antimitochondrial antibodies that **attack antigens in the bile duct** epithelium. **Granulomatous inflammation** is commonly present in the triads. Jaundice is a late feature of the disease.
- **Mid-zonal liver cell necrosis with Councilman bodies** represents yellow fever. **Perivenular fibrosis** of the terminal hepatic venules is a

characteristic finding in alcoholic liver disease owing to acetaldehyde-protein complex stimulation of myofibroblasts to synthesize collagen.

- **"Pipestem" cirrhosis** is the classic finding of schistosomiasis (Schistosoma mansoni) involving the portal vein radicals, which leads to fibrosis of the vessels. Ring (doughnut) granulomas are a feature of Q fever due to Coxiella burnetti. **Interstitial pneumonia** and **granulomatous hepatitis** are two consistent features of the disease.

Ans. 175: (d) Hereditary sensory motor neuropathy
Ref: Read the text below
Sol:

- In view of the family history, **this patient is most likely to have hereditary sensory motor** neuropathy type I.
- **HMSN I** is the most common form of hereditary neuropathy. Severely and uniformly slowed nerve conduction velocities (NCVs) and primary hypertrophic myelin pathology with prominent onion bulbs and secondary **axonal changes are the hallmarks of the disease. Motor symptoms predominate over sensory symptoms.**
- **Often, patients report loss of balance, muscle weakness**, and foot deformities. Onset in the first decade of life is typical, but disease develops in some patients in young or mid adulthood.
- **HMSN II, on the other hand, represents the non**demyelinating neuronal type with relatively normal NCVs and primary axonal pathology. Although nerves are not enlarged in the neuronal form, weakness often is less marked and onset of this neuropathy is delayed. Peripheral nerves are not enlarged clinically, and weakness of feet and leg muscles predominates; hands are less **severely affected than the legs. Patients experience sensory loss in the distal extremities, and f**oot deformities (ie, pes cavus) tend to be less marked than those of HMSN I.

Ans. 176: (c) MELAS
Ref: Read the text below
Sol:

- This patient has **MELAS** (myopathy, encephalopathy, lactic acidosis and stroke like episodes). Lactic acidosis is a very important feature of this disorder, as measured by **a high lactate to pyruvate ratio**.
- However, in general, **lactic acidosis does not lead to systemic metabolic acidosis**, and it may be absent in patients with impressive involvement of the **central nervous system.**
- Patients have a myopathy causing proximal muscle weakness and hypotonia, **seizures and strokelike episodes. It is a mitochondrial inherited disorder.**

Ans. 177: (d) A is false but R is true
Ref: Read the text below
Sol:

- Omalizumab is a blocking antibody that neutralizes circulating IgE without binding to cell-bound IgE; it thus inhibits IgE-mediated reactions.
- This treatment has been shown to reduce the number of exacerbations in patients with severe asthma and may improve asthma control.
- However, the treatment is very expensive and only suitable for highly selected patients who are not controlled on maximal doses of inhaler therapy and have a circulating IgE within a specified range. Patients should be given a 3–4 month trial of therapy to show objective benefit.
- Omalizumab is usually given as a subcutaneous injection every 2–4 weeks and appears not to have significant side effects.

Ans. 178: (b) Both A and R are true and R is not correct explanation of A
Ref: Read the text below
Sol:

- This is very **peculiar about sweat glands that though they** are having sympathetic innervation but the **neurotransmitter is Acetylcholine.**
- Also remember that all postganglionic **parasympathetic and few postganglionic.**
- Sympathetic (sweat glands & some blood vessels) are having **Muscarinic receptors while ganglia of both sympathetic and parasympathetic are having nicotinic receptors**

Ans. 179: (c) A is true but R is false
Ref: Read the text below
Sol:

- COCKAYNE SYNDROME: Autosomal recessive condition with photosensitivity and neurological degeneration.
- It differs from Xeroderma pigmentosa by the lack of freckling and skin cancers and presence of dwarfism, beaked nose, and loss of subcutaneous fat, basal ganglion calcification, retinopathy and deafness. Cockayne described syndrome as dwarfism with retinal atrophy and deafness.
- Derrnatologic features include photodermatitis with telangiectasia, atrophy, and scarring. The hands and feet are large and cyanotic. Microcephaly, sunken eyes, severe flexion contractures, dorsal kyphosis, cryptorchidism, cataracts, growth retardation, mental retardation, hypothalamic and cerebellar dysfunction, and retinitis pigmentosa, optic atrophy may be seen. There is progressive neurologic disturbance with a shortened lifespan.

Ans. 180: (c) A is true but R is false
Ref: Read the text below
Sol:

- **Herpes zoster** is generally limited to 1 dermatome or at most 2 or 3 adjacent dermatomes in normal hosts.
- **The thoracic dermatomes are the most commonly involved sites, followed by the lumbar dermatomes.**

1 The neural **elements of retina are bound together** by glial cells, **called as**:
a. Horizontal cells
b. Amacrine cells
c. Muller cells
d. Bipolar cells

2 The only intervention known to **delay aging is**:
a. Caloric restriction
b. Antioxidants
c. Vitamin supplementation
d. Avoidance of sunlight

3 Sudden distension of the biliary tree **produces**:
a. Steady pain
b. Colicky pain
c. Throbbing pain
d. Pricking pain

4 **Cluster headache** is associated with all, **except**:
a. Unilateral headache
b. Onset typically in 20-50 years of life
c. Affects predominantly females
d. Commonly awakens the patient from sleep

5 A 56-year-old coal mine worker **presented with joint pains, cutaneous nodules and occasional cough with dyspnoea.** His chest X-ray showed multiple small nodules in both lungs with cavitation and calcification. **Most likely** diagnosis is:
a. Silicosis
b. Caplan's syndrome
c. Sjogren's syndrome
d. Sarocidosis

6 A 65-year-old man **with diabetes, on an oral hypoglycemic, presents to the ER with a sports-related right shoulder injury**. His heart rate was noted to be irregular and the following ECG was obtained.

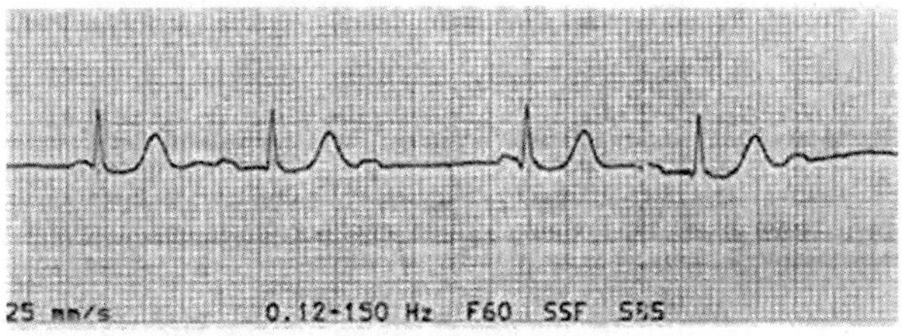

The best immediate therapy is:
a. Atropine
b. Pacemaker
c. Digoxin
d. Observation

7 The patient pictured below presents with **gynecomastia and infertility. On exam, he has small, firm testes.** Which of the following is correct?

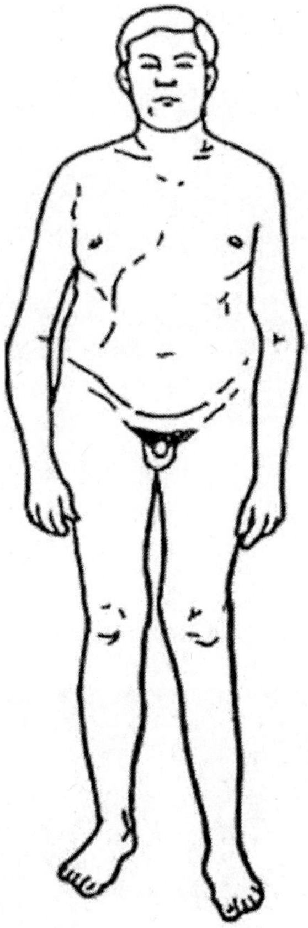

a. The patient is likely to have low levels of gonadotropins
b. The patient has Turner syndrome
c. His most likely karyotype is 47 XXY
d. The patient will have normal sperm count and testosterone

8 **In a case of** first idiopathic venous thromboembolism event; **current recommendations for warfarin therapy is for**:
a. Less than 3 months
b. 3–6 months
c. 6 months
d. 12 months to lifetime

9 **Distal gastrectomy without vagotomy** has traditionally been the procedure of choice for:
a. Type I gastric ulcer
b. Type II gastric ulcer
c. Type III gastric ulcer
d. Hiatal hernia

10 Procedure of **choice** for bleeding gastric ulcer is:
a. Distal gastric resection
b. Vagotomy and drainage
c. Vagotomy and drainage with oversewing of the ulcer
d. Highly-selective vagotomy

11 Retinitis pigmentosa is a hereditary disorder, which affects the photoreceptors (the rods and the cones) in the retina. These photoreceptors are located in which of the numbered layers in the following figure?
a. 2
b. 3

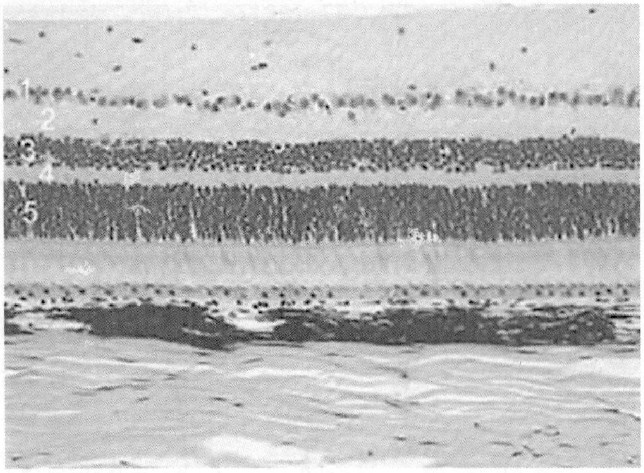

c. 4
d. 5

12 The structure indicated by **arrow 1 in Fig is which** of the following vessels?

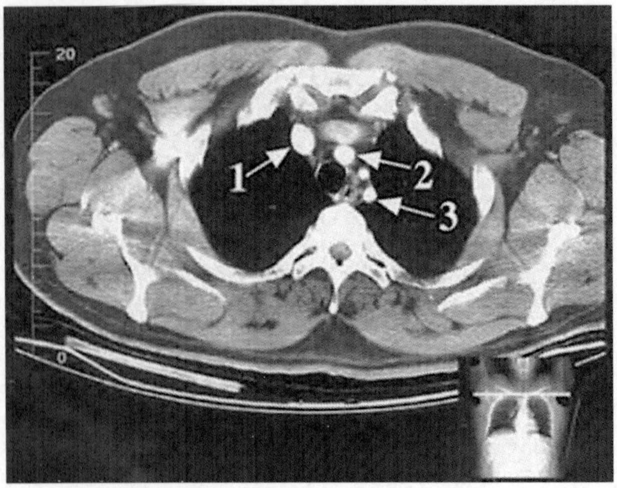

a. Brachiocephalic artery
b. Left brachiocephalic vein
c. Left common carotid artery
d. Right brachiocephalic vein

13 An external fistula (e.g., enterocutaneous fistula or rectovaginal fistula) involves the skin or another external surface epithelium. **High-output fistulas** are those that drain more than:
a. 200 mL of fluid per day
b. 300 mL of fluid per day
c. 400 mL of fluid per day
d. 500 mL of fluid per day

14 Because radiation has its greatest impact on rapidly proliferating cells, the small-intestinal epithelium is acutely susceptible to radiation induced injury, **most frequently affected segment** is:
a. Terminal ileum
b. Terminal duodenum
c. Proximal ileum
d. Proximal duodenum

15 The **most common** presentation associated with **symptomatic meckel's diverticula** in a **5 years old child** is:
a. Bleeding
b. Intestinal obstruction
c. Diverticulitis
d. Carcinoid tumors

16 **Endorectal ultrasound** can reliably differentiate most benign polyps from invasive tumors based upon the integrity of the:
a. Mucosa
b. Submucosa
c. Muscularis propria
d. Perirectal fat

17 Which of the following is **not** a WHO **recommendation for recording blood pressure**?
a. Record BP in sitting position
b. Measure BP thrice at 3 minutes' interval
c. Take the average of three readings as the correct BP
d. Use one arm consistently

18 **Which** of the following syndromes do **not** constitute 'Stroke' as per WHO definition?
a. Transient ischaemic attack (TIA)
b. Subarachnoid haemorrhage
c. Hemiplegia
d. Monoplegia

19 **Angiogram of the cerebral vasculature is given below:**

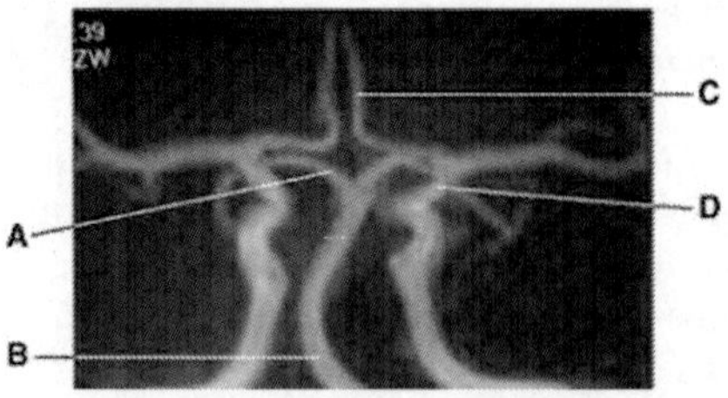

A **large tumor in the foramen magnum** may decrease blood flow in **which artery?**
a. A
b. B
c. C
d. D

20 In relation to epidemiology of cancers, all of the following statements are **true; except**:
a. Occupational exposures account for 5-10% of human cancers
b. Erythroplakia is a precancerous lesion of oral cancer
c. Genital warts act as risk factor for cervical cancer
d. Early menarche and late menopause are risk factors for breast cancer

21 **Which** is the **most** reliable test for screening of the population for diabetes mellitus?
a. Urine examination for glycosuria
b. Fasting blood sugar
c. Random blood sugar
d. Glucose tolerance test

22 Which of the following is the **common** cause of **infant mortality** rate in India?
a. Acute respiratory infections
b. Diarrhoea
c. Congenital anomalies
d. Low birth weight

23 The **maximum number** of students that a classroom should accommodate under the guidelines for school health services is:
a. 40 b. 50
c. 60 d. 70

24 A 14-year-old boy having lost his father a year ago is **caught shoplifting**. The boy will be sent to:
a. Orphanage
b. Remand home
c. Foster home
d. Borstal

25 In **ICDS** scheme, the nutritional supplement for **pregnant and nursing** mothers is aimed at providing:
a. 300 kcals and 15 g proteins
b. 300 kcals and 25 g proteins
c. 500 kcals and 25 g proteins
d. 500 kcals and 15 g proteins

26 **ICDS package** includes all of the following **except**:
a. Immunization
b. Formal education
c. Health check up
d. Nutrition

27 A third-year medical student is asked to review the computerized tomographic (CT) results of a patient with a possible abdominal aortic aneurysm. Which of the following arrows in figure points to the abdominal aorta?
a. 1 b. 2
c. 3 d. 4

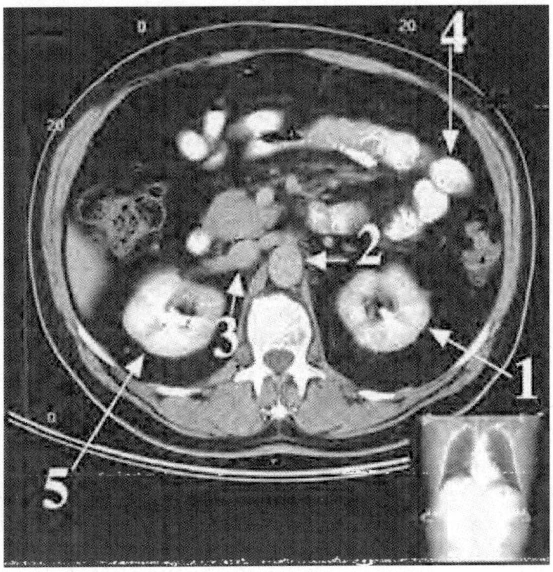

28 The most common complication of **biliopancreatic diversion is**:
a. Anemia
b. Protein-calorie malnutrition
c. Dumping syndrome
d. Hypocalcemia

29 Choose the **incorrect** statement regarding **Campylobacters jejuni**?
a. Campylobacters are motile, curved, oxidasepositive, gram-negative rods
b. C. jejuni grows well only on enriched media under microaerophilic conditions
c. The cells have polar flagella
d. It break down carbohydrates,uses metabolic intermediates for energy

30 **Resection of hemorrhoidal tissue and closure of the w**ounds with absorbable suture is:
a. Ferguson hemorrhoidectomy
b. Open Hemorrhoidectomy
c. Whitehead's Hemorrhoidectomy
d. Stapled Hemorrhoidectomy

31 A patient presents with a **loss of sensation to the skin over the shoulder**. Injury to which of the following nerve cells **would most likely affect the conduction of sensory information to the central nervous system (CNS)?**
a. Multipolar neurons
b. Bipolar neurons
c. Unipolar or pseudounipolar neurons
d. Neurons in the ventral horn

32 A 51-year-old woman came with **rapid and progressive impairment in her vision affecting her left eye over a few days**. Apart from red swollen left optic disc with severely reduced visual acuity to finger **counting and Marcus-Gunn pupil, her examination is totally unremarkable**. Few days later while she is in the way of investigations, she said that her vision is better now. Which one is **the correct statement**?
a. Brain MRI with contrast is not indicated
b. Auto antibody screen is useless
c. The findings are consistent with Foster Kennedy syndrome
d. Gradual and excellent improvement is against giant cell arteritis

33 A 32-year-old man presents with a 2-year **history of left sided headache and ocular pain**. The pain seems to occur in severe bouts for about two hours**, with eye redness and nasal watering, day and night, with no remission, somewhat responsive to phenacetin**. He is non-smoker and non-alcoholic, on no medications or illicit drugs. Examination revealed **only gynecomastia** and soft testes.Which one is the **correct statement**?
a. He has migraine without aura
b. Brain MRI or CT scan should be done

c. Increasing the dose of phenacetin is helpful
d. Reassure and discharge him

34 A 40-year-old man was admitted because of **progressive somnolence over few days**. He has a history of extensive chronic plaque **psoriasis for which he is receiving cyclosporine. Examination revealed fever, neck stiffness and obtundation**. Which one is the correct statement regarding his new presentation?
a. We should increase the dose of cyclosporine
b. Start intravenous cefotaxime and vancomycine
c. Add azathioprine
d. Blood cultures should be avoided

35 A 21-year-old woman, who was **reasonably well and healthy, presents with 4-month history of progressive unsteadiness in stance and gait.** She denied any drug abuse or a back trauma, and there are no risk factors for **HIV infection, and no family history of a similar condition. Examination revealed spastic paraparesis with loss of join position** and vibration sense in the lower limbs and right-sided **primary optic atrophy. No sensory level was detected**. What is your next step?
a. Give high dose pulse intravenous methylprednisolone
b. Give vitamin B_{12} injections
c. Plain X-ray of the lumbosacral spine
d. Brain MRI with contrast

36 A 57-year-old woman with a history **of mitral stenosis presents with sudden onset of right sided weakness and global aphasia**. Brain CT scan revealed **massive infarction covering the whole area supplied by the left middle cerebral artery and midline shif**t. ECG showed rapid atrial fibrillation. Which one is the correct step?
a. Omit anticoagulation for the time being
b. Avoid digoxin
c. Mannitol is hazardous
d. Immediate electrical cardioversion should be done

37 A 60-year-old right-handed man has a **history of embolic stroke, and he is aphasic**. His speech is non-fluent, with impaired **repetition and naming, but relatively intact comprehension**. Where is the site of the lesion that is likely to be **responsible for his aphasia**?
a. Upper posterior temporal gyrus, left hemisphere
b. Left frontal pole
c. Left mesial temporal lobe
d. Lower posterior inferior frontal gyrus, left hemisphere

38 If a **supralevator abscess arises from the upward extension of an ischiorectal abscess,** it should be drained through the ischiorectal fossa. **Drainage** of this type of abscess through the rectum may result in an:
a. Ischiorectal abscesses
b. Intersphincteric abscess
c. Perianal abscess
d. Extrasphincteric fistula

39 In the diagram of a **normal heart shown below, the coronary artery most likely to be involved in a posteroseptal infarct** (as in this patient) is indicated by which letter?

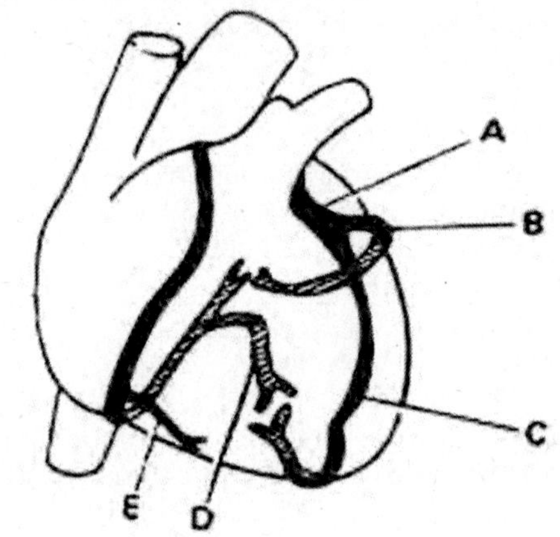

a. A
b. B
c. C
d. D

40 Which of the following structures needs to be **repaired in a fractured penis**?
a. Tunica albuginea
b. Corpus spongiosum
c. Corpora cavernosum
d. Urethra

41 Which of the following is **not an acceptable indication** for open-**chest cardiac massage**?
a. Arrest after penetrating chest trauma with minimal downtime
b. Arrest after blunt trauma with signs of life in the ED
c. Arrest with severe hypothermia
d. Arrest due to myocardial infarction

42 Which of the following findings are consistent with **acute prerenal failure**?
a. BUN to creatinine ratio of <10, fractional excretion of sodium (FeNa) <1, red cells in urine sediment
b. BUN to creatinine ratio of >20, FeNa >1, normal urinalysis
c. Urine osmolality <350, moderate proteinuria, granular casts
d. Urine osmolality >500, red cell casts, proteinuria, FeNa <1

43 The **graph in figure** shows the **pressure-volume curve** of the left ventricle of this patient (shaded area). The pressure-volume curve of a normal **subject is shown for comparison** (broken lines). Compared to normal, which term best **describes this patient's heart**?

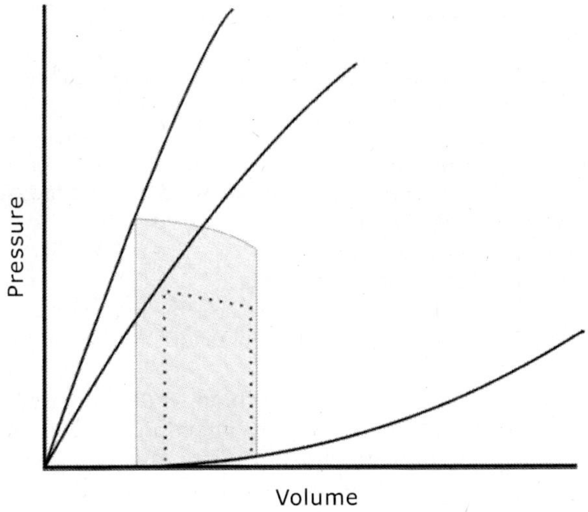

a. Decreased afterload
b. Decreased preload
c. Decreased stroke volume
d. Increased force of contraction

44 A 41-year-old man requests **information concerning vasectomy for sterilization**. In this prcedure, which of the **following statements is true**?
a. The incidence of sexual dysfunction is not influenced in those with dependent personalities
b. The failure rate occurs in 1/400 patients
c. Recanalization of the vas deferens does not occur
d. The procedure is difficult and requires laparotomy

45 A 6-month-old boy was born **with hypos-padias. This** condition is due to failure in the development of which **of the following?**
a. Urogenital fold b. Müllerian system
c. Genital tubercle d. Urachus

46 A 64-year-old woman notes an ulcer on her **left labia majora. Biospy reveals squamous cell carcinoma.** What is the treatment?
a. Preoperative radiotherapy followed by wide local excision
b. Radiotherapy
c. Wide excision and unilateral groin dissection
d. Radical vulvectomy and bilateral groin dissection

47 A 6-year-old healthy appearing girl **is brought for evaluation of bloody vaginal discharge**. The most likely diagnosis is:
a. Squamous cell carcinoma
b. Sarcoma botryoides
c. Carcinosarcoma
d. Clear cell adenocarcinoma

48 A healthy appearing, 8-year-old boy is **evaluated for an abdominal mass,** felt by his mother during a bath. What is the **most likely diagnosis?**
a. Lymphoma
b. Rhabdomyoscarcoma
c. Wilms' tumor
d. Neuroblastoma

49 After undergoing a partial **cystectomy for carcinoma of the rectum, a 76-year-old woman develops a vesicovaginal fistula.** The repair will have a higher chance of success if which of the following occurs?
a. Scare tissue is not excised
b. The bladder wall is closed under tension
c. Repair is performed more than 6 months after the causative operation
d. Repair is performed within 7–14 days of the onset of symptoms

50 After being treated for **ovarian carcinoma, a 65-year-old woman develops complications attributed to cisplatin.** What is a common side effect of cisplatin?
a. Ankylosing spondylitis
b. Megaloblastic anemia
c. Pulmonary fibrosis
d. Peripheral neuropathy

51 Which of the following is **not a concern** about stored **blood products (packed red blood cells)?**
a. Stored red blood cells have depleted 2, 3-diphosphoglycerate, leading to decreased offloading of oxygen at the tissue level
b. Stored blood products exacerbate splanchnic hypoperfusion
c. The increased pliability of stored red blood cells allows them to seep into the interstitium
d. Stored red blood cells are characterized as having decreased deformability

52 A 52-year-old woman has biopsy of a **breast lesion which confirms the mass as malignant**. She is also found to clinically have a **palpable ipsilateral axillary lymph** node. Which of the following would be the most likely pathologic finding in this node?
a. Follicular hyperplasia
b. Paracortical hyperplasia
c. Granulomatous inflammation
d. Sinus histiocytosis

53 A history of which of the following conditions would **result in the greatest increase in the likelihood of developing colon cancer**?
a. Crohn's disease
b. Hamartomatous polyp
c. Pseudomembranous colitis
d. Ulcerative colitis

54 Which of the following is the most **common characteristic of a serous** cystadenocarcinoma of the ovary?
a. It causes pseudomyxoma peritonei
b. It is composed of transitional epithelial cells
c. It is frequently bilateral
d. It often metastasizes to the brain

55 A 28-year-old female shows clinical **manifestations related to secretion of excess androgenic hormones and persistent anovulation**. What would be the most likely finding in the ovary?
a. Endometriosis
b. Polycystic ovary
c. Endometrioid carcinoma of the ovary
d. Granulosa cell tumor of the ovary

56 A small area of abnormality is noted on the **lateral wall of the urinary bladder during a cystoscopy** on a patient being evaluated for asymptomatic microscopic **hematuria.** Biopsy of the lesion is most likely to reveal which of the following?
a. Neuroendocrine carcinoma
b. Rhabdomyosarcoma
c. Squamous cell carcinoma
d. Papillary transitional cell carcinoma

57 What is the most common manifestation of **Coccidioides infection in an immuno-competent host**?
a. Acute pneumonia
b. Asymptomatic seroconversion
c. Hypersensitivity phenomena such as erythema nodosum
d. Meningitis

58 Most likely diagnosis:

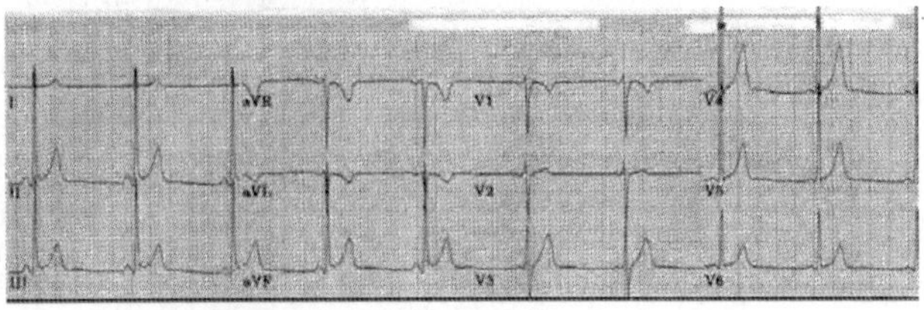

a. Pulmonary embolism
b. Early repolarization
c. Acute pericarditis
d. Acute myocardial infarction

59 What is the best method for **diagnosis of Norovirus**?
a. Acute and convalescent antibody titers
b. Demonstration of Norwalk toxin in the stool
c. Electron microscopy
d. Polymerase chain reaction (PCR)

60 The figure below shows **pressure volume loops for two situations**. When compared with loop A, **loop B demonstrates:**

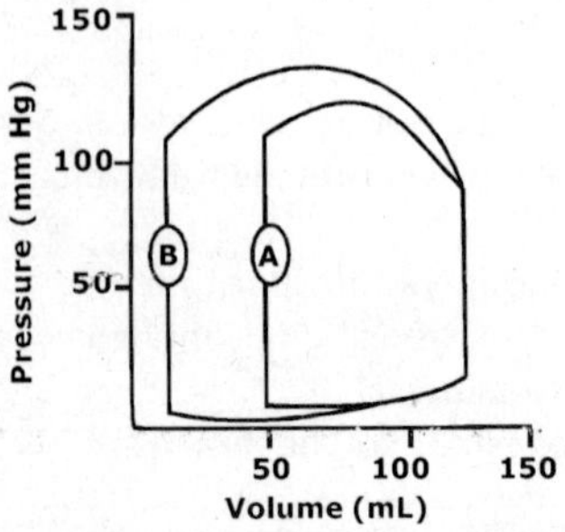

a. Increased preload
b. Decreased preload
c. Increased contractility
d. Increased afterload

61 **Most likely assessment** technique to be clinically useful in predicting the **likelihood of successful resuscitation after cardiac arrest is:**
a. Serial blood gases.
b. End-tidal CO_2 monitoring.
c. Ventricular fibrillation waveform analysis.
d. Invasive hemodynamic pressure monitoring.

62 A 70 kg (154 lb) man on a **fixed NaCl intake (200 mmol/day**) is given daily injections of a potent **mineralocorticoid hormone for 4 days.** He has free access to water and consumes his usual caloric intake. Excretion of **NaCl is as follows**:

Day	NaCl (mmol)
1	30
2	90
3	180
4	200

Assuming that 1 L of 0.9% saline contains 150 mmol of NaCl and weighs 1 kg, how much will this patient weigh (in kg) at the end of day 4?
a. 66
b. 68
c. 70
d. 72

63 A 46-year-old man comes to the **physician because of a 2-week history of intermittent dizziness and difficulty standing up**. His symptoms began after he **started treatment with sildenafil for erectile dysfunction**. Physical examination **shows no abnormalities**. Which of the following is the most likely mechanism of action of sildenafil **causing these adverse effects?**
a. Decreased basal vascular smooth muscle tone
b. Decreased parasympathetic nerve activity
c. Decreased sympathetic nerve activity
d. Increased basal vascular smooth muscle tone

64 A 72-year-old man who is a retired **construction worker comes to the physician because he has had a lesion on his face for 3 months.** Physical examination **shows a 6-mm, red, ulcerated lesion** with heaped borders. A **biopsy specimen of the lesion** shows atypical, dysplastic keratinocytes within the **epidermis and dermis**. Which of the following is the **most likely diagnosis**?
a. Actinic keratoses
b. Discoid lupus erythematosus
c. Melanoma
d. Squamous cell carcinoma

65 Scanning of inhaled, radioactively **labeled aerosols** has been used to study the distribution of pulmonary ventilation. However, **data obtained using aerosols with a particle diameter of 20 μ** do not accurately reflect the **distribution of alveolar ventilation in the lungs**. Which of the following is the best explanation for this finding?

a. Ingestion of these particles by alveolar macrophages occurs nonuniformly
b. The majority of particles this size do not adhere to airway or alveolar walls
c. Many particles are rapidly absorbed into the pulmonary capillary blood
d. Most particles this size are deposited in the conducting airways

66 **Myodesis is contraindicated** in:
a. Children
b. Tumor
c. Ischemia
d. Paralysis

67 **Ring fracture** is present around:
a. Obturator foramen
b. Glenoid cavity
c. Foramen magnum
d. Base of metacarpal bone

68 In the diagram shown, **point X** indicates the **acid base status** of a healthy person. Which of the following is the most likely cause of the condition **indicated by point Y**?

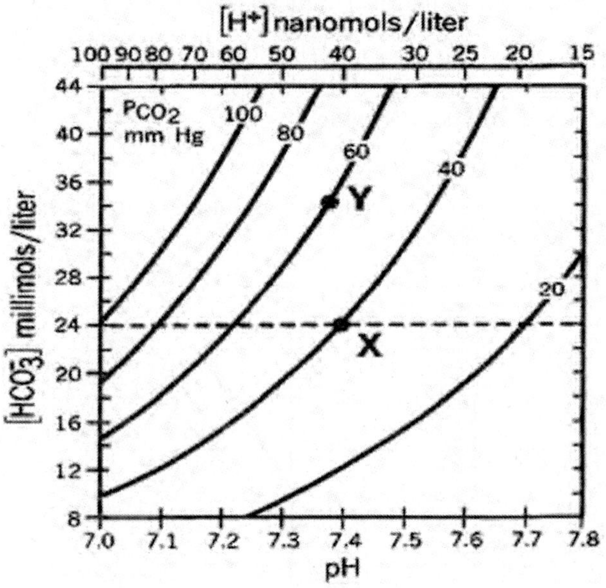

a. Adaptation to high altitude
b. Chronic obstructive pulmonary disease
c. Diarrhea
d. Ingestion of a strong acid

69 The control curve shown in the graph **illustrates the relationship between the initial velocity** of a reaction and the substrate concentration for **any enzyme obeying Michaelis-Menten kinetics**. Which of the following curves best **represents the result that would be obtained** by halving the amount of enzyme?
a. Curve 1
b. Curve 2

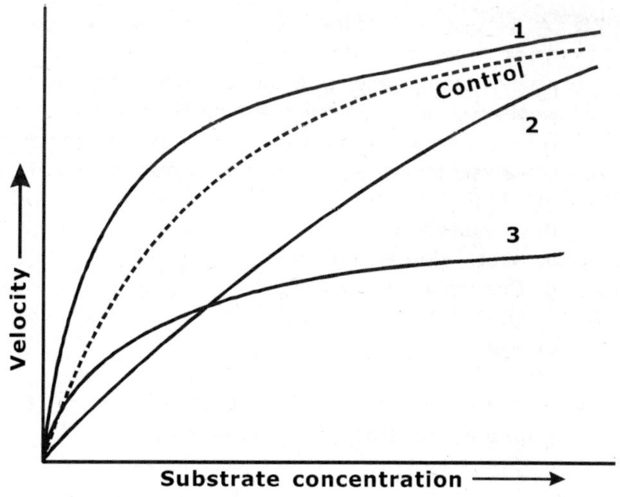

c. Curve 3
d. Control curve

70 A 12-year-old boy presents with **redness and swelling of his left foot for 24 hours**. Three days ago, the boy scraped his foot while **wading in a drainage ditch**. Examination of the left foot shows a purulent abrasion with edema, **erythema, and tenderness on the lateral side**. Infection is most likely to next spread from the lateral side of the foot to the regional lymph nodes in which of the following areas?
a. Lateral surface of the thigh
b. Medial malleolus, posteriorly
c. Popliteal fossa
d. Sole of the foot

71 A slightly drowsy 42-**year-old man is admitted with severe diabetic ketoacidosis, nausea, serum** potassium of 6.1 mEq/L, and a **BUN of 46 mg/dL.** Which of the following statements is correct regarding this patient?
a. The need to initiate potassium replacement is determined primarily by repeated measurements of serum potassium
b. Initial replacement should consist of 120 mEq of potassium given orally over a 4-hour period
c. Administration of bicarbonate to treat the acidosis may hasten the development of hypokalemia and magnify its intensity
d. Intravenous administration of potassium should not exceed 15 mEq/hour

72 A 32-year-old man is brought to the **emergency department because of confusion, wheezing, vomiting, and diarrhea for the past 6 hours**. He is sweating and **salivating profusely**. There is generalized **muscle weakness**. Which of the following substances is the most likely cause of these findings?
a. Glutethimide
b. Heroin
c. Jimson weed (belladonna alkaloids)
d. Parathion

73 A 24-year-old primigravid woman at 28 weeks' **gestation has had nagging headaches, a puffylooking face, and swollen legs** for the past week. Her blood pressure is 180/95 mm Hg; it was within normal **limits earlier in the pregnancy**. Urinalysis shows a protein concentration of 0.6 g/dL. Which of the following is **the most likely diagnosis**?
a. Acute glomerulonephritis
b. Congestive heart failure
c. Eclampsia
d. Preeclampsia

74 For each clinical **description select the appropriate stage of breast cancer**.
a. Stage I b. Stage II
c. Stage III d. Stage IV
e. Inflammatory carcinoma
1. Tumor not palpable, clinically positive lymph nodes fixed to one another, no evidence of metastases **(SELECT 1 STAGE).**
2. Tumor 5.0 cm; clinically positive, movable ipsilateral lymph nodes; no evidence of metastases **(SELECT 1 STAGE).**
3. Tumor 2.1 cm, clinically negative lymph nodes, no evidence of metastases **(SELECT 1 STAGE).**
4. Tumor not palpable but breast diffusely enlarged and erythematous, clinically positive supra-clavicular nodes, and evidence of metastases **(SELECT 1 STAGE).**
5. Tumor 0.5 cm, clinically negative lymph nodes, pathological rib fracture **(SELECT 1 STAGE).**
Option:
a. 1-c; 2-a; 3-b; 4-e; 5-g
b. 1-c; 2-a; 3-b; 4-a; 5-e
c. 1-c; 2-b; 3-b; 4-e; 5-d
d. 1-c; 2-h; 3-b; 4-e; 5-g

75 Match each description with the correct abnormality.
a. Rupture of the diaphragm
b. Paraesophageal hiatal hernia
c. Sliding hiatal hernia
d. Foramen of Bochdalek hernia
e. Foramen of Morgagni hernia
1. The most common congenital diaphragmatic hernia in infants **(SELECT 1 ABNORMALITY).**
2. The hernia most likely to cause acute respiratory distress in infants **(SELECT 1 ABNORMALITY).**
3. A congenital hernia that is most frequently discovered as an incidental finding in adults **(SELECT 1 ABNORMALITY).**
Option:
a. 1-c; 2-e; 3-b
b. 1-d; 2-a; 3-c
c. 1-d; 2-d; 3-e
d. 1-b; 2-c; 3-a

76 **Common** cause of **compartment syndrome** is:
a. Femur fracture
b. Metacarpal fracture
c. Radius fracture
d. Tibia fracture.

77 Which of the following **statement is true**?
a. The most common cause for breast disease in postmenopausal women is fibrocystic disease
b. If the patient is under 30 with a breast mass, then an outpatient ultrasound should be performed with possible needle aspiration
c. Fibrocystic changes of the breast include skin thickening, discoloration, and discharge
d. Patients over the age of 40 with a normal exam do not need a mammogram

78 What **external aids** can be used to help a **myopic eye compensate** for distance vision?
a. A positive (converging) lens placed in front of the eye
b. A negative (diverging) lens placed in front of the eye
c. A cylindrical lens placed in front of the eye
d. Eyeglasses that are partially opaque, to reduce the light intensity

79 A 36-year-old multiparous woman presents with **an episode of vaginal bleeding. Further questioning reveals she is at 31 weeks' gestation, as confirmed by ultrasound scan. Her vital signs are BP 142/78, temperature 36.7°C, pulse 96/minute**. Which of the following is the most likely diagnosis?
a. Cervical cancer
b. Placenta praevia
c. Abruptio placentae
d. Placenta accrete

80 The value of **km for the enzyme** depicted by **curve A** is:

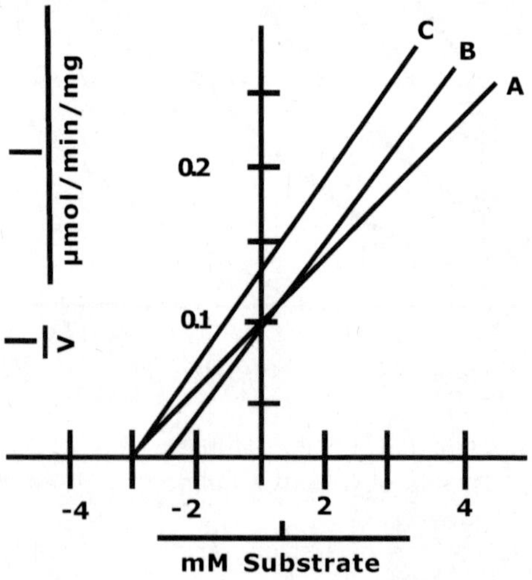

a. 0.5 mM b. 1 mM
c. 2 mM d. 1 μmol/min/mg

81 All of the following are common **manifestations of cytomegalovirus (CMV) infection** following lung transplantation **except:**
a. Bronchiolitis obliterans
b. CMV esophagitis
c. CMV pneumonia
d. CMV retinitis

82 Which of the following statements regarding **severe acute respiratory syndrome (SARS) is true**?
a. SARS displays poor human-to-human transmission
b. SARS is more severe among children than adults
c. The etiologic agent of SARS is in the Adenovirus family
d. There is known environmental reservoir for the virus causing SARS

83 **Helicobacter pylori colonization** is implicated in all of the following conditions except:
a. Duodenal ulcer disease
b. Gastric adenocarcinoma
c. Gastric mucosa-associated lymphoid tissue (MALT) lymphoma
d. Gastroesophageal reflux disease

84 Which of the following statements regarding **Clostridium difficile–associated disease relapses** is true?
a. A first recurrence does not imply greater risk of further recurrences
b. Most recurrences are due to antibiotic resistance
c. Recurrent C. difficile–associated disease has been associated with a higher risk of colon cancer
d. Recurrent disease is associated with serious complications

85 **Staphylococciare** routinely differentiated from **streptococci by:**
a. Coagulase test
b. Testwith hydrogen peroxide
c. Polymerase chain reaction
d. Protein A immune assay

86 Which of the following is a **contraindication to pertussis immunization**?
a. Cerebral palsy
b. Cow's milk protein intolerance
c. Fever to 39.5°C following the first dose
d. Redness of >2.5cm at the injection site after the first dose

87 A 60-year-old man takes **atenolol for hypertension**. Which of the following side effects is he most likely to be aware of two **hours after taking atenolol**?
a. Fatigue
b. Hesitancy of micturition
c. Nausea
d. Orthostatic hypotension

88 Which of the following **is true regarding metformin**?
a. It is associated with hypoglycaemia at normal doses
b. It is safe in patients with renal impairment
c. It may cause metabolic alkalosis
d. It is contraindicated in patients suffering a myocardial infarction

89 A 16-year-old female with **Addison's disease is intolerant of her hydrocortisone treatment** which she takes at a dose **of 20mg in the morning and 10mg in the evening**. Which of the following doses of prednisolone would **provide an equivalent daily dose as her hydrocortisone**?
a. 5 mg b. 7.5 mg
c. 10 mg d. 12.5 mg

90 Which of the following reactions is involved in the **metabolism of paracetamol under normal conditions?**
a. Cytochrome p450 dependent oxidation
b. Hydrolysis
c. Conjugation to glucuronic acid
d. Conjugation to glutathione

91 A diagnosis of diabetes mellitus is being **considered in 32-year-old woman who is 16 weeks pregnant. Her body mass index (BMI) was 22 kg/m² (18-25).** A 75g oral glucose tolerance test revealed:

Time	Plasma glucose concentration
• 0 hr	6.0 mmol/l (3.0-6.0)
• 2hr	12.5 mmol/l (<11.1)

Which of the following is the most appropriate step **in the management of this patient**?
a. A low calorie diet
b. Metformin therapy
c. Repeat her oral glucose tolerance test in four weeks
d. Insulin therapy

92 The changes seen in **the kidney shown in figure** were an incidental finding in **the autopsy of a 39-year-old woman**. The most likely cause is which of the following?

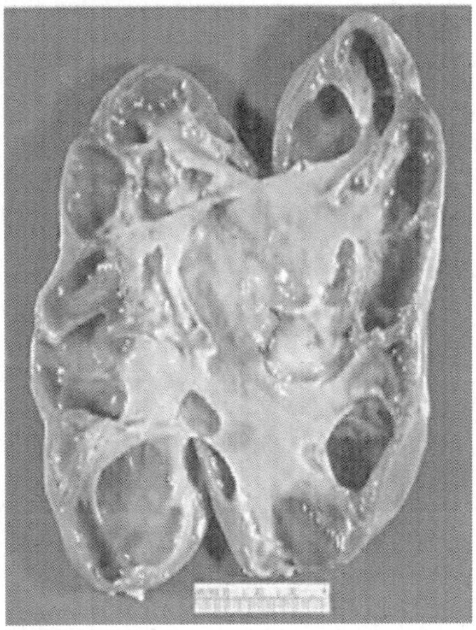

a. Abuse of analgesics
b. Hypertension
c. Postrenal obstruction
d. Renal infarct

93 Which statement about **monoamine oxidase inhibitor (MAOI) overdose** is true?
a. The tyramine reaction typically starts 8-10 hours after ingestion of foods high in tyramine
b. Once an irreversible MAOI has been stopped, a 2-week "washout" period is necessary before MAO activity returns
c. Use of epinephrine and norepinephrine are contraindicated in patients with an MAOI overdose
d. For severe hypertension, metoprolol is considered first-line therapy and should be given in 5 mg boluses every 10 minutes until the mean arterial pressure is decreased by 25-30%

94 Which of the following **side effects of neuroleptic medications** is paired incorrectly with its **clinical presentation**?
a. Dystonic reaction facial grimacing and oculogyric crises
b. Akathisia motor restlessness
c. Neuroleptic malignant syndrome cogwheel rigidity
d. Tardive dyskinesia choreoathetoid movements

95 Which of the following statements about **cocaine is true**?
a. Cocaine has no antiarrhythmic effect on cardiac conduction
b. Cocaine accelerates conduction of nerve impulses via fast sodium channel activation in the cell membrane
c. Neuromuscular blocking agents may have a long duration of effect in patients who have ingested cocaine
d. Neuroleptics like haloperidol or droperidol are very effective at calming the agitation or psychosis of cocaine intoxication and should be considered second-line therapy after benzodiazepines

96 Which description of the **pathophysiology of salicylate toxicity is false**?
a. As systemic pH decreases, salicylate concentrations in the brain will be higher than plasma concentrations
b. While salicylates can mobilize glycogen stores, resulting in hyperglycemia, they are also potent inhibitors of gluconeogenesis
c. The centrally mediated increased respiratory rate seen in salicylate poisoning is partially offset by a salicylate-induced decrease in carbon dioxide production
d. Despite its antiplatelet activity, hemorrhage from acute, massive salicylate poisoning is an uncommon occurrence

97 Which of the following substances is **not well adsorbed by activated charcoal**?
a. Acetaminophen
b. Tricyclic antidepressant
c. Iron
d. Calcium channel blockers

98 A 32-year-old man presents with jaundice **and malaise. He is found to have acute hepatitis B with positive hepatitis B virus (HBV) DNA and E antigen**. Which of the following antiviral agents are approved as part of a therapeutic regimen **for mono-infection with hepatitis B**?
a. Efavirenz
b. Ganciclovir
c. Lamivudine
d. Rimantadine

99 **Vascular Supply of** "Free TRAM flap" is:
a. Superior epigastric artery
b. Thoracodorsal
c. Deep inferior epigastric artery
d. Inferior gluteal artery

100 **"Winter shunt"** is related with:
a. Peyronie's disease
b. Erectile dysfunction
c. Hydronephrosis
d. Priapism

101 **Assertion A**: Patients with acute, severe and life threatening asthma are treated with parenteral steroids.
Reason R: Steroids are the most potent bronchodilators available.
a. Both A and R are true and R is correct explanation of A
b. Both A and R are true and R is not correct explanation of A
c. A is true but R is false
d. A is false but R is true

102 **Assertion A:** Some strains of clostridium perfringens type A can cause food poisoning.
Reason R: Clostridium perfringens type A produce heat-stable toxin
a. Both A and R are true and R is correct explanation of A
b. Both A and R are true and R is not correct explanation of A
c. A is true but R is false
d. A is false but R is true

103 Choose **incorrect** statement regarding **"hydrocele"**:
a. Communicating hydroceles in newborns should generally be observed
b. In pediatric patients, the surgery should be performed through an scrotal incision
c. In pediatric patients, the processus vaginalis should be ligated
d. In adults, hydroceles most commonly form as a consequence of local inflammation

104 Surgical procedure of choice during the **first and second trimesters of pregnancy with breast cancer is**:
a. Modified radical mastectomy
b. Radical mastectomy
c. Lumpectomy with axillary node dissection
d. Only lumpectomy

105 During the **sixth week of fetal development**, the midgut grows too rapidly to be accommodated in the abdominal cavity. If rotation is **incomplete,** the cecum remains in the epigastrium, but the **bands fixing the duodenum to the retroperitoneum and cecum** continue to form. **This results in (Ladd's) bands extending from the cecum to the**:
a. Duodenum
b. Lateral abdominal wall
c. Anterior abdominal wall
d. Posterior abdominal wall

106 An 80-year-old man presented with **impairment of higher intellectual function and alterations in mood and behavior.** His family reported progressive disorientation and memory loss over the last six months. There is no family **history of dementia. The patient was tentatively diagnosed with Alzheimer disease.** Which of the following **best** describes the disease?
a. It is associated with b-amyloid-an abnormal protein with an altered amino acid sequence
b. It results from accumulation of denatured proteins that have random conformations
c. It is associated with the accumulation of amyloid precursor protein
d. It is associated with the deposition of neurotoxic amyloid peptide aggregates

107 Following statement concerning the **binding of oxygen by hemoglobin** is **correct**?
a. The Bohr effect results in a lower affinity for oxygen at higher pH values
b. Carbon dioxide increases the oxygen affinity of hemoglobin by binding to the amino terminal groups of the polypeptide chains
c. The oxygen affinity of hemoglobin increases as the percentage saturation increases
d. The hemoglobin tetramer binds four molecules of 2, 3-BPG

108 A 67-year-old man presented to the **emergency department with a one week history of angina and shortness of breath**. He complained that his face and extremities had a "blue color". His medical history included chronic stable **angina treated with isosorbide dinitrate and nitroglycerin. Blood obtained for analysis was chocolate-colored**. The **most likely** diagnosis is:
a. Sickle cell disease
b. Carboxyhemoglobinemia
c. Methemoglobinemia
d. β-Thalassemia

109 Many antimicrobials inhibit **protein transla-tion. Which** of the following antimicrobials is **correctly** paired with its **mechanism of action?**
a. Tetracyclines inhibit peptidyltransferase
b. Puromycin inactivates eEF-2
c. Clindamycin binds to the 30S ribosomal subunit
d. Erythromycin binds to the 50S ribosomal subunit

110 **Which** of the following is required for **both** prokaryotic and eukaryotic protein synthesis?
a. Binding of the small ribosomal subunit to the Shine-Dalgarno sequence
b. Movement of the mRNA out of the nucleus and into the cytoplasm
c. Recognition of the 5'-cap by initiation factors
d. Translocation of the peptidyl-tRNA from the A site to the P site

111 A physician would like to determine the global **patterns of gene expression in two different types** of tumor cells in order to **develop the most appropriate form of chemotherapy for each patient.** Which of the following techniques would be **most appropriate** for this purpose?
a. Southern blot
b. Western blot
c. ELISA
d. Microarray

112 Which is **not** required for hydroxylation of proline in **collagen synthesis**?
a. Oxygen
b. Fe^{+2}
c. a-ketoglutarate
d. Thiamine

113 A newborn baby has a sibling with sickle cell anemia and is at risk for the disease. The **appropriate diagnostic test** for sickle cell anemia in this baby will include:
a. DNA amplification
b. Hemoglobin antibodies
c. DNA restriction
d. DNA fingerprinting

114 **Xeroderma pigmentosum** is an inherited human skin disease that causes a variety of phenotypic changes in skin cells exposed to sunlight. The **molecular basis of the disease** appears to be:
a. Rapid water loss caused by defects in the cell membrane permeability
b. The inactivation of temperature-sensitive transport enzymes in sunlight
c. The inability of the cells to synthesize carotenoid-type compounds
d. A defect in an excision-repair system that removes thymine dimers from DNA

115 Which of the following results is provided by **northern blot analysis**?
a. Detects DNA molecules
b. Detects RNA molecules
c. Detects proteins
d. Determines chromosome structure

116 New proteins destined for secretion are **synthesized in the**:
a. Golgi apparatus
b. Smooth endoplasmic reticulum
c. Free polysomes
d. Rough endoplasmic reticulum

117 A 20-year-old woman presents **with bilateral conductive deafness, palpable purpura on the legs and hemoptysis.** Radiograph of the **chest shows a thin-walled cavity in left lower zone. Investigations reveal total leukocyte count 12000/mm, red cell casts** in the urine and 12,000/mm3 serum creatinine 3 mg/dL. What is the most probable diagnosis? (Question as given in Question Paper)
a. Henoch-Schönlein purpura
b. Polyarteritis nodosa
c. Wegener's granulomatosis
d. Disseminated tuberculosis.

118 An 18-year-old boy presents with **digital gangrene in third and fourth fingers for last 2 weeks. On examination the blood pressure is 170/110 mm of Hg and all peripheral pulses were palpable. Blood and urine examinations were unremarkable.** Antinuclear antibodies, antibody to double stranded DNA and anti neutrophil cytoplasmic antibody were negative. The most likely diagnosis is:
a. Wegener's granulomatosis
b. Polyarteritis nodosa
c. Takayasu's arteritisv
d. Systemic lupus erythematosus (SLE)

119 A 10-year-old boy has a fracture of femur. **Biochemical evaluation revealed Hb 11.5 gm/dl and ESR 18 mm 1st hour, Serum calcium 12.8 mg/dl, serum phosphorus 2.3 mg/dl, alkaline phosphatase 28 KA units and Blood urea 32 mg/dl**. Which of the following is the most probable diagnosis in his case?
a. Nutritional rickets
b. Renal rickets
c. Hyperparathyroidism
d. Skeletal dysplasia

120 The first investigation of choice in a **patient with suspected subarachnoid haemorrhage should be:**
a. Non-contrast computed tomography
b. CSF examination
c. Magnetic resonance imaging (MRI)
d. Contrast-enhanced computed tomography

121 **Presentation** not consistent with **"Legg-Calve-Perthes Disease"**:
a. Loss of abduction
b. Painful limp
c. Loss of internal rotation of the hip
d. Flexion contracture of 0-30 degrees

122 An 8-year-old patient presented **with fever, sore throat & cervical lymphadenopathy. On examination generalised lymphadenopathy** with maculopapular rashes are found. Peripheral blood smear shows absolute **lymphocytosis with large atypical lymphocytes having pale blue cytoplasm & eccentric nucleus.** The **most likely** diagnosis is:
a. Infectious mononucleosis
b. Tuberculosis
c. Acute lymphoblastic leukemia
d. Influenza

123 A 5-year-old-child of normal **intelligence presents with hypotonia. On examination, there is generalised weakness, absent DTR, fasciculations in tongue are seen and patient ke**eps his body in a frog like posture. Serum CPK is mildly elevated and motor nerve conduction velocity is normal. The **diagnosis** is:
a. Down's syndrome
b. GB syndrome
c. Spinal muscular atrophy
d. Limb girdle atrophy

124 A pregnant female was **found to be Hepatitis B positive in second trimester. The risk of transmission of hepatitis B infection** to fetus in utero from the mother is:
a. 30% b. 50%
c. 45% d. 10%

125 The **best** investigation **for staging endometrial cancer** is:
a. Non Contrast CT
b. Contrast enhanced CT
c. MRI
d. MRS

126 Which type of **MRI demonstrates best anatomical detail?**
a. T1 weighted
b. T2 weighted
c. Spin-Echo sequences
d. Fat suppressed imaged

127 The paintbrush metaphysis are **features** of:
a. Rickets b. Scurvy
c. Acromegaly d. Flurosis

128 **'Silver Dollar Vertebra'** is characteristic feature of:
a. Eosinophilic granuloma
b. Brown's tumor
c. Ankylosing spondylitis
d. Metastases

129 Hemophiliac pseudo - tumors are **most common** in:
a. Ilium b. Dorsal vertebrae
c. Lumbar vertebrae d. Calcaneum

130 **Most precise** way of determining gestational age is:

a. Crown rump length
b. Biparietal diameter
c. Femur length
d. Head circumference

131 In figure which labeled bracket spans a sarcomere?

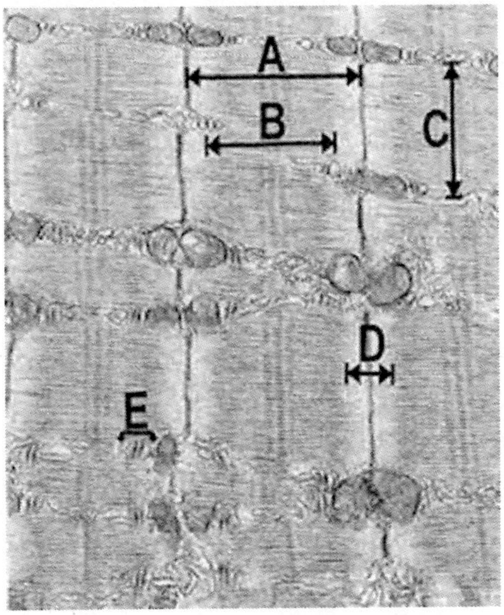

a. A
b. B
c. C
d. D

132 The action potentials shown in figure **represent those of which kind of cells**?

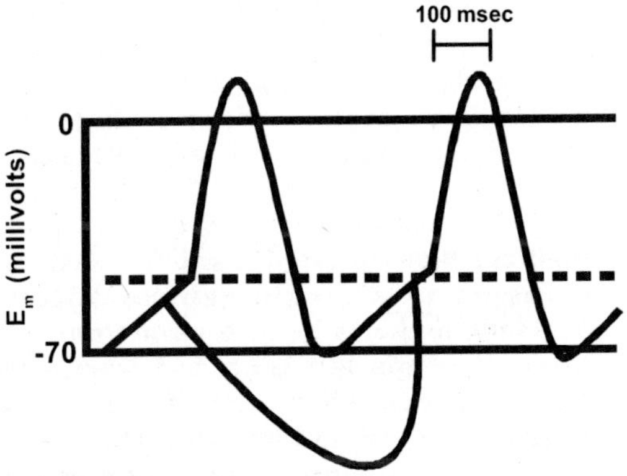

a. Cardiac nodal cells
b. Myelinated motor axons
c. Sensory neurons
d. Skeletal muscle cells

133 A 25-year-old male athlete **has just completed a long distance bicycle race during a hot, humid day**. At the conclusion of the race, **he provides a urine sample for testing. Assuming that his fluid intake during the race was zero, in what portion** of the nephron shown in Figure is the tubular fluid osmolality the lowest?

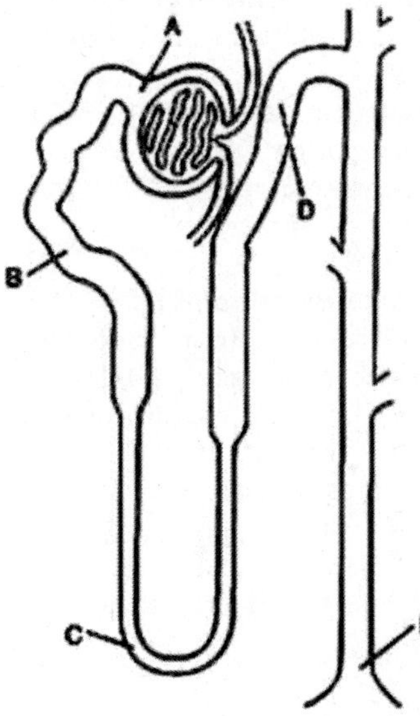

a. A
b. B
c. C
d. D

134 With respect to figure, which of the following will decrease the GFR?

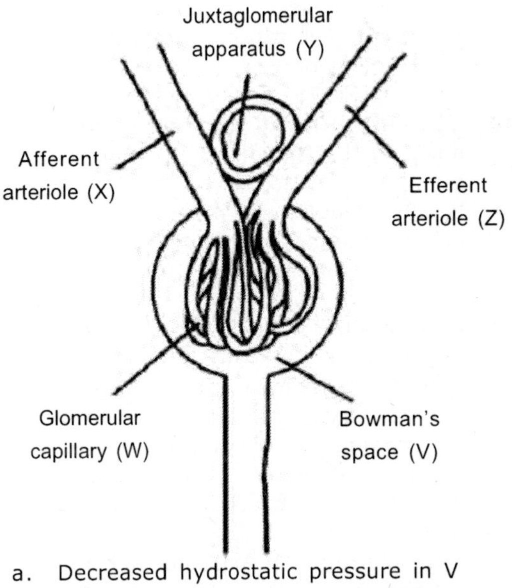

a. Decreased hydrostatic pressure in V
b. Decreased plasma protein concentration in W
c. Dilation of X
d. Dilation of Z

135 Which of the following factors is **the most important determinant of the rate of disease** progression from initial HIV **infection to clinical diagnosis of AIDS?**

a. CD4+ lymphocyte count 6 months after infection
b. Cytomegalovirus (CMV) IgG status
c. HIV resistance panel at infection
d. HIV viral load set point 6 months after initial infection

136 The **lesser sac (omental bursa)** is directly continuous with which of the **following recesses or spaces?**
a. Infracolic compartment
b. Left colic gutter
c. Left subphrenic recess
d. Hepatorenal recess

137 With regard to **development of the kidney**:
a. Kidney is derived from endoderm
b. The transcription factor WT-1 is necessary for induction of the mesenchyme's competence
c. There are two phases of kidney development
d. The kidneys descend during development to their final site

138 How many bullets are fired in **tandem bullets**?
a. One
b. Two
c. Three
d. None of the above

139 In patients with tibial **plateau fractures** which of the **following nerves** is most likely to be damaged as a result **of the injury**?
a. Common peroneal nerve
b. Tibial nerve
c. Sciatic nerve
d. Femoral nerve

140 What is the **most common systemic disease** affecting the spine?
a. Multiple sclerosis
b. Rheumatoid arthritis
c. Amyotrophic lateral sclerosis
d. Malignancy

141 **Most common finding** seen in **cauda equina syndrome**?
a. Urinary retention
b. Decreased anal sphincter tone
c. Weakness or numbness in the lower extremities
d. Saddle anesthesia

142 A 38-year-old man presents with intensely **itchy elbows and knees. He states that this has been going on for the past 2 weeks** and is interfering with his life to the point that he cannot take it any longer. Systemic enquiry **reveals past episodes of malabsorption relieved by a wheatfree diet. He is not allergic to any medication and maintains a gluten-free diet**. The most likely cause of his itch is:
a. Atypical eczema
b. Psoriasis
c. Dermatitis herpetiformis
d. Scabies

143 A 35-year-old male presents with a 4 **cm laceration to his left cheek 2 cm below** his lower eyelid. You explain to him that you would like to **perform regional anesthesia to numb his face**. Which of the following describes the appropriate procedure?
a. A mental block can be performed by injecting 2 cc of lidocaine with epinephrine near the mental foramen
b. An infraorbital block can be performed by injecting 8 cc of lidocaine with epinephrine near the infraorbital foramen
c. A mental block can be performed by injecting 6 cc of lidocaine with epinephrine near the mental foramen
d. An infraorbital block can be performed by injecting 3 cc of lidocaine near the infraorbital foramen

144 **Most frequently** used approach for **the drainage of felon** is?
a. A J-type or "hockey stick" incision
b. Through and through lateral incision
c. "Fishmouth" incision
d. Unilateral longitudinal incision

145 The **after hyperpolarization** phase of the action **potential is caused by:**
a. An outward calcium current
b. An inward chloride current
c. An outward potassium current
d. An outward sodium current

146 **Saltatory conduction** in myelinated axons results from the fact that
a. Salt concentration is increased beneath the myelin segments
b. Nongated ion channels are present beneath the segments of myelin
c. Membrane resistance is decreased beneath the segments of myelin
d. Voltage-gated sodium channels are concentrated at the nodes of Ranvier

147 A 21-year-old unrestrained driver with **a past medical history significant for asthma was involved in a single-vehicle automobile accident and has severe pain from an open fracture of his left tibia and fractured ribs**. He is **hypotensive with an initial blood pressure of 80/50 mmHg. The patient is currently receiving a liter bolus of lactated Ringer's solution**. Which of the following analgesic agents is a reasonable choice in this setting of hypotension?
a. Meperidine 50 mg intravenously
b. Morphine 10 mg intravenously
c. Fentanyl 100 mcg intravenously
d. Propofol 50 mg intravenously

148 The **unlabeled solid curve in** the graph shown represents the loading behavior of normal human hemoglobin at a pH of **7.35 as a function of oxygen concentration**. Which of the following labeled curves best represents the most likely change **after addition of carbon dioxide**?

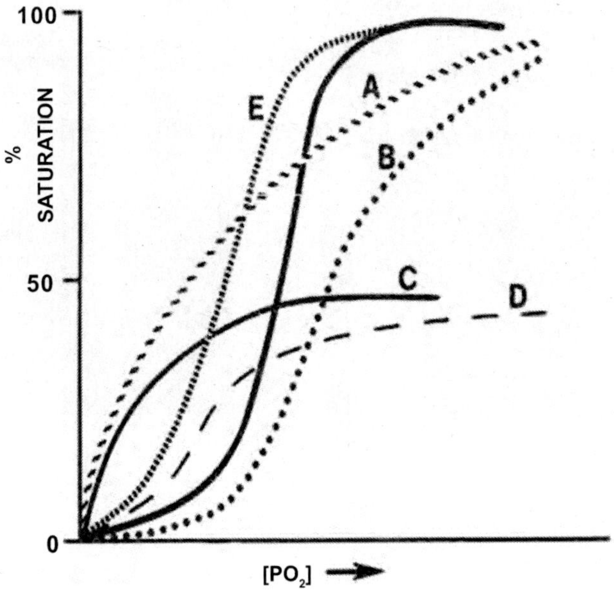

149 Fetal biophysical profile **used for the assessment of fetal** well being **does not** includes:
a. Fetal breathing movements
b. Fetal tone
c. Amount fluid volume
d. Fetal blood PH

150 Which of the following drugs is both **effective** and **safe** to use in a **pregnant patient** suffering from **bipolar disorder** ?
a. Carbamazepine
b. Chlorpromazine
c. Olanzapine
d. Valproic acid

151 A new drug, **becaplermin** is of good use in diabetics. It is attributed to which of the given uses:
a. For control of sugar level
b. For retinopathy treatment
c. As a topical gel for ulcers
d. For treatment of gastroparesis

152 A 50-year-old male suffering from **rheumatoid arthritis**, well controlled with celecoxib, develops angina. The most **suitable NSAID in the light of patient's history** and the recent controversy about **COX-2 selective inhibitors** is:
a. Paracetamol
b. Diclofenac
c. Ibuprofen
d. Nimesulide

153 Which of the following effects is **unlikely** to occur during treatment with **imipramine** ?
a. Alpha adrenoceptor blockade
b. Elevation of the seizure threshold
c. Mydriasis
d. Urinary retention

154 **Human interleukin-11** based drug **oprelvekin (Neumega)** is used in patients for **non-myeloid malignancies** to prevent:
a. Neutropenia
b. Anemia
c. Thrombocytopenia
d. Eosinophilia

155 **Which** of the following conditions is normally caused by sympathetic stimulation of the heart?
a. Acetylcholine release at the sympathetic endings
b. Decreased rate of conduction of the cardiac impulse
c. Decreased force of contraction of the atria
d. Increased force of contraction of the ventricles

156 A decrease in which of the following **would be** expected to occur in response to a direct increase in renal arterial pressure ?
a. Water excretion
b. Sodium excretion
c. Extracellular fluid volume
d. Glomerular filtration rate

157 In normal kidneys, **which** of the following is **true of the osmolarity of renal tubular** fluid that flows through that early distal tubule in the region of the macula densa ?
a. Usually isotonic compared with plasma
b. Usually hypotonic compared with plasma
c. Usually hypertonic compared with plasma
d. Hypertonic, compared with plasma, in antidiurasis

158 In a patient with very high levels of aldosterone and otherwise normal kidney function, approximately **what** percentage of the filtered load of sodium would be reabsorbed by the distal convoluted tubule and collecting duct ?
a. 40 to 60 percent
b. 20 to 40 percent
c. 10 to 20 percent
d. Less than 10 percent

159 A 26-year-old man **received a blade cut. What substance is the major cause** of pain in this acute inflammatory response?
a. Platelet-activating factor
b. Bradykinin
c. Interleukin-1
d. Tumor necrosis factor

160 **Which** of the following blood units carries the **least risk of inducing an immediate transfusion** reaction in a type B, Rh-positive recipient ?
a. Type A-positive whole blood
b. Type O-positive whole blood
c. Type AB-positive whole blood
d. Type O-positive packed red cells

161 **Which** of the following statements concerning the transmission of pain signals into the central nervous system is correct ?

a. The "fast" pain fibers that conduct at about 6 to 30 m/sec are classified as type C fibers
b. Type Ad pain fibers are responsible for the localization of a pain stimulus
c. Upon entering the spinal cord dorsal horn, the fast and slow pain fibers synapse with the same populations of neurons
d. The paleospinothalamic tract is specialized to rapidly conduct pain signals to the thalamus

162 **Which** is the Brodmann number designation for the primary somatosensory cortex ?

a. 4 b. 6
c. 3, 1, 2 d. 41, 42

163 **Which** of the following correctly pairs a small molecule rapidly acting transmitter with its most common source or action ?

a. Glutamate – inhibition
b. Glycine – inhibition
c. Serotonin – locus ceruleus
d. Dopamine – Choroid plexus

164 For the eye to adapt to intense light, **which** of the following may occur ?

a. Bipolar cells continuously transmit signals at the maximum rate possible
b. Photochemicals in both rods and cones are reduced to retinal and opsins
c. Levels of rhodopsin are very high
d. Pupil size increase

165 A 40-year-old diabetic male is experiencing **painless progressive decrease in vision since 1 year. The decrease in vision is more for day time and glare at night**. His father also had similar problems at 60 years age. The most likely diagnosis is:

a. Open angle glaucoma
b. Closed angle glaucoma
c. Diabetic retinopathy
d. Cataract

166 **Early** glaucomatous field defects can be diagnosed on:

a. Humphrey perimetry
b. Frequency double perimetry
c. Goldman perimetry
d. Short wave automated perimetry

167 **Posner-schlossmann syndrome** has all **except**:

a. Decrease in IOP
b. Uveitis
c. Unilateral
d. Males affected more than females

168 The angiogram depicted below **is most typical of the patient whose history** includes:

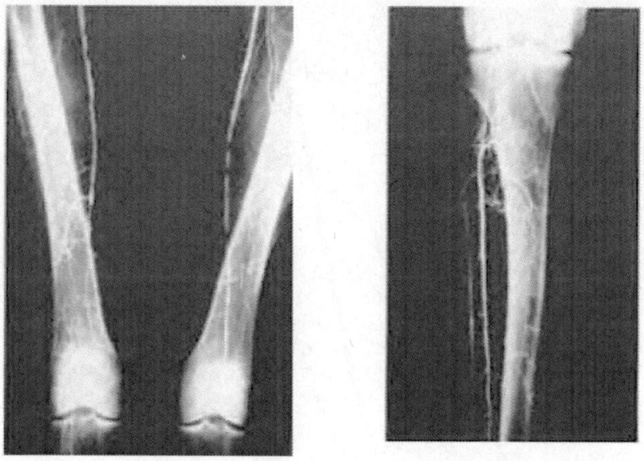

a. Cigarette smoking
b. Alcoholism
c. Hypertension
d. Diabetes

169 A 43-year-old woman with a 1-year history of **episodic leg edema and dyspnea is noted to have clubbing of the fingers. Her ECG is** shown below:

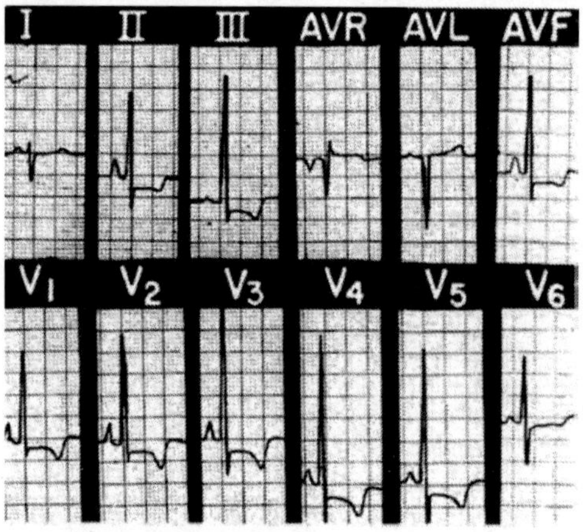

The **correct diagnosis** is:

a. Inferior wall myocardial infarction
b. Right bundle branch block
c. Acute pericarditis
d. Cor pulmonale

170 For each patient with **skin abnormalities, choose the most likely disorder:**

a. Superficial spreading melanoma
b. Basal cell carcinoma
c. Squamous cell carcinoma
d. Bowen's disease
e. Actinic keratoses
f. Seborrheic keratoses
g. Leukoplakia
h. Erythroplasia of Queyrat

1. A 50-year-old construction worker presents with a slowgrowing eroded papule on his lower lip. He has a history of leukoplakia and was a heavy smoker. He has a small, tender supraclavicular node. **(CHOOSE 1 DISORDER)**

2. A 46-year-old man presents with a large, well-demarcated, erythematous, glistening plaque on his glans penis. **(CHOOSE 1 DISORDER)**
3. A 42-year-old man presents with a single, shiny, red nodule on his nose that appears to glisten and shine. **(CHOOSE 1 DISORDER)**

Option:
a. 1-c; 2-h; 3-b
b. 1-a; 2-h; 3-c
c. 1-c; 2-g; 3-b
d. 1-b; 2-h; 3-a

171 For each area of the mediastinum, select **masses found in that compartment of the mediastinum**:
a. Thymoma
b. Teratoma
c. Thyroid adenoma
d. Parathyroid adenoma
e. Bronchogenic cyst
f. Pericardial cyst
g. Neurogenic tumor
h. Menigocele
1. Anterior mediastinum **(CHOOSE 4 MASSES)**
2. Middle mediastinum **(CHOOSE 2 MASSES)**
3. Posterior mediastinum **(CHOOSE 2 MASSES)**

Option:
a. 1-a,b,c,f; 2-b,f; 3-a,h
b. 1-a,c,d,e; 2-c,f; 3-a,h
c. 1-a,b,c,d; 2-e,f; 3-a,h
d. 1-a,b,c,d; 2-e,f; 3-g,h

172 Match each clinical scenario with the appropriate type of tumor.
a. Medulloblastoma
b. Oligodendroglioma
c. Optic glioma
d. Carcinomatous meningitis
e. Schwannoma
f. Choriocarcinoma
g. Metastatic carcinoma
h. Pineocytoma
i. Primary CNS lymphoma
1. A 30-year-old man with the **acquired immune deficiency syndrome (AIDS)** develops headaches and left hemiparesis and is found to have a **right frontal white matter homogeneously enhancing lesion. (SELECT 1 TUMOR)**
2. A 4-year-old boy presents with ataxia, lethargy, and **obstructive hydrocephalus. (SELECT 1 TUMOR)**
3. A 16-year-old boy with café au lait spots and **cutaneous nodules complains of decreased vision in his left eye. (SELECT 1 TUMOR)**
4. A 55-year-old woman presents with mild **unsteadiness, tinnitus, and hearing loss. (SELECT 1 TUMOR)**
5. A 13-year-old girl has headaches and diplopia. On examination, she has impaired upward gaze, lid retraction, and convergence-retraction nystagmus. **Her pupils react on convergence but not to light. (SELECT 1 TUMOR)**

Option:
a. 1-h; 2-a; 3-b; 4-e; 5-a
b. 1-b; 2-a; 3-c; 4-e; 5-i
c. 1-a; 2-g; 3-c; 4-e; 5-b
d. 1-i; 2-a; 3-c; 4-e; 5-h

173 For each stage in the treatment of the patient below, select the appropriate next step.
a. Left hemicolectomy
b. Right hemicolectomy
c. Subtotal colectomy
d. Total colectomy
e. Hepatic wedge resection
f. External beam irradiation
g. 5-fluorouracil and leucovorin
h. External beam irradiation and chemotherapy
i. Abdominal MRI
j. No further treatment
1. A 65-year-old man is admitted to the hospital with complaints of intermittent constipation and microcytic anemia. Barium enema reveals a nonobstructing "applecore" lesion of the proximal sigmoid colon. Colonoscopy confirms the location of the mass and reveals no other synchronous lesions. **(SELECT 1 STEP)**
2. The patient undergoes surgery and recovers uneventfully. Pathology of the resected specimen is reported as Dukes C with negative surgical margins. **(SELECT 1 STEP)**
3. In 6-mo follow-up an abdominal CT scan shows a 2 cm isolated lesion in the right lobe of the liver. Repeat colonoscopy shows no evidence of recurrent or metachronous lesions. Chest X-ray and bone scan are normal. **(SELECT 1 STEP)**

Option:
a. 1-c; 2-h; 3-b
b. 1-a; 2-h; 3-c
c. 1-a; 2-g; 3-e
d. 1-b; 2-h; 3-a

174 A 75-year-old woman has increasing **shortness of breath on exertion**. Findings on physical examination are **unremarkable. X-rays of the chest show no abnormalities** of the heart or lungs. Pertinent laboratory findings include:
- Hematocrit 28%
- Hemoglobin 9 g/dL
- Mean corpuscular volume 70 μm3

Which of the following is the most **likely basis for these findings**?
a. Acquired hemolytic anemia
b. Chronic blood loss
c. β-Thalassemia minor
d. Pernicious anemia

175 Which of the following is **true** regarding **perilunate and lunate dislocations**?
a. All require emergent intervention
b. Associated carpal bone fractures are rare

c. Complications of these injuries include avascular necrosis and median nerve compression
d. Patients present with obvious hand deformity

176 A 40-year-old diabetic male **patient presents with sudden painless loss of vision right eye. No history of trauma.** Patient had undergone cataract surgery 2 years back and gained good vision post op.
Vision: hand movement close to face (HMCF) PR accurate. Intraocular pressure = 10 mmHg [normal 16-18 mm Hg]
History of retinal detachment in other eye 4 yrs back.
The likely diagnosis is:
a. Sympathetic ophthalmia
b. Retinal detachment
c. Diabetic vitreous hemorrhage
d. Diabetic macular edema

177 All are true about posterior keratoconus **except**:
a. Unilateral
b. Progressive
c. Anterior surface is normal
d. Vision is minimally affected

178 **Assertion A: Hyperacute rejection** occurs within minutes to hours.
Reason R: Hyperacute rejection is due to preformed antibodies.
a. Both A and R are true and R is correct explanation of A
b. Both A and R are true and R is not correct explanation of A
c. A is true but R is false
d. A is false but R is true

179 **Assertion A:** Endometrial carcinoma usually presents with postmenopausal bleeding.
Reason R: Endometrial carcinoma usually have a adnexal mass.
a. Both A and R are true and R is correct explanation of A
b. Both A and R are true and R is not correct explanation of A
c. A is true but R is false
d. A is false but R is true

180 **Assertion A**: Microtubules are made up of two globular protein subunits; α and β-tubulin.
Reason R: Microtubule assembly is prevented by colchicines and vinblastine.
a. Both A and R are true and R is correct explanation of A
b. Both A and R are true and R is not correct explanation of A
c. A is true but R is false
d. A is false but R is true

Ans. 1: (c) Muller cells
Ref: G20 - 145
Sol:

- The processes **of mullar cells form an internal limiting membrane** on the inner surface of ratina and an external limiting **membrane in the receptor layer.**

Ans. 2: (a) Caloric restriction
Ref: Read the text below
Sol:

- To date, the only **intervention known to delay aging is caloric restriction. The salutary** effect of restricting caloric intake by 30 to 40% has been **documented in multiple species, from single-cell organisms to rodents.**

Ans. 3: (a) Steady pain
Ref: Read the text below
Sol:

- **Sudden distension of the billiary** tree produced a steady rather than colicky type of pain; hence the term **biliary colic is misleading.**

Ans. 4: (c) Affects predominantly females
Ref: Read the text below.
Sol:
Cluster headache:

- Affects **predominantly males (7-8 times more than females).**
- **Also known as Raeder's syndrome, histamine cephalalgia, and** sphenopalatine neuralgia.
- **Lateralized.**
- Peak at 30-50 years.
- Excruciating, **deep, explosive pain which begins without** warning, reaches it's peak within 5 minutes and lasts for 45 minutes and commonly awakens the patients from sleep and is associated with homolateral **lacrimation and reddening of eye and ptosis and nasal stuffiness.**

Ans. 5: (b) Caplan's syndrome
Ref: Read the text below.
Sol:

- **Caplan's syndrome** is a rare condition characterized by the presence of necrobiotic nodules in the **periphery of the lung in coal workers with** rheumatoid arthritis (Coal worker's pneumoconiosis + Rheumatoid arthritis)

Ans. 6: (d) Observation
Ref: Read the text below
Sol:

- This ECG **shows Mobitz type I second-degree AV block, also known** as Wenckebach phenomenon, characterized by progressive **PR interval prolongation prior to block of an atrial impulse.**
- **This rhythm generally does not require therapy.**
- It may be seen in normal individuals; **other causes include inferior MI and drug** intoxications such as from digoxin, beta blockers, or calcium channel blockers.
- Even in the post-MI setting, it is usually stable, although **it has the potential to progress to higher-degree AV block with consequent need for pacemaker.**

Ans. 7: (c) His most likely karyotype is 47 XXY
Ref: Read the text below
Sol:

The picture of infertility, **gynecomastia, and tall stature is consistent with Klinefelter syndrome and an XXY karyotype.**

The patient has abnormal gonadal development with hyalinized testes that result in low testosterone levels and elevated levels of gonadotropin.

Turner syndrome refers to the **45 karyotype that result in abnormal sexual** development in a female.

Ans. 8: (c) 6 months
Ref: Read the text below
Sol:
Current ACCP recommendations for duration of warfarin therapy

Recommendations for Long-Term Anticoagulation

Indiction	Durtion
First VTE event with reversible risk factor (transient immobilization, estrogen use, surgery, trauma)	3–6 months
First idiopathic VTE event	6 months
Recurrent VTE or first VTE event in patient with irreversible risk factors (cancer or hypercoagulable state)	12 months to lifetime
VTE=Venous tromboembolism	

Ans. 9: (a) Type I gastric ulcer.
Ref: Sch8- 962-963
Sol:
Distal Gastrectomy

- **Distal gastrectomy without vagotomy** (usually about a 50% gastrectomy to include the ulcer) has traditionally been the procedure of choice for **type I gastric ulcer.**
- Reconstruction may be done as a **Billroth I (preferable) or Billroth II.**
- **Truncal vagotomy is added for type II and III gastric ulcers**, or if the patient is believed to be at increased risk for recurrent ulcer, and should be considered if **Billroth II reconstruction is contemplated.**

Ans. 10: (a) Distal gastric resection

Ref: Sch8- 967
Sol:
Bleeding Gastric Ulcer

- **Bleeding gastric ulcers tend to occur in older and/or medically complicated patients, and this fact tends to increase the operative** risk.
- Patients with gastric ulcer bleeding who are most likely to require surgery have bled more than **6 units and have presented in shock.**
- Endoscopically, their ulcers tend to be on **the lesser curvature with the usual stigmata of recent hemorrhage.**
- Distal gastric resection to include the **bleeding ulcer is the procedure of choice for bleeding gastric ulcer.**
- **Second best is vagotomy and drainage with oversewing** and biopsy of the ulcer.

Ans. 11: (d) 5
Ref: Read the text below
Sol:

- The retina **contains three layers of cells.**
- **They are, from top to bottom, the ganglion cells (choice** A), the bipolar cells (choice C), and the photoreceptor cells (rods and cones, choice E).
- The internal plexiform layer (**choice B) contains the synapses between the bipolar cells and the ganglion cells.**
- **The external plexiform layer (choice D) contains the synapses between the photoreceptors and the bipolar cells.**
- Remember that light enters from the **top and traverses all the layers to reach the photoreceptors in the bottom layer.**

Ans. 12: (d) Right brachiocephalic vein
Ref: Read the text below
Sol:

- Remember that in viewing axial or transverse CT scans through the body, the right side of the patient is to your left and the left side to your **right.**
- **In other words, the feet of the patient are toward you and the head awa from you.**
- **The back of the patient is at the bottom of the image and the** front of the patient toward the top. Directional terms are always in reference to the patient. The insert at the bottom right indicates the level of the section.
- **Arrow 1 indicates the right brachiocephalic vein. The left brachiocephalic vein (choice B) is seen as the elongated structure immediately posterior to the manubrium of the sternum and to the left of the right brachiocephalic vein.**
- **Immediately posterior to the left brachiocephalic vein is the** brachiocephalic artery (choice A, arrow 2). To the left of the latter are the left common carotid artery (choice C) and the left subclavian artery (arrow 3).
- **The superior vena cava (choice E) is not seen at this level because the right and left brachiocephalic veins are still separate.**

Ans. 13: (d) 500 mL of fluid per day
Ref: Read the text below
Sol:

- A fistula is **defined as an abnormal communication between** two epithelialized surfaces. The communication occurs between two parts of the gastrointestinal tract or adjacent organs in an internal fistula (e.g., **enterocolonic fistula or colovesicular fistula).**
- **Enterocutaneous fistulas that drain less than 200 mL of fluid per day are known as low-**output fistulas, whereas those that drain more than **500 mL of fluid per day are known as high-output fistulas.**
- More than 80% of **enterocutaneous fistulas represent iatrogenic complications** that occur as the result of enterotomies or intestinal anastomotic dehiscences.
- Fistulas that arise spontaneously without **antecedent iatrogenic injury are usually manifestations of progression of underlying Crohn's disease** or cancer.

Ans. 14: (a) Terminal ileum
Ref: Sch8- 1042
Sol:
RADIATION ENTERITIS

Radiation therapy is a component of multimodality therapy for many intra-abdominal and pelvic cancers,such as those of the **cervix, endometrium, ovary, bladder, prostate, and rectum.**

Pathophysiology

- **Radiation induces cellular injury** directly and through the generation of free radicals.
- The principal mechanism of radiation-induced cell death is believed to be apoptosis resulting from free radical-induced breaks in **double-stranded DNA.**

Clinical Presentation

- The **most common manifestations** of acute radiation enteritis are nausea, vomiting, diarrhea, and crampy abdominal pain.
- **The terminal ileum is the most frequently affected segment**.
- Other manifestations of chronic radiation enteritis include complete bowel obstruction, acute or chronic intestinal hemorrhage, and abscess or fistula formation.

Ans. 15: (a) Bleeding
Ref: Sch 8-1043
Sol:

- **Meckel's diverticula** are asymptomatic unless associated complications arise.
- The most common presentations associated with

symptomatic Meckel's diverticula are **bleeding, intestinal obstruction, and diverticulitis.**

- **Bleeding is the most common** presentation in children with Meckel's diverticula, representing more than 50% of Meckel's diverticulum-related complications among patients who are younger than 18 years of age.
- **Bleeding associated with Meckel's diverticula** is rare among patients who are older than 30 years of age.
- **Intestinal obstruction is the most common presentation in adults with Meckel's diverticula**.
- **Diverticulitis,** present in 20% of patients with symptomatic Meckel's diverticula, is associated with a clinical syndrome that is indistinguishable from acute appendicitis.
- **Neoplasms, most commonly carcinoid tumors**, are present in 0.5 to 3.2% of symptomatic Meckel's diverticula that are resected.

Ans. 16: (b) Submucosa
Ref: Read the text below
Sol:
ENDORECTAL ULTRASOUND

- **Endorectal ultrasound** is primarily used to evaluate the depth of invasion of **neoplastic lesions in the rectum.**
- The **normal rectal wall appears as a five-layer structure**.

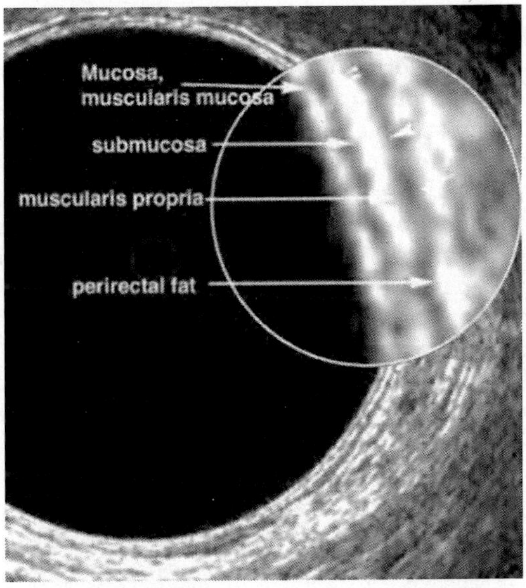

Normal endorectal ultrasonography

- **Ultrasound can reliably differentiate most benign polyps from invasive tumors based upon the integrity of the submucosal layer**.
- Ultrasound can also differentiate superficial **T1-T2 from deeper T3-T4 tumors**.
- Overall, the accuracy of ultrasound in detecting depth of mural invasion ranges between **81 and 94%.**
- This modality also can detect enlarged **perirectal lymph nodes**, which may suggest nodal metastases;accuracy of detection of pathologically positive lymph nodes is **58 to 83%.**
- **Ultrasound may also prove useful for early detection of local recurrence after surgery.**

Ans. 17: (a) Record BP in sitting position
Ref: Read the text below
Sol:

- The **lowest** of the **three** readings recorded is taken as the BP of the person.

Ans. 18: (a) Transient ischaemic attack (TIA)
Ref: Read the text below
Sol:

- **WHO** definition of stroke is, "**Rapidly developed** clinical signs of **focal** (or global) disturbance of **cerebral function**; lasting **more** than **24 hours** or leading to death with no apparent cause other than vascular origin.
- "**TIAs** are typically of **less** than **24 hour** duration.

Ans. 19: (b) B
Ref: Read the text below
Sol:

- The **basilar artery** is formed by the union of the two vertebral arteries at the lower border of the pons.
- A **large tumor in the foramen magnum** compresses the vertebral arteries, resulting in decreased blood flow in **the basilar artery.**

Ans. 20: (a) Occupational exposures account for 5-10% of human cancers
Ref: Read the text below
Sol:

- **Occupational exposures** account for **1-5%** of all human cancers.

Ans. 21: (d) Glucose tolerance test
Ref: Read the text below.
Sol:

- The **sensitivity** of urine examination varies between **10 and 50%**, hence likely to yield numerous **'false negatives'**.
- Fasting blood sugar test is **not** reliable as **true fasting cannot be assured and considerable false positives** may occur.
- Random blood sugar can **only** give a crude estimation of frequency of diabetes in the population.
- Therefore, for epidemiological purposes, **2-hour value after 75 g of oral glucose** is ideal either alone or with fasting value.

Ans. 22: (d) Low birth weight
Ref: Read the text below
Sol:

- **Neonatal deaths** make a **major** contribution to the infant mortality.
- In **developing** countries, the high infant mortality is due to **low birth weight** and the combined effects of **infections** (diarrhoea and respiratory infections) and **malnutrition**.
- In the developed countries, it is due to **congenital anomalies**, and **anoxia** and **hypoxia**.

Ans. 23: (a) 40
Ref: Read the text below
Sol:

- Under the same guidelines, the recommended **per capita space** in a classroom should **not be less than 10 sq. ft., doors and windows** area should **not** be **less than 25%** of the floor space; **ventilators** should not be less than **2% of the floor area**.

Ans. 24: (b) Remand home
Ref: Read the text below
Sol:

- In a **remand** home, the children are placed under the **care** of doctor, psychiatrist, psychologist and medicalsocial worker, etc.
- Effort is made to **improve** the **physical and mental well being** of the child.
- Facilities for **elementary schooling** and **recreation** are available.

Ans. 25: (c) 500 kcals and 25 g proteins
Ref: Read the text below
Sol:

- **Similar** supplement is given to **adolescent** girls. Child up to **6 years** of age gets **300 kcal** and **8-10 g** of **proteins**.
- Each **malnourished** child gets **600 kcal and 16-20 g proteins**. Supplementary nutrition is given for **300 days** in a year.

Ans. 26: (b) Formal education
Ref: Read the text below
Sol:

- Only **non-formal** education is to be provided to **pre-school** children in the **Anganwadi** under the **ICDS** scheme.

Ans. 27: (b) 2
Ref: Read the text below
Sol:

- **Arrow 2 points** to the abdominal aorta, located anterior to the lumbar vertebra.
- Arrows 1 (choice **A) and 5 (choice B) indicate the left and right kidneys respectively.**
- Arrow 3 points to the inferior vena cava; the junctions of the left **and right renal veins to the inferior vena cava are seen in this CT scan.**
- Arrow 4 points to a loop of the small intestine, filled with **contrastenhancing material.**

Ans. 28: (a) Anemia
Ref: Read the text below
Sol:
BILIOPANCREATIC DIVERSION
Mechanism of Action

- The procedure **combines gastric restriction with an intestinal malabsorptive procedure.**
- A 50 **to 100 cm common absorptive alimentary** channel is created proximal to the ileocecal valve; digestion and **absorption are limited to this segment of bowel.**

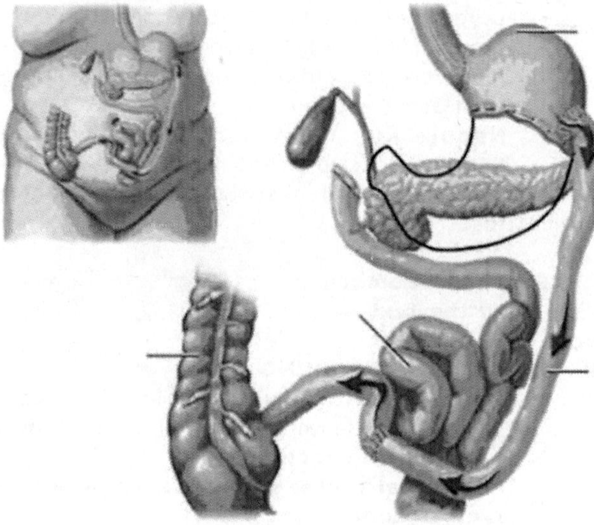

Indications

- This **procedure is primarily indicated for the superobese** or for those who have failed restrictive bariatric procedures.

Contraindications

- Patients with **anemia, hypocalcemia, and osteoporosis, and** those who are not motivated to comply with stringent postoperative supplementation regimens may not be appropriate for this procedure.

Complications

- The most common **morbidities include anemia (30%), protein-calorie malnutrition** (20%), dumping syndrome,and marginal ulceration (10%).
- The duodenal switch **modification is associated with a lower ulceration rate (1%) and a lower incidence of dumping syndrome.**
- **Other complications include vitamin B12** deficiency, hypocalcemia, fat-soluble vitamin deficiencies, osteoporosis,night blindness, and prolongation of prothrombin time.

Ans. 29: (d) It break down carbohydrates, uses metabolic intermediates for energy
Ref: Medical microbiology by C. George ray—379
Sol:

Campylobacters jejuni

- Campylobacters are **motile, curved, oxidase-positive, Gram-negative** rods similar in morphology to vibrios.
- The cells have **polar flagella** and are often are attached at their ends giving pairs **"S" shapes or a "seagull" appearance.**
- C. jejuni grows well only on enriched media under **microaerophilic conditions**. That is, it requires oxygen at reduced tension (5 – 10%), presumably due to vulnerability of some of its enzyme systems to superoxides.
- **Growth usually requires 2 to 4 days, sometimes as much as a week.**
- C. jejuni has the **structural components** found in other Gram-negative bacteria (eg, outer membrane,LPS).
- In contrast to the vibrios, **it does not break down carbohydrates, but uses amino acids and metabolic intermediates for energy.**

Ans. 30: (a) Ferguson hemorrhoidectomy
Ref: Sch 8-1102
Sol:

Closed Submucosal Hemorrhoidectomy

- The **Parks or Ferguson hemorrhoidectomy** involves resection of hemorrhoidal tissue and closure of the wounds with absorbable suture.

Open Hemorrhoidectomy

- This technique, often called the **Milligan and Morgan hemorrhoidectomy**, follows the same principles of excision described above, **but the wounds are left open** and allowed to heal by secondary intention.

Whitehead's Hemorrhoidectomy

- **Whitehead's hemorrhoidectomy** involves **circumferential excision of the** hemorrhoidal cushions just proximal to the dentate line.
- After excision, the rectal mucosa is then advanced and sutured to the dentate line.
- While some surgeons still use the Whitehead hemorrhoidectomy technique, most have abandoned this approach because of the **risk of ectropion (Whitehead's deformity).**

Stapled Hemorrhoidectomy

- **Stapled hemorrhoidectomy** has been proposed as an alternative surgical approach.
- Unlike excisional hemorrhoidectomy, **stapled hemorrhoidectomy does not aim to excise redundant hemorrhoidal tissue.**
- Instead, stapled hemorrhoidectomy removes a short circumferential segment of rectal mucosa proximal to the dentate line using a circular stapler.

Ans. 31: (c) Unipolar or pseudounipolar neurons
Ref: Read the text below
Sol:

- **Sensation from the skin** is carried by general somatic afferent (GSA) fibers, and their cells are unipolar **or pseudounipolar types located in the dorsal root ganglia**.
- **Multipolar neurons** and neurons in the ventral horn and in sympathetic chain ganglia are motor neurons.
- **Bipolar neurons are sensory neurons, but they are not somatic sensory neurons.**

Ans. 32: (d) Gradual and excellent improvement is against giant cell arteritis
Ref: Read the text below
Sol:

- The picture is **of an acute left sided papillitis**, which has a broad differential diagnosis and causes.
- The pace and severity of **the clinical picture, physical findings, and careful investigations and follow up are very important.**
- **Vasculitides, infectious agents, sarcoidosis**...etc all can produce this picture, and multiple sclerosis (MS) although unlikely it is worthy to exclude it.
- The **visual loss in giant cell arteritis is irreversible**, and a rapid spontaneous improvement goes with MS.
- **Foster Kennedy** gives a slowly progressive optic atrophy in one side and papilloedema in the other side.

Ans. 33: (b) Brain MRI or CT scan should be done
Ref: Read the text below
Sol:

- Notice that the overall **picture is of a cluster headache-like, but** the picture is atypical given the 2 years of non-**remission and occurrence during day and night, and there are features of hypogonadism.**
- All of them might indicate an intracranial space-**occupying lesion in and around the sella**. Actually, MRI of this patient revealed a large sellar mass with supra-sellar extension and impingement upon the left carotid artery, which explains both the hyperprolactinemia and the dysautonomia affecting the left side of **the face (eye redness and nasal discharge) by affecting the sympathetic fibers around the left carotid artery**.
- It was a **prolactimona by histopathological examination** after successful surgical debulking.

Ans. 34: (b) Start intravenous cefotaxime and vancomycine
Ref: Read the text below
Sol:

- This patient is immune **suppressed because of cyclosporine**.
- Given the presence of **impaired consciousness**, fever, and neck stiffness, meningitis (or meningoencephalitis) is the most **likely diagnosis.**
- We should stop cyclosporine, and start broad-spectrum antibiotics and do CSF examination.

- **Blood cultures** can be done, and adding another immune suppressant (azathioprine) would be a silly step.

Ans. 35: (d) Brain MRI with contrast
Ref: Read the text below
Sol:

- She has two **sites of involvements: spinal cord and optic.**
- Both are of **white matter signs. The** pace is somewhat rapid, and although she did not report an improvement, **B12 deficiency and heredito-familial degenerative conditions are highly unlikely.**
- Instead, one should **exclude multiple sclerosis by having this clinical picture** and should be differentiated from anti-phospholipid syndrome**, SLE, vasculitis...etc.**
- Therefore, Brain imaging would **be a reasonable step here.**

Ans. 36: (a) Omit anticoagulation for the time being
Ref: Read the text below
Sol:

- This is most **likely an embolic stroke to the main stem of the left middle cerebral artery**. The infracted area is large with mass **effect and midline shift.**
- So, measures to reduce the raised intracranial pressure should be instituted without any delay like high **concentration O_2, mannitol infusion**...etc; while anticoagulation is definitely indicated, it is should be omitted for the time being as there is a very high risk of hemorrhagic transformation in **this large friable infarcted area, and starting it after 1-2 weeks is reasonable.**
- **Her atrial fibrillation is rapid and she needs** measures to slow it like giving digoxin, and an echo study is needed to evaluate her heart.
- A DC shock is not indicated as we don't know the duration of the AF; besides, given the presence of mitral **stenosis, there is a very high risk of recurrence and emboli showering in the presence of no anticoagulation coverage.**

Ans. 37: (d) Lower posterior inferior frontal gyrus, left hemisphere
Ref: Read the text below
Sol:

- This is **Broca's aphasia in a right-handed** man; the posterior part of the lower left frontal gyrus is **the culprit site.**

Ans. 38: (d) Extrasphincteric fistula
Ref: Sch8- 1107
Sol:
Supralevator Abscess
Digital rectal examination may reveal an indurated, bulging mass above the anorectal ring.

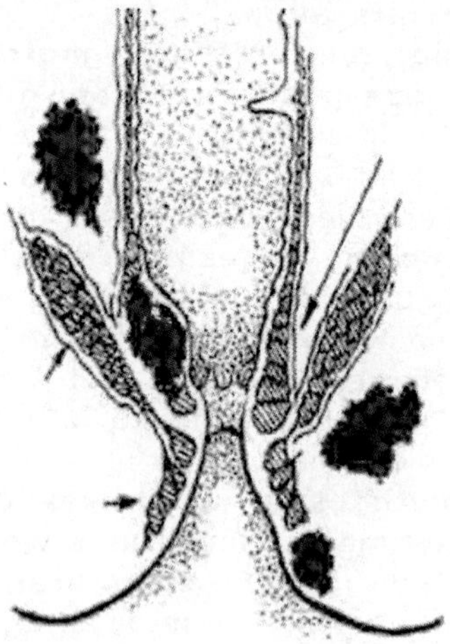

Treatment
It is essential to identify the origin of **a supralevator abscess** prior to treatment.

1. If the **abscess is secondary to an upward extension** of an intersphincteric abscess, it should be drained through the rectum.
2. If it is **drained through the ischiorectal fossa**, a complicated, suprasphincteric fistula may result.
3. If a **supralevator abscess arises from the upward extension of an ischiorectal abscess,** it should be drained through the ischiorectal fossa. D**rainage** of this type of abscess through the rectum may result in an extrasphincteric fistula.
4. If the **abscess is secondary to intra-abdominal disease**, the primary process requires treatment and the abscess is drained via the most direct route (transabdominally, rectally, or through the ischiorectal fossa).

Ans. 39: (d) D
Ref: Read the text below
Sol:

- The **artery labeled D in the diagram** accompanying the question represents the posterior interventricular (descending) artery, which supplies blood to the posterior portions of the **interventricular septum as well as to the posterior wall of the right ventricle.**
- This **artery usually is a branch of the right coronary artery**, and the diagnosis of this patient's disorder is consistent with the results of the ECG, which indicates a posterior septal infarct.
- The **anterior interventricular artery (C) arises** from the left coronary artery (A) and supplies the anterior portion of the interventricular septum and the anterior walls of both ventricles.
- The **posterior interventricular artery (D)** usually anastomoses with the anterior interventricular artery (C) near the apex of the heart.
- The **circumflex artery (B)** circles toward the back of the heart in the coronary sulcus and

may occasionally give rise to the posterior interventricular artery (D).

Ans. 40: (a) Tunica albuginea
Ref: Read the text below
Sol:

- **Tear of the penile tunica albuginea**, the thick fascial layer around the corpora cavernosum, can **occur during sexual intercourse or other sexual activity.**
- The urethra is rarely injured, but a retrograde urethrogram may be necessary for full evaluation. The tunica **albuginea should be surgically repaired.**

Ans. 41: (d) Arrest due to myocardial infarction
Ref: Read the text below
Sol:

- **Emergency thoracotomy** accompanied by open-chest cardiac compressions should be considered in patients who arrest after penetrating trauma to the chest or abdomen or after blunt trauma, although **recommendations vary with regard to downtime**.
- **Outcome is better after penetrating trauma**, when a reversible cause is identified. Arrest from severe hypothermia is also an acceptable indication for emergency thoracotomy, allowing for aggressive **mediastinal rewarming and open cardiac massage.**
- **Emergency thoracotomy** and open cardiac massage is not recommended after cardiac arrest from most medical conditions, including ischemic heart disease.

Ans. 42: (b) BUN to creatinine ratio of >20, FeNa >1, normal urinalysis
Ref: Read the text below
Sol:

- **Prerenal failure is due to volume loss, decreased cardiac output, or renal artery and small vessel disease.**
- When the clinical picture is not clear, chemistry and urinalysis can aid in distinguishing prerenal from **intrinsic and postobstructive renal failure**.
- **Prerenal failure** is associated with a BUN to creatinine ratio of >20, urine osmolality of >500, FeNa of >1, and normal urinalysis.
- **In postrenal failure, urine osmolality is <350. Active urine sediment and FeNa of >1 are associated with intrinsic renal failure.**

Ans. 43: (d) Increased force of contraction
Ref: Read the text below
Sol:

- Note **that the end-diastolic volume of this patient** is the same as that of a normal subject. **Because the patient's stroke volume** is larger than that of a normal subject, the force of contraction must also be larger.
- This could be due to increased sympathetic tone or to the fact that the patient took inotropic medications. **The volume remaining after the ventricular contraction is correspondingly smaller compared to normal.**
- **Preload equals end-diastolic volume** and is the same in the patient and normal subjects. Afterload is equal to arterial pressure.
- Both **afterload and stroke volume** are larger in this patient compared to normal.

Ans. 44: (b) The failure rate occurs in 1/400 patients
Ref: Read the text below
Sol:

- The failure rate of **1/400 patient has been reported.**
- Since there is **no alteration in the level of testosterone** production, there is no reported sexual dysfuntion attributed to vasectomy.
- The success rate for reversal of **vasectomy greatly depends on the time since the vasectomy was performed.**
- Failure rates for vasovasostomy has **been reported to be >80% after 10 years**.

Ans. 45: (a) Urogenital fold
Ref: Read the text below
Sol:

- Embryologically, the **genital tubercule develops into the penis**.
- The edge of the cloacal **membrane forms the urogenital fold** and by the process of invagination forms the urethral groove and **finally the penile urethera**.
- The severity of hypospadias depends on the location of the anomalous opening onto the penile urethra. The mildest degree is **where the opening is on the glans and the most severe form at the penoscrotal junction.**

Ans. 46: (d) Radical vulvectomy and bilateral groin dissection
Ref: Read the text below
Sol:

- Similar to penile cancer, radical **vulvectomy and bilateral groin dissection have improved survival in patients with carcinoma of the vulva.**
- The deep and superficial nodes are removed. If the **lymph nodes are not involved, the cure rate exceeds 70%.**
- **The overall survival is approximately 50%. Radiotherapy has not** offered additional benefit pregnancy.

Ans. 47: (b) Sarcoma botryoides
Ref: Read the text below
Sol:

- **Sarcoma botryoides** usually occurs as a grape-like polypoid mass in the vagina of young girls.
- **Clear-cell adenocarcinoma** occurs at an older age, in the second decade of life. It is associated with the administration of DES to patient's mothers during pregnancy.
- **Squamous carcinoma** is the most common tumor of the vagina in postmenopausal patients. However, **malignant tumors of the vagina are rare in children.**

Ans. 48: (c) Wilms' tumor
Ref: Read the text below
Sol:

- Typically **Wilms' tumor is noted in well appearing children in the** second half of their first decade of life.
- These masses are usually felt or visually noted **by parents during routine daily activities. Children with neuroblastoma are usually younger and appear quite** sick.
- Although unlikely, renal cell carcinoma has been reported in children and diagnosis is only based on final pathology results.
- Lymphoma should be ruled out based on **CT scan findings and subsequent needle-guided biopsy, since treatment is usually nonsurgical.**

Ans. 49: (c) Repair is performed more than 6 months after the causative operation
Ref: Read the text below
Sol:

- **Repair of vesicovaginal fistula** is recommended after enough time has passed, to allow a reduction in the inflammatory reaction and even spontaneous closure to occur. To promote spontaneous closure, **a Foley catheter is inserted for bladder drainage**.
- It is advised to perform meticulous repair, **excision of previous fistulous tract, and tension-free anastomosis.**
- Frequently an **omental interposition** helps to separate overlapping suture lines.

Ans. 50: (d) Peripheral neuropathy
Ref: Read the text below
Sol:

- **Peripheral neuropathy, ototoxicity, and nephrotoxicity** may be encountered following cisplatinum treatment.
- **Nephrotoxicity can be minimized** by hydrating the patient well prior and during the treatment.

Ans. 51: (c) The increased pliability of stored red blood cells allows them to seep into the interstitium
Ref: Read the text below
Sol:

- **Red blood cells** are actually rendered less pliable when they have been stored for a long period of time.
- **Currently employed preservatives allow packed red blood cells to be stored and last approximately 42 days.**
- Despite improvements in blood storage, **2,3-diphosphoglycerate is diminished. The lack of 2, 3-diphosphoglycerate shifts the oxygen-hemoglobin dissociation curve to the left, which allows less oxygen to be delivered to tissues.**
- **Red blood cells** stored over 2 weeks have been associated with mesenteric hypoperfusion.
- Stored red blood cells are less deformable and consequently **can get lodged in capillaries.**

Ans. 52: (d) Sinus histiocytosis
Ref: Read the text below
Sol:

- **Sinus histiocytosis** represents hyperplasia of the endothelial lining of the sinusoids, **which become dilated and contain many histiocytes.**
- This reaction, which is also called reticular hyperplasia, becomes very prominent in lymph nodes **when they are draining a cancerous process. This is particularly common in the axillary nodes when cancer of the breast has been detected.**
- It is thought to **represent an immune response** to the host against the tumor products.

Ans. 53 : (d) Ulcerative colitis
Ref:Read the text below
Sol:

- **Ulcerative colitis** is an inflammatory disease of uncertain etiology that has a relapsing course.
- Patients with **ulcerative colitis have a higher than normal incidence** of developing colon carcinoma, **approximately 10%.**

Ans. 54 : (c) It is frequently bilateral.
Ref:Read the text below
Sol:

- **Serous cystadenocarcinoma of the ovary** is the most common malignant ovarian tumor and is frequently bilateral. Microscopically, they show a variegated **appearance with papillary pattern**.
- **Different degrees of anaplasia of the cuboidal** to columnar cells cover the papilla and occasional calcified concretions (Psammoma bodies) are present.
- These tumors almost **never metastasize to the brain and they are not seen in children or young adults.**

Ans. 55: (b) Polycystic ovary
Ref: Read the text below
Sol:

- Polycystic ovary syndrome is characterized by clinical manifestations related to the secretions of excess of androgen hormones.
- There is usually a persistent anovulation, resulting clinically in irregular or absent menstruation.
- The ovaries are moderately enlarged and contain many small cysts located in the cortex.

Ans. 56: (d) Papillary transitional cell carcinoma
Ref: Read the text below
Sol:

- **Papillary cancer arises** most frequently from the lateral and posterior bladder walls.
- At cystoscopy, tumors may be small, delicate, lowgrade papillary lesions limited to the mucosal **surface or larger high grade, solid, and invasive which are often ulcerated.**
- **Papillary and exophitic cancers** tend to be better differentiated.
- Infiltrating tumors are usually more anaplastic. Nonurothelial forms of bladder cancer are **squamous cell carcinomas, adenocarcinomas, neuroendocrine carcinomas, and rhabdomyosarcomas. The frequency of these tumors is much lower.**

Ans. 57: (b) Asymptomatic seroconversion
Ref: Read the text below
Sol:

- **Coccidioidomycosis is** amazingly diverse in terms of its scope of clinical presentation, as well as clinical severity. **60% of infections as determined by serologic conversion are asymptomatic.**
- The **most common clinical syndrome** in the other 40% of infected patients is an acute respiratory illness characterized by fever, cough, and pleuritic pain. Skin manifestations, such as erythema nodosum, **are also common with Coccidioides infection.**
- Coccidioides infection can cause a severe and difficult to- treat meningitis in AIDS patients, other immunocompromised **patients, and occasionally immunocompetent hosts, and can occasionally cause acute respiratory distress syndrome and fatal multilobar pneumonia.**

Ans. 58: (b) Early repolarization
Ref: Read the text below
Sol:

- One must be able to **distinguish acute pericarditis from normal early repolarization**. This pattern is most common in teenaged **boys and men in their 20s.**
- These individuals **differ from pericarditis patients in that the clinical syndrome of pain and dyspnea is absent, PR-segment depression** is present in some patients but uncommon, and, most important, the ECG does not, **over time, evolve a pattern of return of the ST segment to baseline followed by T-wave inversion**

Ans. 59: (d) Polymerase chain reaction (PCR)
Ref: Read the text below
Sol:

- **Norovirus, or the so-called Norwalklike agent, was initially described as a cause of food-borne illness in Norwalk, Ohio.**
- The initial **detection of the Norwalk agent was poor**, relying on electron microscopy or immune electron microscopy. Using these techniques, the Norwalk agent was identified as the causative agent in 19–42% of **nonbacterial diarrheal outbreaks.**
- With the development of more sensitive molecular assays (reverse transcriptase PCR, enzyme-linked immunosorbent assay**), Norwalk-like viruses are being found as increasingly frequent causes of diarrheal outbreaks.**
- **Treatment is supportive as symptoms improve within 10–51 h.** Rotavirus is the most common cause of viral diarrhea in infants but is uncommon in adults.
- **Salmonella, shigella, and E. coli present with more colonic and systemic manifestations.**

Ans. 60: (c) Increased contractility
Ref: Read the text below
Sol:

- **Loop B shows increased contractility because stroke volume is increased at a constant preload and afterload.**
- When loop **B is compared to loop A**, preload is not increased or decreased because there is no change in the pressure or volume at which the mitral valve closes and isovolumetric contraction begins.
- **Afterload** is not changed because there is no change in the pressure or volume at which the aortic valve opens and ejection begins.
- The **evidence that stroke volume is increased is the larger volume difference between the point at which the aortic valve opens and closes—that is, between isovolumetric contraction** and relaxation.

Ans. 61: (b) End-tidal CO_2 monitoring
Ref: Read the text below
Sol:

- **In order for a technique** to be clinically useful in assessing the likelihood of successful resuscitation, it should **be rapid, require few resuscitative resources, be cost effective, and correlate with clinical outcome.**
- So far, no technique has overwhelmingly met these criteria; however, endtidal CO_2 has shown some promise. **One small prospective observational study of adult, nontraumatic, prehospital arrest victims correlated**

higher CO_2 levels on arrival with successful return to spontaneous circulation.

- Although **arterial blood gas parameters** are often abnormal in critically ill patients, serial blood gases are difficult to obtain in the arrest patient, and results are delayed, so information obtained **is unlikely to affect clinical outcome**.
- **Ventricular fibrillation waveform analysis** is intended to summarize attempts to identify characteristics of the fibrillation waveform that correlate with the likelihood of successful defibrillation.
- **Waveform analysis** has been shown in a small retrospective study to possibly correlate with the likelihood of successful defibrillation, but in order to be effective, waveform analysis would need to be done in real time.
- **Invasive hemodynamic pressure** monitoring with central venous and aortic catheters provides the most direct measurement of coronary perfusion pressure; however, the procedure is time consuming, **requires significant resuscitative resources, and provides data far into the arrest period unlikely to affect clinical outcome.**

Ans. 62: (d) 72
Ref: Read the text below
Sol:

- Typically, **body NaCl level is constant: NaCl** excretion equals NaCl intake. However, administration of mineralocorticoid will cause the body to reabsorb more NaCl.
- For each day, the difference between **NaCl intake and NaCl excretion** equals NaCl retention. On day 1 he **retains 170 mmol NaCl; on day 2 he retains an additional 110** mmol NaCl; on day 3 he retains an additional 20 mmol NaCl.
- On day 4, NaCl excretion equals NaCl intake, showing he has reached a new steady-state. Thus, overall he has retained **170 + 110 + 20 = 300 mmol NaCl. With** free access to water and usual caloric intake, the retained NaCl is equivalent to addition of isotonic fluid.
- Given that **150 mmol NaCl weighs 1 kg, 300 mmol NaCl therefore weighs 2** kg. This 70-kg man will weigh 72 kg at the end of day 4.

Ans. 63: (a) Decreased basal vascular smooth muscle tone
Ref: Read the text below
Sol:

- **Sildenafil (Viagra) is a commonly-used medication for erectile dysfunction and increasingly pulmonary hypertension.**
- The drug is a potent **cGMP phosphodiesterase 5 (PDE5) inhibitor**. Thus, it blocks PDE5, which increases cellular cGMP **in the corpus cavernosum**.
- The increased **cGMP promotes smooth muscle relaxation and vasodilitation**, facilitating an erection. A major side effect of sildenafil is that the above cascade can also occur in the general circulation at the level of the arteriole, thus causing systemic vasodilitation. This may result in dizziness and orthostatic hypotension.
- Such symptoms are especially worsened by nitrates such as nitroglycerin, which is contraindicated in patients **taking sildenafil or other PDE5 inhibitors.**

Ans. 64: (d) Squamous cell carcinoma
Ref: Read the text below
Sol:

- **Skin cancer comes in three major forms** - squamous cell carcinoma (SCC), basal cell carcinoma (BCC), and melanoma. This patient's presentation and histology suggest squamous cell carcinoma.
- In **general, a lesion described as ulcerated** or with heaped borders is cancerous until proven otherwise. The **atypical and dysplastic keratinocytes** indicate a squamous cell origin. **Actinic keratosis** is a thick, scaly lesion that a predecessor lesion to SCC.
- It would be fair to consider in this patient except that the clinical presentation describes a lesion that has progressed much further.
- **Melanoma is a neoplasm of melanocytes**. Melanoma should be associated with ABCDE - Asymmetry, irregular Borders, multiple Colors, Diameter greater than 5mm, and Evolution of a pre-existing nevus.
- **Melanoma is more common in younger people.**

Ans. 65: (d) Most particles this size are deposited in the conducting airways
Ref: Read the text below
Sol:

- The test is attempting to measure the **alveolar ventilation**, or the amount of gas reaching the alveoli that is capable of gas exchange. **The 20 micrometer particles** are not arriving as they are too large to pass through **the 10+ levels of conducting airways.**
- One can reach this answer through elimination of the others:

a. Macrophage ingestion takes a long time, and would not affect a quick scan such as this. There is no evidence that nonuniform ingestion, if it exists, can explain the problem with this aerosol.

b. If the particles adhered to the walls, the more distal parts of the lung would be less ventilated by the particles, which would exacerbate the problem with the aerosol.

c. This would happen uniformly throughout the lung, which would not affect the measurement of alveolar ventilation.

Ans. 66: (c) Ischemia
Ref: Read the text below
Sol:
Myoplasty and myodesis
There are 2 approaches to managing the muscle in the limb during amputation: myodesis and myoplasty.
With a myodesis, the muscles and fasciae are sutured directly to the distal residual bone through drill holes. The objective of this technique is to provide a structurally stable residual limb, with the insertions of the residual muscles securely attached to maintain their function; this ultimately results in better prosthetic control and function. Myodesis is not always performed, because when attempted by even the most **experienced surgical hands it often fails. Myodesis is contraindicated in patients with severe peripheral vascular disease, because the blood supply to the muscle may be compromised.**
Myoplasty requires the surgeon to suture the opposing muscles in the residual limb to each other and to the periosteum or to the distal end of the cut bone. Sufficient muscle stretch must be provided to maintain active muscle control of the residual limb following amputation, but without producing so much muscle tension that the blood supply is compromised. A well-performed myoplasty can provide some distal soft-tissue padding over the residual bone and result in a stable, functional residual limb. On occasion, some myoplasties will not securely anchor to the distal residual **limb, resulting in a movable soft-tissue sling, with a bursa developing between the soft tissues and the underlying bone. Some of this bursa can become symptomatic and painful.**

Ans. 67: (a) Obturator foramen
Ref: Read the text below
Sol:
- **Obturator Foramen** is seen in association with **pelvic ring disruptions**.

Ans. 68: (b) Chronic obstructive pulmonary disease
Ref: Read the text below
Sol:
- **Point Y shows** an elevated **pCO_2, but the pH** is slightly below normal, indicating that the patient has compensated and is thus **experiencing a chronic acid/base imbalance**.
- In chronic obstructive pulmonary disease, **patients retain CO_2** and thus are in a state of chronic respiratory acidosis; the renal compensation is to retain bicarbonate and secrete **H+ to correct the pH.**
- **Adaptation to high altitude** would lead to a higher than normal pH, as a person would try to breathe in more oxygen would hyper-ventilate, blowing off CO_2 and become alkalotic. In diarrhea, the patient experiences metabolic acidosis, but the respiratory compensation would lower the pCO_2, not raise it.
- **Similary, in the case of ingestion of a strong acid, the patient would hyper-ventilate to blow off CO_2 to compensate for the metabolic acidosis, lowering the pCO_2, not raising it.**

Ans. 69: (c) Curve 3
Ref: Read the text below
Sol:
- In Michaelis-Menten kinetics, halving the amount of enzyme decreases the maximum velocity (Vmax) in half.
- The Vmax is how quickly a given amount of enzyme can work if provided with unlimited substrate, thus decreasing the amount of enzyme decreases the Vmax.
- Choices a, b, and d are thus incorrect because the Vmax is not decreased.

Ans. 70: (c) Popliteal fossa
Ref: Read the text below
Sol:
- The boy's **wound appears to be superficial** - he "scraped" his foot which is now infected (likely by a Gram **positive organism such as Strep A or Staph**).
- The **superficial lymphatic drainage** of the lower extremity roughly follows the superficial vessels.
- In this case of the lateral **foot, the lymphatics drain** along the path of the small saphenous vein to the **popliteal fossa.**

Ans. 71: (c) Administration of bicarbonate to treat the acidosis may hasten the development of hypokalemia and magnify its intensity
Ref: Read the text below
Sol:
- **Hypokalemia** is magnified by bicarbonate treatment of acidosis, which causes potassium to enter cells. Patients with **severe diabetic ketoacidosis** always have a depletion of their total body potassium even though the **serum potassium may be elevated.**
- This **patient's hyperkalemia**, however, still represents a risk because of its potential to produce cardiac arrest, a risk that may be greatly accentuated if potassium replacement is begun too early.
- **Patients should be monitored very carefully** to obtain unequivocal evidence that serum potassium has begun to fall before potassium therapy is started. Oral potassium is unwise in a drowsy, nauseated patient.
- **The electrocardiogram is more reliable than serum potassium levels to assess the need for potassium replacement.**
- **Potassium can be administered at 30 mEq/hour with caution if potassium deficiency becomes severe.**

Ans. 72: (d) Parathion

Ref: Read the text below
Sol:

- This patient has been poisoned by **the organophosphate parathion**.
- Organophosphates inh**ibit acetylcholinesterase (AChE), leading to toxic build-up of acetylcholine (ACh)** and resulting in the symptoms listed above.
- Remember the mnemonic **DUMBELS associated with cholinergic toxicity**: Defecatioin, Urination, Miosis, Bronchorrhea/ Bronchospasm/Bradycardia, Emesis, Lacrimation, Salivation.

Ans. 73: (d) Preeclampsia
Ref: Read the text below
Sol:

- **Proteinuria, edema, and hypertension** after 20 weeks' gestation in a previously normotensive woman **are pathognomonic for preeclampsia**.
- This disease is associated **with the HELLP syndrome** (Hemolysis, Elevated LFTs, Low Platelets.) When the above presentation includes seizures, a diagnosis of eclampsia is made.
- In this case, this **woman's headaches are caused by hypertension**, while her edema is secondary to the reduced plasma oncotic pressure following protein loss in the urine.
- Acute **glomerulonephritis** can cause hypertension, but is less likely to cause edema, Congestive heart failure does not cause orbital edema.

Ans. 74: (c) 1-c; 2-b; 3-b; 4-e; 5-d
Ref: Read the text below
Sol:

- The American Joint **Committee on Cancer has defined a four-tiered staging system** for breast cancer based on the clinical criteria of tumor size, involvement of lymph nodes, and metastatic **disease. In one version of this system, a separate category is reserved for inflammatory breast cancer. While the grouping of breast cancers into stages provides useful shorthand for expressing** a patient's survival probability, it is noteworthy that considerable heterogeneity exists both with respect to tumor size and nodal characteristics among tumors that are classified within a given stage.
- The **TNM stage of breast cancer is assigned by measuring** the greatest diameter of the tumor ("T"), assessing the axillary and clavicular lymph nodes for enlargement and fixation ("N"), and judging whether metastatic disease is present ("M"). In general, the worst of the three **TNM parameters will determine the s**tage assignment.
- Tumors that are not palpable are classified T0; tumors 2 cm or less, T1; tumors greater than 2 but not more than 5 cm, T2; **tumors greater than 5 cm, T3; and tumors with extension into the chest wall or skin, T4.**
- **Clinically negative lymph nodes are classified N0; positive, movableipsilateral axillary nodes, N1; fixed ipsilateral axillary nodes, N2; and clavicular nodes, N3.**
- **Absence of evidence of metastatic disease is clas**sified M0; distant metastatic disease, M1.
- The patient in question **1 has a T0, N2,** M0 lesion. This is stage III (fixed or matted nodes are a poor prognostic sign).
- The patient in **question 2 has a T2, N1, M0 lesion. This is stage II.**
- The patient in question 3 has a T2, **N0, M0 lesion. Though smaller than the tumor in** question 2 and without clinically involved nodes, this tumor is also stage II.
- The patient in question 4 has findings compatible with inflammatory breast cancer. A biopsy of the involved skin and a mammogram would confirm the **diagnosis.**
- **The patient in question 5 has a T1, N0, M1 lesion. This is stage IV (stage IV is any T, any N, M1).**

Ans. 75: (c) 1-d; 2-d; 3-e
Ref: Read the text below
Sol:

- **Paraesophageal hernias, generally** thought to be acquired, involve herniation of any portion or all of the stomach into the thoracic cavity via the esophageal hiatus. These hernias are usually repaired **electively because of a high incidence of complications. In these dangerous hernias, the cardioesophageal junction is in its normal position below the diaphragm.**
- **Diaphragmatic ruptures usually affect adults** and result from blunt trauma to the abdomen. Unless such ruptures are repaired, the negative intrathoracic pressure associated with each respiratory **effort tends to such the abdominal contents into the chest with consequent loss of necessary space for lung expansion and substantial risk of damage to the intrathoracic bowel.**
- Sliding hiatal hernias, the most frequent type of hernia found in adults, are generally acquired.
- The significance of this type of hernia rests in its association with gastroesophageal reflux, a condition that may lead to **reflux esophagitis. Because sliding hiatal hernias frequently do not exhibit significant gastroesophageal reflux, it is likely that other factors may be more important in the pathophysiology** of that disorder.
- The foramen of Bochdalek hernia is a congenital hernia of the posterolateral aspect of the diaphragm in which abdominal viscera enter

the thorax and cause acute respiratory distress in infants. This hernia requires emergency repair.

- The foramen of Morgagni hernia, **although also congenital, is not usually detected until adulthood. It is usually an incidental finding on chest X-ray, where it appears as a low anterior mediastinal mass. However, on rar**e occasions it can produce acute respiratory distress in infants.

Ans. 76: (d) Tibia fracture
Ref: Read the text below
Sol:

- **Specific injuries** are at particular risk for developing compartment syndrome.
- These include **tibial and forearm fractures, crush and burn injuries, and ischemic-reperfusion injuries.**

Ans. 77: (b) If the patient is under 30 with a breast mass, then an outpatient ultrasound should be performed with possible needle aspiration
Ref: Read the text below
Sol:

- **Fibrocystic breast disease** is the most common cause for benign breast disease in **premenopausal women.**
- It includes **nodularity and tenderness** that occurs as a result of breast tissue response to hormonal cycling. **Fibrocystic changes** do not include skin thickening, edema, discoloration, nipple retraction, or discharge.
- **All patients with a palpable mass** with or without other symptoms should be referred to a breast specialist. **All women over the age of 40 with a normal exam** should also be referred to a breast specialist.
- If the **patient is under 30 with a breast mass**, then an outpatient ultrasound should be performed with possible needle aspiration. For patients in their 30s, the management is not clear.
- It is **clear that the risk factors for breast cancer** in young women include the inheritance of the **BRCA1 or BRCA2 genes**, a history of childhood malignancy, and a history of childhood irradiation.
  For **women 30 and older the risks factors** also include a first-degree relative with breast cancer, increased exposure **to endogenous estrogens, and biopsy-confirmed atypical hyperplasia of the breast.**

Ans. 78: (b) A negative (diverging) lens placed in front of the eye
Ref: Read the text below
Sol:

- **A myopic eyeball is too long, and light rays coming from great distances focus in front of the retina.**
- The **range of motion** available to the lens is not sufficient to provide accommodation **regardless of the effort made.**
- A **negative lens placed in front of the eye** corrects the eye's refractive power, and the rays will now focus on the retina. A **positive lens** would only worsen matters, and a cylindrical lens (which has two foci, depending on the orientation considered) would not compensate satisfactorily.
- **Reducing the light intensity** also would not help; the pupils would dilate and admit more peripheral rays **that would be further out of focus.**

Ans. 79: (b) Placenta praevia
Ref: Read the text below
Sol:

- The condition **placenta praevia** occurs **when the placenta abnormally implants in the lower segment** of the uterus.
- **Bleeding is usually** painless unlike the other common cause of antepartum haemorrhage, **abruptio placentae (placental abruption).**
- Physical signs are usually few. Breech or oblique presentation is occasionally seen due to the mechanical obstruction to birth canal outflow. Routine ultrasound scans may over-estimate the prevalence of this condition as the lower segment grows cephalically late in the **last trimester and it is estimated that up to 10% of placentae are low-lying before 37 weeks.**
- **Cervical cancer** would otherwise be a diagnosis not to be dismissed; however, as cervical smears are usually recommended as part of antenatal care, this makes this option unlikely.
- **Placenta accreta is usually encountered at Caesarean section, often with catastrophic effect, and does not usually present with antepartum haemorrhage.**

Ans. 80: (a) 0.5 mM

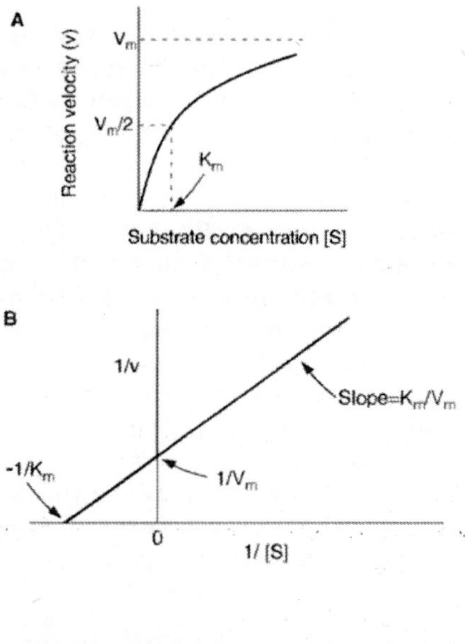

Ref: Read the text below
Sol:
Lineweaver-Burk equation
V-$_m$ = maximum velocity, and **Km** = substrate concentration at 1/2 **V-$_m$**.

a. **The intercept on the x axis is -1/ Km = -2.Therefore, Km = 0.5 mM.**

Ans. 81: (d) CMV retinitis
Ref: Read the text below
Sol:

- **CMV retinitis, a common CMV infection in HIV patients**, occurs very rarely in solid organ transplant patients.
- CMV does affect the lung in a majority of transplant patients if either donor or recipient is CMV-**seropositive pretransplant. CMV disease in transplant recipients typically develops 30–90 days posttransplant.**
- It rarely occurs within 2 weeks of transplantation. CMV very commonly causes a pneumonitis that clinically is **difficult to distinguish from acute rejection. Prior CMV infection has been associated with bronchiolitis obliterans syndrome (chronic rejection) in lung transplant recipients.**
- As **with HIV, the gastrointestinal tract is commonly involved** with CMV infection. Endoscopy with biopsy showing characteristic giant cells, not serum polymerase chain reaction (PCR), is necessary to **make this diagnosis. The CMV syndrome is also common in lung transplant patients.**
- Serum CMV PCR should be sent as part of the workup for all nonspecific fevers, worsening lung function, liver **function abnormalities, or falling leukocyte counts occurring more than a couple of weeks after transplant.**

Ans. 82: (d) There is known environmental reservoir for the virus causing SARS
Ref: Read the text below
Sol:

- **In 2002, an outbreak of a severe systemic illness, named severe acute respiratory syndrome, or SARS, began in China.**
- Ultimately 8000 cases were recorded in 28 countries. The etiologic agent proved to be a virus associated with the **Coronavirus family, now named SARS-CoV. The natural reservoir appears to be the horseshoe bat, though human exposure may have come from domesticated animals such as the palm civet.**
- While some patients acquired the virus from animals or the environment, the majority appear to have contracted the illness **from other people. Human-tohuman transmission, either by aerosol or fecaloral routes, is efficient.**
- Environmental transmission (water, sewage) may also have played a role, particularly in the outbreak centered in an apartment complex. In the outbreak, children had a much less severe clinical course compared to adults.
- In 2003 the outbreak ceased, and no **new cases have arisen since 2004. Many unanswered questions linger in the wake of this illness.**

Ans. 83: (d) Gastroesophageal reflux disease
Ref: Read the text below
Sol:

- **Helicobacter pylori is thought to colonize** ~50% (30% in developed countries, >80% in developing countries) of the **world's population.**
- The organism induces a direct tissue response in the stomach, with evidence of mononuclear **and polymorphonuclear infiltrates in all of those with colonization, regardless of whether or not symptoms are present.**
- **Gastric ulceration and adenocarcinoma of the stomach arise** in association with this gastritis. MALT is specific to H. pylori infection and is due to prolonged B cell activation in the stomach.
- Though **H. pylori do not directly infect the intestine**, it does diminish somatostatin production, indirectly contributing to the development of duodenal ulcers.
- **Gastroesophageal reflux disease** is not caused by H. pylori, and some early, controversial research may suggest that it is in fact protective against this condition.

Ans. 84: (d) Recurrent disease is associated with serious complications
Ref: Read the text below
Sol:

- **Clostridium difficile–associated disease recurrences** are most often due to reinfection (because patients carry similar risk **factors as they did before first infection) or relapse (due to persistence of spores in the bowel).**
- Approximately 15–30% of **patients have at least one relapse**. Recurrent disease has been associated with ~10% risk of serious complications including shock, megacolon, perforation, colectomy, or death at 30 days.
- Metronidazole resistance occurs but **is actually a very rare event**. Metronidazole and vancomycin have a similar efficacy in a first episode of recurrence. Repeated courses of metronidazole should be avoided due to neurotoxicity.
- Unfortunately, patients who recur **are more likely to recur again, and many patients receive multiple cycles of antibiotics and are even candidates for more extreme measures such as intravenous**

immunoglobulin or fecal transplant via stool enema. Testing for clearance is not likely to be informative.

- A negative stool antigen would not change management, as symptomatic improvement is the true goal of therapy.
- A **positive stool antigen** and toxin test in a patient whose symptoms have improved after standard therapy implies colonization, not disease. It can therefore be needlessly discouraging to patients and again does not impact clinical management.
- There is **no known association between C. difficile–associated disease and colon cancer**.

Ans. 85: (b) Testwith hydrogen peroxide
Ref: Read the text below
Sol:

- The **catalase test** is carried out with hydrogen peroxide. The **other tests do not differentiate.**

Ans. 86: (c) Fever to 39.5°C following the first dose
Ref: Read the text below
Sol:
True contraindications to pertussis immunisation include:

- **Acute illness** - Until recovered.
- **Previous reaction to pertussis:**
  - **Local:** an extensive area of redness and swelling which becomes indurated, involving most of the anterolateral surface of the thigh or a major part of the circumference of the upper arm.
  - **General**: fever equal to or more than 39.5°C within 48 hours of vaccine, anaphylaxis, bronchospasm, laryngeal oedema, generalised collapse, prolonged hyporesponsiveness, prolonged inconsolable or high-pitched screaming of >4 hours, convulsions or encephalopathy occurring within 72 hours.

A personal family history of allergy is not a contraindication, nor is stable neurological conditions such as cerebral palsy or spina bifida. In patients who have had a previous reaction, immunisations should be completed with DT vaccine, and acellular vaccine considered.

Ans. 87: (a) Fatigue
Ref: Read the text below
Sol:

- **Atenolol is a water soluble beta blocker**, taken once daily and is not associated with **drowsiness/sleep disturbance like the lipid-soluble beta-blockers**.
- It is not associated with nausea or **hesitancy of micturition** and would be unlikely to produce significant postural hypotension in a hypertensive subject.
- However, **fatigue is a frequent side effect** which typically is felt two hours and beyond after taking the drug.

Ans. 88: (a) It is associated with hypoglycaemia at normal doses
Ref: Read the text below
Sol:

- **Metformin is a biguanide** which acts to improve insulin sensitivity through mechanisms that involve **hepatic gluconeogenesis** and improved muscle glucose utilization.
- Thus, some insulin must **be produced for it to have an effect**. It is associated with hypoglycaemia **although this side effect is unusual.**
- It is **contra-indicated in subjects with renal failure, hepatic failure and heart failure** due to the association with lactic acidosis.

Ans. 89: (b) 7.5 mg
Ref: Read the text below
Sol:

- The equivalent ratio of **prednisolone to hydrocortisone is 1:**4. For **Dexamethasone to hydrocortisone the ratio is roughly 1:40.**

Ans. 90: (c) Conjugation to glucuronic acid
Ref: Read the text below
Sol:

- **Paracetamol is conjugated to glucuronic acid and sulphate** under normal conditions.
- In overdose these processes become **saturated and the drug is then conjugated** with glutathione.
- If the **glutathione supply** is depleted then a toxic **metabolite is formed**.

Ans. 91: (d) Insulin therapy
Ref: Read the text below
Sol:

- The result confirms a **diagnosis of gestational diabetes mellitus with the 2hr OGTT result above 11.1 mmol/l.**
- To minimise **the fetal consequences of GDM (**macrosomia, fetal malformations, still birth, IUGR etc), the patient's glycaemia should be strictly controlled with insulin.
- A low calorie diet is **inappropriate and neither metformin nor glipizide are licenced for use in pregnancy.**
- There is **no point in repeating the OGTT in 4 weeks as control is required now.**

Ans. 92: (c) Postrenal obstruction
Ref: Read the text below
Sol:

- The **kidney in Figure 5-16 demonstrates** severe hydronephrosis characterized by dilation of the renal pelvis at the expense of the subadjacent renal medulla and cortex. Post renal obstruction, such as a ureteral **stone, is the most likely etiology.**

- **Abuse of analgesics** may be associated with necrosis of the renal papillae. The papillae in the photo are not necrotic.
- **Hypertension mainly affects the blood vessels of the renal cortex**, sparing the pelvic region of the kidney.
- An acute renal infarct demonstrates a pale, wedge-shaped area with its base along the renal capsule. A **chronic infarct** shows either fibrous scarring or cyst formation. The renal pelvis is usually unaffected by renal infarcts.

Ans. 93: (b) Once an irreversible MAOI has been stopped, a 2-week "washout" period is necessary before MAO activity returns.
Ref: Read the text below
Sol:

- **MAOIs have mostly been supplanted by newer antidepressants due to MAOI toxicity and the availability of safer alternatives like selective serotonin reuptake inhibitors.**
- Commercially available **MAOIs irreversibly block both subtypes of MAO**, leading to the accumulation of aminated neurotransmitters in the **presynaptic terminals. MAOIs,** however, have a minimal role on the effect of circulating catecholamines, which are metabolized by a different enzyme system.
- The **tyramine reaction** occurs about 15-90 minutes after the ingestion of foods high in tyramine (aged or pickled foods), causing headache, hypertension, neck stiffness, and palpitations.
- **Hypertension is typically treated with phentolamine or nitroprusside. Beta-blockers are contraindicated in MAOI ingestions** due to the resulting unopposed alpha effect, causing worsening hypertension.

Ans. 94: (c) Neuroleptic malignant syndrome–cogwheel rigidity
Ref: Read the text below
Sol:

- **Neuroleptics can cause numerous side effects. Dystonic reactions are involuntary muscle contractions commonly seen after a first dose.**
- **Muscles of the neck and jaw** are commonly affected, as are ocular muscle (oculogyric crises). **Akathisia is motor restlessness** combined with agitation and can often be mistaken for worsening psychosis.
- **Tardive dyskinesia** is a result of chronic neuroleptic use, taking months to years to appear. It is characterized by rhythmic choreoathetoid movements of the face and limbs; lip smacking and **rhythmic tongue protrusion are classic signs.**
- **Neuroleptic malignant syndrome (NMS)** is a rare idiosyncratic reaction characterized by muscle rigidity, hyperthermia, autonomic instability, and alterations in mental status.
- **The rigidity of NMS is characterized as a "lead-pipe" rigidity. Parkinsonism (also seen with neuroleptic use) is classically associated with "cogwheel" rigidity.**

Ans. 95: (c) Neuromuscular blocking agents may have a long duration of effect in patients who have ingested cocaine.
Ref: Read the text below
Sol:

- **Cocaine is a sympathomimetic agent with local anaesthetic and central nervous system stimulant properties.**
- Its stimulant activity comes mainly from **blockade of presynaptic uptake of dopamine, serotonin, and norepinephrine.**
- Like other local anesthetics, cocaine inhibits conduction of nerve impulses by blocking fast-**acting sodium channels in neural tissue.**
- Cocaine has many effects on the heart. Its **ability to cause widened QRS complexes and QTc prolongation comes from a type 1A quinidine-like effect** on cardiac conduction tissue.
- **Cocaine is metabolized by plasma cholinesterase** so neuromuscular blocking agents (both depolarizing and nondepolarizing) should be used with some caution–they may have a prolonged effect as **a result of decreased metabolism**.
- **Haloperidol and droperidol** can cause hyperthermia, dysrhythmia, and lowered seizure threshold in patients **who have ingested cocaine, and they should be avoided in the cocaine-intoxicated patient.**

Ans. 96: (c) The centrally mediated increased respiratory rate seen in salicylate poisoning is partially offset by a salicylate-induced decrease in carbon dioxide production
Ref: Read the text below
Sol:

- **Salicylates have multiple effects on the body, and an understanding of the mechanisms of their toxicity is the key to understanding the treatment principles.**
- **Salicylates are mostly ionized at a physiologic pH.** However, as acidemia progresses, more of the salicylate molecules will be ionized and will be free to cross the blood-brain barrier, allowing for relatively higher **concentrations of salicylates in the brain with larger ingestions.**
- This higher degree **of ionization is also the key to the principle of ion trapping in the kidney used to treat the condition**. Salicylates have profound effects on glucose homeostasis. While they do cause mobilization of glycogen stores, they can also inhibit gluconeogenesis.

- **Normoglycemia, hyperglycemia, or hypoglycemia can be seen in the salicylate-poisoned patient. Hemorrhage** is a surprisingly rare complication of acute massive salicylate poisoning, although it is slightly more common with chronic salicylate poisoning. Although it is true that the respiratory stimulation of salicylates is centrally mediated, salicylates also cause increased metabolism of skeletal muscle, thereby increasing the amount of carbon dioxide in the blood.
- Once the **buffering capacity is overcome and the ventilatory compensation can no longer keep up with carbon dioxide production, a respiratory acidosis superimposes upon the anion gap metabolic acidosis.**

Ans. 97: (c) Iron
Ref: Read the text below
Sol:

- **Activated charcoal is generally agreed upon as the most appropriate agent to decontaminate the gastrointestinal (GI) tract.**
- It is formed by heating charcoal in an anhydrous environment, making it porous and increasing its **surface area, allowing toxic agents in the GI tract to be adsorbed to the charcoal more effectively.**
- **Maximal benefit for the use of charcoal** is generally agreed upon as being within 2 hours of ingestion, although benefit may still exist beyond that time frame.
- **Reasons not to use charcoal include a risk of aspiration without airway protection, ileus, caustic ingestions (charcoal may accumulate in burned areas), and drugs that do not adsorb to activated charcoal.**
- Substances that do not bind to activated charcoal include metals (like iron and lead), small molecules (such as lithium and borates), hydrocarbons (particularly long-chain molecules), liquids (i.e., alcohols, methylsalicylate), organophosphates and carbamates, quinidine, meprobamate (**which forms gastric concretions), DDT, cyanide, and hydroxides of sodium and potassium.**

Ans. 98: (c) Lamivudine
Ref: Read the text below
Sol:

- **Lamivudine is a pyrimidine nucleoside** analogue that has activity against HIV and hepatitis B. In acute hepatitis B**, lamivudine results in suppression of HBV DNA and loss of hepatitis E antigen in 30% of patients.**
- Tenofovir is a nucleotide **analogue with activity against HIV and hepatitis B.** It is not approved for initial treatment for HBV but may be used for HIV/HBV co-infection or for HBV resistant to lamivudine.
- Efavirenz has activity only **against HIV and not hepatitis B.** Ganciclovir has activity against herpes viruses and is mostly used for **treatment of cytomegalovirus.**
- Rimantadine has **antiviral activity only against influenza A.**

Ans. 99: (c) Deep inferior epigastric artery
Ref: Sch8- 1816
Sol:

Breast Reconstruction: Autogenous Choices

	Vascular Supply	Advantages	Disadvantages
Pedicled TRAM flap	Superior epigastric artery	Ease of elevation	Occasional partial flap loss
Pedicled latissimus dorsi flap	Thoracodorsal	Ease of elevation	Needs an implant for volume; some limitation of upper extremity function possible
Free TRAM flap	Deep inferior epigastric artery	More robust blood supply than pedicled TRAM (less affected by radiation)	Slightly longer procedure than pedicled TRAM
Deep inferior epigastric artery perforator flap	Perforating arteries of the deep inferior epigastric artery	No rectus muscle taken with flap	Tedious dissection of perforators; possible higher incidence of fat necrosis
Superficial inferior epigastric artery flap	Superficial inferior epigastric artery	No violation of rectus fascia	Smaller volume of soft tissue for reconstruction: vessels not always present or suitable for anastomosis
Gluteal artery flap	Inferior gluteal artery	Useful if prior surgery has compromised abdominal tissue	Donor-site irregularity and possible gait disturbance
Deep circumflex iliac artery flap	Deep circumflex iliac artery	Useful if other donor sites are compromised	Donor-site hernia, pain
Anterolateral thigh flap	Descending branch of the profunda femoris artery	Useful if other donor sites are compromised	Depending on patient anatomy, less volume of soft tissue, possible need to skin-graft donor site

Ans. 100: (d) Priapism
Ref: Sch8- 1557
Sol:
Priapism

- **Priapism** refers to an erection that is unrelated to sexual activity or persists beyond sexual activity.
- **Priapism can be classified as low-flow (ischemic) or high-flow (nonischemic).**
- The management of low-flow priapism should be dictated by the duration of the priapism.
- **Within 36 hours of onset of low-flow priapism**, intracorporal irrigation with an alpha-adrenergic agonist may be effective.

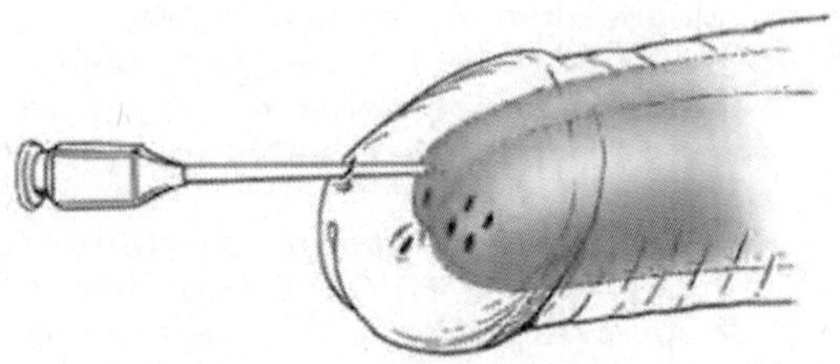

Winter shunt

- **If this is ineffective, or if the priapism has been present for more than 36 hours, a distal shunt should be performed under anesthesia**. A commonly performed distal shunt is the **Winter shunt**, in which a biopsy needle is inserted through the penile glens into the corpora cavernosa to create a shunt.
- **If this** procedure is unsuccessful, a **more proximal shunting procedure, between the corpora**
- **cavernosum and the corpora spongiosum, should be performed**.

Ans. 101: (c) A is true but R is false
Ref: Read the text below
Sol:

- Patients **with acute, severe and life threatening** asthma are treated with parenteral steroids.
- Steroids are **not bronchodilators**

Ans. 102: (c) A is true but R is false
Ref: Read the text below
Sol:

- Some **strains of Clostridium perfringens type A can** cause food poisoning by producing a heat labile enterotoxin which like the **enterotoxins of V. cholera and entero-toxigenic E. coli leads to fluid accumulation in the intestine.**
- Staphylococcal enterotoxin is a heat-stable toxin inactivated only slowly at 100 C in 10-40 mins depending on the toxin **concentration and nature of the medium.**
- **Bacillus cereus can produce a heat-stable enterotoxin** which is responsible for the emetic form of the disease and a heat labile toxin which causes diarrhea.
- Many strains of Yersinia enterocolitica **that cause food poisoning produce a heat-stable enterotoxin like E. coli.**

Ans. 103: (b) In pediatric patients, the surgery should be performed through an scrotal incision
Ref: Sch8- 1550
Sol:

- In **infants, hydroceles are fluid collections** within the tunica vaginalis or processus vaginalis.
- **Surgical repair is reserved for tense hydroceles** that may interfere with testicular circulation or large hydroceles that may cause discomfort.
- **Communicating hydroceles in newborns should generally be observed.**
- Spontaneous closure of the processus vaginalis and resolution of the hydrocele is common; however, **hydroceles that persist beyond the first year of life are unlikely to resolve**.
- **In pediatric patients, the surgery should be performed through an inguinal incision. The processus vaginalis should be ligated** and the distal hydrocele sac should be excised.
- In adults, hydroceles most commonly form as a consequence of local inflammation and the process vaginalis is almost never patent. Consequently, surgery is performed through a scrotal incision. The hydrocele sac is decompressed and then either plicated or excised to prevent recurrence.

Ans. 104: (a) Modified radical mastectomy
Ref: Read the text below
Sol:
Breast cancer during pregnancy

- Because of the deleterious effects of **radiation therapy** on the fetus, **a modified radical mastectomy** is the surgical procedure of choice during the **first and second trimesters of pregnancy**, even though there is an increased risk of spontaneous abortion following **first trimester anesthesia.**
- During the **third trimester**, lumpectomy with **axillary node dissection** is considered if adjuvant radiation therapy is deferred until after delivery.

Ans. 105: (b) Lateral abdominal wall
Ref: Read the text below
Sol:
MALROTATION AND MIDGUT VOLVULUS

- During the **sixth week of fetal development**, the midgut grows too rapidly to be accommodated in the abdominal cavity, and it therefore prolapses into the umbilical cord.
- **Between the tenth and twelfth week**, the midgut returns to the abdominal cavity, undergoing **a 270 degree counterclockwise rotation** around the superior mesenteric artery.

- Because the duodenum also rotates caudal to the artery, it acquires a C-loop which traces this path.
- The **cecum rotates cephalad to the artery,** which determines the location of the transverse and ascending colon.
- Subsequently, **the duodenum becomes fixed retroperitoneally** in its third portion and at **the ligament of Treitz,** while the cecum becomes fixed to the lateral abdominal wall by peritoneal bands.
- If rotation is incomplete, the cecum remains in the epigastrium, but the bands fixing the duodenum to the retroperitoneum and cecum continue to form. **This results in (Ladd's) bands extending from the cecum to the lateral abdominal wall and crossing the duodenum, which creates the potential for obstruction.**

Ans. 106: (d) It is associated with the deposition of neurotoxic amyloid peptide aggregates
Ref: Read the text below
Sol:

- **Alzheimer disease** is associated with long, fibrillar protein assemblies consisting of b-pleated sheets found in the brain and **elsewhere. The disease is associated with abnormal processing of a normal protein.**
- The accumulated altered protein **occurs in a b-pleated sheet configuration that is neurotoxic.**
- The **Ab amyloid that is deposited** in the brain in Alzheimer disease is derived by proteolytic cleavages from **the larger amyloid precursor protein-a single** transmembrane protein expressed on the cell surface in the brain and other tissues.
- Most cases of Alzheimer disease are sporadic, **although at least five to ten percent of cases are familial.**

Ans. 107: (c) The oxygen affinity of hemoglobin increases as the percentage saturation increases
Ref: Read the text below
Sol:

- The binding of **oxygen at one heme group increases** the oxygen affinity of the remaining heme groups in the same molecule.
- Carbon dioxide decreases oxygen **affinity because it lowers the pH; also, binding of carbon dioxide stabilizes the taut, deoxy form**.
- Hemoglobin binds one molecule of 2, **3-BPG. Deoxyhemoglobin has a greater affinity for protons and, therefore, is a weaker acid.**

Ans. 108: (c) Methemoglobinemia
Ref: Read the text below
Sol:

- **Oxidation of the heme component** of hemoglobin to the ferric ($Fe3+$) state forms methemoglobin.
- This may be caused by **the action of certain drugs, such as nitrates.**
- The methemoglobinemias are characterized by **chocolate cyanosis (a brownish-blue coloration of the skin and membranes), and chocolate-colored blood as a result of the darkcolored methemoglobin.**
- Symptoms are related to tissue hypoxia, and include **anxiety, headache, dyspnea. In rare cases, coma and death can occur.**

Ans. 109: (d) Erythromycin binds to the 50S ribosomal subunit
Ref: Read the text below
Sol:

- **Tetracyclines inhibit the 30S ribosomal subunit** (chloramphenicol inhibits peptidyl transferase). Puromycin has **structure similar to that of aminoacyl-tRNA.**
- It is incorporated into the growing chain, and inhibits **further elongation of the peptide chain.**
- **Clindamycin and erythro**mycin both bind the 50S ribosomal subunit.

Ans. 110: (d) Translocation of the peptidyl-tRNA from the A site to the P site
Ref: Read the text below
Sol:

- In both **prokaryotes and eukaryotes,** continued translation (elongation) requires movement of the **peptidylt RNA from the A site to the P site to allow t**he next tRNA~amino acid to enter the A site.
- Only prokaryotes have a Shine-**Dalgarno sequence and use fmet, while o**nly eukaryotes have a nucleus and **posttranscriptionally process their mRNA.**

Ans. 111: (d) Microarray
Ref: Read the text below
Sol:

- **Microarray analysis** allows the determination of mRNA production (thus, gene expression) from thousands of genes at once.
- A Northern blot **only measures mRNA production from one gene at a time.**
- Western blots and ELISA measure protein production (also gene expression), but only from one gene at a time. Southern blots are used to **analyze DNA, not gene expression.**

Ans. 112: (d) Thiamine
Ref: Read the text below
Sol:

- **Hydroxyproline and hydroxylysine** arise from proline and lysine, but only after these amino acids have been incorporated in peptides.

- **Hydroxylation of peptide bound prolyl and lysyl residues** is catalyzed by prolyl hydroxylase and lysyl **hydroxylase of tissues, including skin and skeletal muscles and of granulating wounds.**
- The hydroxylases are mixed function oxidases that require substrate, molecular oxygen, ascorbate, **Fe+2 and** a-**ketoglutarate**.
- For every mol of proline or lysine hydroxylated, one mole of a-ketoglutarate is decarboxylaed to succinate. One **atom of oxygen is incorporated into proline or lysine, the other into succinate.**

Ans. 113: (a) DNA amplification
Ref: Read the text below
Sol:

- Sufficient **DNA** for analysis can be obtained by **amplification of leukocyte DNA** using the **polymerase chain reaction (PCR)**.
- **Newborns have fetal hemoglobin (α and γ -globin)** with little expression of hemoglobin A (α and β globin genes) **until 3 to 6 months of life, so testing for anemia or** for abnormal hemoglobin with antibodies would not be helpful.
- If the sequence variation affects the recognition **site for a restriction endonuclease, the altered segment size produced by endonuclease digestion allow detection of the sequence change.**
- If the nucleotide changes causing the **RFLP** is adjacent to (linked with) or coincident with a disease mutation, then one size variant of the **RFLP** may be diagnostic.

Ans. 114: (d) A defect in an excision-repair system that removes thymine dimers from DNA
Ref: Read the text below
Sol:

- **Xeroderma pigmentosum** appears to be due to **the inability of an excision-repair system to remove thymine dimers**, which are formed on exposure of DNA to ultraviolet radiation.
- This results in a **deficiency** in the **ability to repair the damaged DNA**.

Ans. 115: (b) Detects RNA molecules
Ref: Read the text below
Sol:

- **Northern blotting** is analogous to **Southern blotting**, a technique that was first described by **Edward Southern**. **DNA fragments** are separated on agarose gels by electrophoresis **and then transferred to nitrocellulose filters. The filters** are then exposed to labeled probes, which hybridize to the DNA fragments.
- **Northern blotting** is an analogous procedure that uses more powerful denaturing substances to extend the **RNA molecules** and ensure that their electrophoretic migration is inversely proportional to their length.
- **Labeled RNA or DNA segments** (probes) are used to identify particular **RNA species** within the size separated array.
- **Western blotting** is a technique for detecting proteins. It uses a different type of denaturing gel and labeled antibodies as probes to detect **specific proteins.**

Ans. 116: (d) Rough endoplasmic reticulum
Ref: Read the text below
Sol:

- **Protein synthesis** occurs in the cytoplasm, on groups of free ribosomes called **polysomes**, and on ribosomes associated with membranes, termed the **rough endoplasmic reticulum**.
- However, proteins **destined for secretion are only synthesized on ribosomes of the endoplasmic reticulum** and are synthesized in **such a manner that they end up inside the lumen of the endoplasmic reticulum.**
- From there **secretory proteins** are packaged in vesicles.
- The **Golgi apparatus** is involved in the **glycosylation and packaging of macromolecules into membranes for secretion.**

Ans. 117: (c) Wegener's granulomatosis
Ref: Read the text below
Sol:

- **Wegener's granulomatosis** is a distinct clinicopathologic entity characterized by granulomatous vasculitis of the upper and lower respiratory tracts together with glomerulonephritis. In **addition, variable degrees of disseminated vasculitis involving both small arteries and veins may occur.**
- **Typically Paranasal sinus pain and drainage**
  - Nasal mucosal ulceration, Nasal septal perforation, Saddle nose deformity, Serous otitis media may occur as a result of eustachian tube blockage, Subglottic stenosis.
- **Pulmonary involvement**
  - Asymptomatic infiltrates or may be clinically expressed as cough, hemoptysis, dyspnea, and chest discomfort.
- **Eye involvement**
  - Mild conjunctivitis, dacryocystitis, episcleritis, scleritis, granulomatous sclerouveitis, ciliary vessel vasculitis, and retroorbital mass lesions leading to proptosis.
- **Skin lesions**
  - Papules, vesicles, **palpable purpura**, ulcers, or subcutaneous nodules; biopsy reveals vasculitis, granuloma, or both.
- **Cardiac involvement**
  - Pericarditis, coronary vasculitis, or, rarely, cardiomyopathy.
- **Nervous system manifestations**
  - Cranial neuritis, Mononeuritis multiplex, Cerebral vasculitis and/or granuloma.

- **Renal disease (77% of patients) generally** dominates the clinical picture and, if left untreated, accounts directly or indirectly for most of the mortality in this disease. Although it may smolder in some cases as a mild glomerulitis with proteinuria, hematuria, and red blood cell casts, it is clear that once clinically detectable renal functional impairment occurs, rapidly progressive renal failure usually ensues unless appropriate treatment is instituted.
- While the **disease is active, most patients have nonspecific symptoms and signs such as malaise, weakness, arthralgias**, anorexia, and weight loss.
- Fever may indicate activity of the underlying disease but more often reflects secondary infection, usually of the upper airway.
- **Characteristic laboratory findings include a markedly** elevated ESR, mild anemia and **leukocytosis**, mild hypergammaglobulinemia (particularly of the IgA class), and mildly elevated rheumatoid factor. **Thrombocytosis may be seen as an acute-phase reactant. In typical Wegener's granulomatosis with granulomatous vasculitis of the respiratory tract and glomerulonephritis, approximately 90% of patients have a positive c-ANCA. However, in the absence of renal disease, the sensitivity** drops to approximately 70%.
- The specificity of **a positive c-ANCA titer for Wegener's granulomatosis is** very high, especially if active glomerulonephritis is present. However, the presence of c-ANCA should be adjunctive and, with very rare exceptions, should not substitute for a tissue diagnosis. False-positive ANCA titers have been **reported in certain infectious and neoplastic diseases.**

Ans. 118: (b) Polyarteritis nodosa
Ref: Read the text below
Sol:

- The **vascular lesion in classic PAN is a necrotizing** inflammation of small and medium-sized muscular arteries.
- The lesions are segmental and **tend to involve bifurcations and branchings of arteries. They may spread circumferentially to involve adjacent veins.**
- **However, involvement of venules is not seen in classic PAN and, if present, suggests microscopic polyangiitis or the polyangiitis** overlap syndrome (see below).
- In the acute stages of disease, polymorphonuclear neutrophils infiltrate all layers of the vessel wall and perivascular areas, which results in intimal proliferation and degeneration of the vessel wall. Mononuclear cells **infiltrate the area as the lesions progress to the subacute and chronic stages.**
- **Fibrinoid necrosis of the vessels ensues with** compromise of the lumen, thrombosis, infarction of the tissues supplied by the involved vessel, and, in some cases, hemorrhage.
- As the lesions heal, there is collagen deposition, which may lead to further occlusion of the vessel lumen. **Positive ANCA titers (usually of the p-ANCA type) are found in a low percentage (<20%) of patients with classic PAN**.

Ans. 119: (c) Hyperparathyroidism
Ref: Read the text below
Sol:

1. Nutritional rickets presens with lowered or normal Serum Calcium.
2. Renal rickets presents with abnormal renal parameters.
3. Hyperparathyroidism fits in with the picture given.
4. Skeletal dysplasia may not have increased Serum Calcium.

The classification of Hyperparathyroidism and hypoparathyroidism merits recapulation

- Primary Hyperparathyroidism
  - Due to a disease of Parathyroid
    - o Ademoma of Parathyroid
    - o Carcinoma of Parathyroid
    - o Primary Chief Cell Hyperplasia of Parathyroid
- **Secondary Hyperparathyroidism**
  - Presents with Mild Hypocalcemia
  - Due to a disease elsewhere producing Hypocalcemia and the Parathyroid compensates
    - o Chronic Renal Insufficiency
    - o Vitamin D Deficiency
    - o Intestinal Malabsorption
- **Tertiary Hyperparathyroidism**
  - o Complication of Secondary Hyperparathyroidism
  - o Hyperfunction persists inspite of removal of the cause
    - o Probably a hyperplastic nodule has turned into adenoma
- **Primary Hypoparathyroidism**
  - Due to disease of Parathyroid
    - o Surgery
- Of Thyroid
- Radical neck Dissection
    - o Auto immune diseases
- **Pseudo Hypoparathyroidism**
  - Tissues fail to respond to Parathyroid hormone though Parathyroid may be normal
  - Inherited as Autosomal Dominant
  - Signs and symptoms of Hypoparathyroidism
    - o Short Stature
    - o Short Metacarpals and Metatarsals
    - o Flat Nose
    - o Round Face
    - o Multiple Exostoses
    - o Hypercalciuria
    - o Hypocalcemia
    - o Hyperphosphatemia

- Pseudo Pseudo Hypoparathyroidism
  - Probably an incomplete form of Pseudo Hypoparathyroidism.
  - Clinical features of Pseudo Hypoparathyroidism, but tissues respond normally.

Ans. 120: (a) Non-contrast computed tomography
Ref: Read the text below
Sol:

- **Intracranial hemorrhage** is often discovered on non contrast CT imaging of the brain during the acute evaluation of stroke.
- CT is more sensitive than routine MRI **for acute blood. The location of hemorrhage narrows the differential diagnosis to a few entities.**

Ans. 121: (b) Painful limp
Ref: Current diagnosis and treatment-orthopedics 4th edition—608-610
Sol:
Legg-Calve-Perthes Disease

- The clinical presentation of **LCP** in a child age **4-10 years** is usually a painless limp.
- **Physical examination** discloses atrophy of the thigh on the affected side and, usually, limited hip motion.
- The typical patient has a **flexion contracture of 0-30 degrees, loss of abduction compared with the opposite side** (in severe cases, no abduction beyond 0 degrees), and loss of internal rotation of the hip.

Ans. 122: (a) Infectious mononucleosis
Ref: Read the text below
Sol:

- **Infectious mononucleosis** - Causative agent is Epstein-Barr virus (DNA virus). Incubation period is 4-5 weeks.
- There is **fever, malaise, sore throat and loss of appetite. 1-2 weeks** later there is generalized lymphadenopathy with hepatomegaly.
- In most cases maculopapular **rash develops. There may be enanthems in** oral cavity.
- Splenomegaly is seen in more **than half of cases.**

Ans. 123: (c) Spinal Muscular atrophy
Ref: Read the text below
Sol:

- **Spinal Muscular atrophy** - cardinal features are severe hypotonia, generalised weakness absent DTR,thin muscle mass, involvement of tongue, face and jaw muscles.
- **Fasciculations are seen in tongue, deltoid, biceps**. There is sparing of extraocular muscles and sphincters.
- Heart is not involved. Intelligence is normal. **CPK is normal / mild increased. NCV is** normal. **EMG shows fibrillation potentials.**

Ans. 124: (d) 10%
Ref: Read the text below
Sol:

- **HBsAg positive mothers** may infect the fetus in the 3rd trimester or during early post partum period.
- Only 5-10% are **infected in utero, rest at the time of delivery**.
- Association of HBeAg in maternal blood is correlated with a high **transmission rate.**

Ans. 125: (c) MRI
Ref: Read the text below
Sol:
MRI is **currently** the **best** investigation for staging cervical and endometrial cancer and for anorectal sepsis.
Other salient features of MRI:

- Non-radiation.
- Excellent soft tissue contrast.

Ans. 126: (a) T1 weighted
Ref: Read the text below
Sol:

- T1 images **usually demonstrate exquisite anatomical** detail because of the high soft-tissue discrimination. Most pathological processes increase T2 relaxation times, producing a higher signal than the **surrounding normal tissue on T2 weighted scans.**
- **T2 weighted images have higher T repetition time and T echo time than T1 weighted images.**
- Intravenous **gadolinium acts as a contrast agent for MRI.**
- T1 reflects **the time taken to return to the axis of the original** field and T2 reflects the time the protons take to dephase.

Ans. 127: (a) Rickets
Ref: Yochum and Rowe's - Essentials of skeletal radiology 3-1515
Sol:
Radiological feature of rickets are:

- Generalized osteopenia.
- Coarse trabecular changes.
- Widened growth plates.
- Frayed and cupped paintbrush metaphysis.
- Absent zone of provisional calcification.
- Bowing deformities.
- Fractures.
- Decreased bony length.
- Scoliosis.
- Pseudo fractures.

Ans. 128: (a) Eosinophilic granuloma
Ref: Yochum and Rowe's - Essentials of skeletal radiology 3-1536.
Sol:

- **'Silver Dollar vertebra'** is the extreme **flattening of lumbar vertebral body with** preserved disc spaces and posterior arch structures.

- It is characteristic of **eosinophilic granuloma**.

Ans. 129: (a) Ilium
Ref: Yochum and Rowe's – Essentials of skeletal radiology 3-1437
Sol:

- Hemophiliac pseudo-tumors are **most common** in the ilium.
- 80% of the **bleeding occurs solely in the joints.**
- Knee is the most common side **of hemophiliac arthropathy. The** joint space is maintained until late in the disease.

Ans. 130: (a) Crown rump length
Ref: Read the text below
Sol:

- Estimation of **gestational age** by Crown rump length is **most precise** (variation ±5 days).

Ans. 131: (a) A
Ref: Read the text below
Sol:

- An **individual sarcomere, the** unit of contraction in striated muscle, spans the interval between **successive Z lines.**
- Each sarcomere **encompasses an A-band (choice B) and half of each of two I bands (choice D).**
- Each myofibril **(choice C) of a striated muscle fiber is composed of a tandem series of sarcomeres.**
- **Coupling of excitation and** contraction is a critical function of the triad, which is composed of a T tubule **interposed between two cisternae of the sarcoplasmic reticulum.**

Ans. 132: (a) Cardiac nodal cells
Ref: Read the text below
Sol:

- The action **potentials illustrated must be those of cardiac nodal cells (SA node or AV node).**
- **The duration of these action** potentials is too long for motor axons, (choice B), sensory neurons (**choice C), or skeletal muscle fibers (choice D).**
- Also, the configuration is different and a pacemaker potential is clearly present.
- They cannot be ventricular Purkinje action potentials because these have a more negative diastolic component that does not gradually depolarize, **a longer duration (200 msec) and a plateau region.**

Ans. 133: (d) D
Ref: Read the text below
Sol:

- The bicycle racer is likely **dehydrated from his exercise and ADH would be secreted by** the posterior pituitary in response to increased extracellular osmolality.
- The area of the nephron with the lowest **osmolality will be the early distal tubule (choice D), a nephrondiluting segment.**
- **The fluid in Bowman's capsule (choice A) will be at the same** osmolality as the plasma entering the glomerular capillaries.The fluid **at the end of the proximal tubule (choice B) is isoosmotic with the Bowman's capsule fluid while the fluid in the thin descending loop of Henle (choice C) is greatly concentrated due to** water reabsorption into the hyperosmotic medullary interstitium.
- The fluid at the end of the collecting duct **can be very concentrated or very dilute, but since ADH greatly increases water reabsorption in this segment, the fluid becomes very concentrated.**

Ans. 134: (d) dilation of Z
Ref: Read the text below
Sol:

- These choices **revolve around the Starling forces that directly regulate glomerular filtration.**
- **Choice D is correct and choice** C is incorrect because glomerular capillary pressure is regulated by **the ratio of upstream (afferent arteriole) and downstream (efferent arteriole) resistance to flow.**
- **Dilation of the afferent arteriole (choice C) will increase glomerular capillary pressure and increase filtration, whereas dilation of the efferent arteriole (choice D) will decrease the pressure and thus decrease** filtration.
- Choice A is incorrect because Bowman's space pressure normally acts to oppose filtration, hence a decreased pressure will increase filtration. Choice B is incorrect because the osmotic **pressure of the plasma proteins opposes filtration, so a decreased plasma protein concentration will predictably increase filtration.**
- **Choice E is incorrect, first** of all because the juxtaglomerular apparatus does not secrete aldosterone, but instead secretes renin, which **ultimately can trigger aldosterone secretion from the adrenal cortex via** angiotensin II.
- Secondly, **aldosterone is likely to trigger salt and water** retention by an action on the distal nephron of the kidney, which is **likely to alter the Starling forces in favor of increased glomerular filtration.**

Ans. 135: (d) HIV viral load set point 6 months after initial infection
Ref: Read the text below
Sol:

- **Rate of progression from initial HIV infection to AIDS** is likely determined by many factors, but viral load set point,

measured ~2–6 months after acute infection, is the most predictive factor.

- Most persons have a median time of 10 years, but rapid progressors with high viral loads can develop AIDS over 5 years whereas some "long-term nonprogressors" with low viral load set points can **be asymptomatic with HIV infection for decades.**
- CD4+ lymphocyte count is a measure of how close one is to developing AIDS rather than a measure of rate of progression: it tends to be close to normal once viral load set point is achieved.
- Resistance of the virus is more of a determinant of response to specific therapies than disease progression in the absence of **therapy. CMV serology is important as a predictor for CMV disease once a person reaches a CD4+ lymphocyte count < 50/uL.**

Ans. 136 : (d) Hepatorenal recess
Ref: Read the text below
Sol:

- The **omental (epiploic) foramen** connects the lesser sac with the hepatorenal (subhepatic) recess of the greater sac.
- The **hepatorenal recess** then communicates with the right subphrenic recess and right paracolic gutter.
- The **subhepatic recess** is perhaps the most frequently infected intra-abdominal space as a result of appendicitis, liver abscess, perforated duodenal and gastric ulcers, or **perforation of the biliary tree.**

Ans. 137 : (b) The transcription factor WT-1 is necessary for induction of the mesenchyme's competence
Ref: Read the text below
Sol:

The **kidney** develops from the **intermediate column of mesoderm**. There are three phases of kidney development; the definitive kidney **develops in the last phase:**

- **Stage 1**: Pronephros – primitive tubules.
- **Stage 2**: Mesonephros – functional in the embryo, producing a dilute urine that is important in maintaining the composition of the amniotic fluid; also contributes to the male genital system.
- **Stage 3:** metanephros – true, hind kidneys.

The transcription factor and tumour suppressor gene, WT-1, is expressed in metanephric blastema, making it competent to receive signals from the ureteric bud that are essential for its induction. Mutations in the gene are associated with a cancer of the kidney in children known as Wilms' tumour.

Ans. 138: (b) Two
Ref: Read the text below
Sol:

- **Multiple entrance wounds and multiple exit wou**nds maybe observed sometimes.
- A single soft nosed bullet hitting a victim after ricochet can produce a number of entrance wounds.
- **Tandem cartridge** if used could result in multiple entrance wounds in a single fire.
- If the first bullet fails to leave the barrel and is ejected by the subsequent fired bullets,**the bullets are ejected one before the other and are called as tandem bullets.**

Ans. 139: (a) Common peroneal nerve
Ref: Read the text below
Sol:

- The **common peroneal nerve consists of branches of L4–S1.**
- Its **motor supply** is to the anterior compartment of the calf including tibialis anterior and extensor hallucis longus.
- The **sensory component** supplies the 1st web space and the dorsum of the foot and front side of the leg.
- This nerve winds around the head of the tibia and in certain tibial plateau fractures its **integrity may become compromised.**

Ans. 140: (d) Malignancy
Ref: Read the text below
Sol:

- **Malignant neoplasm** is the most common systemic disease affecting the spine, 80% of which occurs in **patients 50 years of age or** older.

Ans. 141: (a) Urinary retention
Ref: Read the text below
Sol:

- **Urinary retention** with overflow incontinence is the **most common symptom of cauda** equina syndrome, with a sensitivity of 90% and a specificity of about 95%.

Ans. 142: (c) Dermatitis herpetiformis
Ref: Read the text below
Sol:

- **Dermatitis herpetiformis forms crops of itchy blisters that are commonly found on elbows, knees and scalp.**
- **Dermatitis herpetiformis** is associated with coeliac disease and as the risk of lymphoma is greatly increased by having both conditions, regular surveillance is recommended.
- **Psoriasis** does commonly affect the elbows but usually does not present with itch and eczema may present in such sites and with pruritus but is not strongly associated with coeliac disease.
- **Scabies should always** be kept in mind when considering itch, usually in children in the web spaces of the hands and feet. Track marks from the burrowing Sarcoptes scabiei mite can often

be **seen and harvested for microscopic diagnosis.**

Ans. 143:(d) An infraorbital block can be performed by injecting 3 cc of lidocaine near the infraorbital foramen
Ref: Read the text below
Sol:

- An **infraorbital block** may be performed by either an intraoral or extraoral route. The duration of **anesthesia appears to be longer by an intraoral route**.
- The region of anesthesia includes **the ipsilateral cheek, lower eyelid, upper lip, and lateral aspect of the nose**. Infraorbital nerve block should be performed without epinephrine because of the **proximity of the facial artery.**
- It is recommended to limit **infiltration to 2-3 cc of local anesthetic**. A mental nerve block supplies anesthesia to the lower lip and chin and will not provide anesthesia to the area of concern.
- The mental nerve can be anesthetized by an intraoral or extraoral route. Lidocaine with epinephrine is acceptable; however**, the recommended volume should be limited to 1-2 cc.**

Ans. 144: (d) Unilateral longitudinal incision
Ref: Read the text below
Sol:

- The **unilateral longitudinal incision**, distal to the distal interphalangeal crease, is most commonly used **and spares the sensate volar pad**.

Ans. 145:(c) An outward potassium current
Ref: Read the text below
Sol:

- **Voltage-gated potassium channels** open with a delay relative to voltage-gated sodium channels in response to depolarization.
- **Concomitantly,there is a delay** in their closing relative to the sodium channels. During the **afterhyperpolarization phase of the action potential**, the sodium channels are closed, but the potassium channels remain open.
- Because **there is a strong driving force for K^+ to leave the cell**, the cell hyperpolarizes.
- An outward calcium current, an outward sodium current, or an inward chloride current could conceivably hyperpolarize the **cell, but these currents are not the basis for this phase of the action potential.**

Ans. 146 :(d) Voltage-gated sodium channels are concentrated at the nodes of Ranvier
Ref: Read the text below
Sol:

- A **specialization occurs in myelinated axons** in which the voltage-gated sodium channels are preferentially distributed to the **axonal membrane beneath the nodes of Ranvier.**
- Since these channels are required for the generation of an action potential, the action potential **jumps from node to node.**
- This **process is facilitated by an increased membrane** resistance and a decreased capacitance associated with **the myelinated regions of the axon**, both of which promote the electrotonic spread of the positive charge that accumulates beneath one node of Ranvier at the peak of the action potential.
- **Nongated ion channels are not involved in the generation of action potential.**

Ans. 147: (c) Fentanyl 100 mcg intravenously
Ref: Read the text below
Sol:

- **Fentanyl is a potent opioid** with approximately 100 times the potency of morphine but with a shorter half-life and lack of histamine release.It is uncommonly associated with hypotension. **This patient's injury demands attention to the airway, breathing, circulation, and pain.**
- **Meperidine is a synthetic opioid** with multiple side effects including histamine release. Histamine release has been associated with hypotension as it does cause vasodilation. **The assessment of this patient can be confounded by the hyperexcitability associated with meperidine administration.**
- Morphine is a well-known drug, and many clinicians feel comfortable with administering it in various situations. **Morphine is associated with histamine release.**
- **This patient's history of asthma and current hypotension coupled with the high dose could potentially be harmful in this individual. Propofol is an anesthetic agent that is currently being evaluated in the emergency setting.**
- Its role in procedural sedation is still being defined. However, propofol has significant cardiovascular depressive **effects, which should be avoided in this patient**.

Ans. 148: (b) Curve B
Ref: Read the text below
Sol:

- **Increased carbon dioxide shifts the oxygen-dissociation curve** to the right, leading to an increase in oxygen unloading.
- **Curve B** is the only option that depicts this right-shift while maintaining the shape of the curve.

Other factors you should know that can shift the curve to the right include higher temperature, **increased 2,3-BPG, and lower pH.**

Ans. 149: (d) Fetal blood PH
Ref: Read the text below
Sol:
Fetal biophysical profile considers several parameters, which includes:
- Non Stress test.
- Fetal breathing movements.
- Gross body movements.
- Fetal muscle tone.
- Amniotic fluid volume.

Ans. 150: (c) Olanzapine
Ref: Read the text below
Sol:
- **Carbamazepine**, **lithium**, and **valproic acid** are effective in bipolar disorder but are contraindicated in the **pregnant patient** because of possible effects on fetal development.
- Unlike **olanzapine, chlorpromazine** has no proven efficacy in **bipolar disorder**.

Ans. 151: (c) As a topical gel for ulcers
Ref: Read the text below
Sol:
- **Becaplermin (Regranex)** is a platelet derived growth factor **(rhPDGF)**. It is a topically aplicable gel used particularly for big **non-healing diabetic ulcers**.
- The dosage required is **proportional to the size of the ulcers.**
- It is particularly help in **treating lower limb** ulcers **refractory** to common treatment.

Ans. 152: (b) Diclofenac
Ref: Read the text below
Sol:
- The potency of **diclofenac against COX-2** is substantially higher than other **NSAIDs** and resembles that of **celecoxib**.

Ans. 153: (b) Elevation of the seizure threshold
Ref: Read the text below.
Sol:
- **Tricyclics** modify peripheral sympathetic effects in **2 ways** : through blockade of **NE reuptake** at neuroeffector junctions and through a-**adrenoceptor blockade**.
- **Sedation** and **atropine-like** side effects are common with tricyclics.
- In contrast to sedative-hypnotics, **tricyclics lower the threshold to seizures**.

Ans. 154: (c) Thrombocytopenia
Ref: Read the text below
Sol:
- **Oprelvekin** is approved for use in patients undergoing chemotherapy for **nonmyeloid malignancies** that displayed severe **thrombocytopenia (platelet count <20000 /ml)** on a prior cycle of the same chemotherapy and is administered until the platelet count returns to more than **100,000/ml.**

Ans. 155: (d) Increased force of contraction of the ventricles
Ref: Read the text below
Sol:
- **Sympathetic stimulation of the heart normally causes** an increased heart rate, increased rate of conduction of the **cardiac impulse, and increased force of contraction in the atria and ventricles.**
- However, it **does not cause acetylcholine release at the sympathetic endings, because they contain norepinephrine**.
- Parasympathetic **stimulation causes acetylcholine release.**
- The sympathetic nervous system firing increases the **permeability of the cardiac muscle fibers, the sinoatrial node, and the atrio-ventricular node** to sodium and calcium.

Ans. 156: (c) Extracellular fluid volume
Ref: Read the text below
Sol:
- An increase in renal arterial **pressure results in pressure natriuresis and diuresis.**
- The loss of sodium and water tends to **decrease extracellular fluid volume.**
- Glomerular filtration rate would be normal or slightly **increased in response to an increase in renal artery pressure.**

Ans. 157: (b) Usually hypotonic compared with plasma
Ref: Read the text below
Sol
- As **water flows up the ascending limb of the loop of Henle,** solutes are reabsored, but this segment is relatively impermeable to water; progressive dilution of the tubular fluid occurs so that the osmolarity decreases to **approximately 100 mOsm/L by the time the fluid reaches the early distal tubule.**
- Even during maximal antidiuresis, this **portion of the renal tubule is relatively impermeable to water and is therefore called the diluting segment of the renal tubule**.

Ans. 158: (d) Less than 10 percent
Ref: Read the text below
Sol:
- **Although aldosterone is one of the body's most potent sodium**-retaining hormones, it stimulates sodium reabsorption only in the late **distal tubule and collecting tubules, which** together reabsorb much less than 10 percent of the filtered load of sodium.
- Therefore, the maximum percentage of the filtered load of sodium **that could be reabsorbed in the distal convoluted tubule and collecting duct, even in** the presence of high levels of aldosterone, would be less than 10 percent.

Ans. 159: (b) Bradykinin
Ref: Read the text below
Sol:

- There are several **factors that can cause and initiate pain**. These include histamine, bradykinin and prostaglandins.
- Platelet-activating factor **activates platelets during the clotting process.**
- Interleukin and tumor necrosis factor are involved in the **inframmatory response and control of macrophages.**

Ans. 160: (d) Type O-positive packed red cells
Ref: Read the text below
Sol:

- In any patient, **transfusion of type O paked cells would minimize** the chance of a transfusion reaction because the antibodies **are removed along with the plasma.**
- If the Rh **factor is matched, this would also minimize the possibility of** a transfusion reaction.
- Therefore, in a B-positive patient, an O-**positive transfusion (as well as a B-positive transfusion) would elicit no transfusion reaction.**

Ans. 161: (d) Type Ad pain fibers are responsible for the localization of a pain stimulus
Ref: Rebd the text below
Sol:

- **Type Ad fibers, not type C fibers, are are responsible for the localization.**

Ans. 162: (c) 3, 1, 2
Ref: Read the text below
Sol:

- **The Brodmann number designation for the primary somatosensory cortex 3, 1, 2.**

Ans. 163: (b) Glycine - inhibition
Ref: Read the text below
Sol:

- Glycine **typically evokes inhibitory responses.**
- Norepinephrine is associated with **the locus ceruleus, and serotonin with the raphe nuclei.**

Ans. 164: (b) Photochemicals in both rods and cones are reduced to retinal and opsins
Ref: Read the text below
Sol:

- The reduction of **rhodopsin and cone pigments by light decreases the concentrations** of photosensitive chemicals in rods and cones.
- Thus, the sensitivity of **the eye to light is correspondingly reduced.**
- **This is called light adaptation.**

Ans. 165: (d) Cataract
Ref: Read the text below
Sol:
Here the important points are:

- Age: 40 years, not senile enough for cataract history of diabetes, which causes early cataract.
- Glare at night: associated with **posterior subcapsular** cataract which is common in diabetic. They have classically snow flake cataracts father had similar complains : its just to confuse the students. He also had cataract, big deal!
- This particular question is not simple and can framed in at least 10 different manners and the ans will be different if certain parameters are changed or added.

Ans. 166: (d) Short wave automated perimetry
Ref: Read the text below
Sol:

- **Short wave automated perimetry detects** damage to parvocellular cells (P-cells). P-cells are the earliest to be damaged in glaucoma.
- The test is done **with blue stimulus on yellow background.**

Ans. 167: (a) Decrease in IOP
Ref: Read the text below
Sol:

- Posner-schlossmann syndrome is characterised by trabeculitis, uveitis, increased Intraocular pressure.
- **Males** affected more than females.
- Also called **hypertensive uveitis.**
- Treatment is: topical steroids.

Ans. 168: (a) Cigarette smoking
Ref: Read the text below
Sol:

- The angiogram presented in the **question demonstrates an isolated** segment of atherosclerotic occlusion of **the superficial femoral artery.**
- Patients who have **isolated femoropopliteal disease tend to be** smokers, whereas those who have isolated tibioperoneal **disease frequently are diabetic.**
- Hypertension and hyperlipidemia predispose **to accelerated atherosclerosis.**
- On the other hand, type I hyperlipoproteinemia (hyperchylomicronemia), which is associated with dramatic levels of plasma triglyceride and **formation of xanthomas, does not cause accelerated vascular disease.**

Ans. 169: (d) Cor pulmonale
Ref: Read the text below
Sol:

- **Cor pulmonale is characterized by the presence** of pulmonary hypertension and consequent right ventricular dysfunction.
- Its causes include diseases leading to hypoxic vasoconstriction, as in cystic fibrosis; occlusion

of the pulmonary vasculature, as in pulmonary thromboembolism; and parenchymal destruction**, as in sarcoidosis.**

- **In the presence of a chronic increase in afterload**, the right ventricle becomes hypertrophic, dilates, and fails.
- The electrocardiographic findings, as illustrated in the question, include tall, peaked P waves in leads II, III, and a VF, **which indicate right atrial enlargement; tall R waves in leads V1 to V3 and a deep S wave in V6 with associated ST-T wave changes,which indicate right ventricular hypertrophy; and right axis deviation.**
- **Right bundle branch block occurs in 15%** of patients.

Ans. 170: (a) 1-c; 2-h; 3-b
Ref: Read the text below
Sol:

- Oral **leukoplakia** is a white, macular **lesion found in the buccal mucosa. Predisposing** factors include tobacco use, alcohol use, human papillomavirus, **and syphilis. It may lead to squamous cell carcinoma.**
- **Actinic** (**solar**) **keratoses** are dry, rough, adherent, scaly lesions occurring in sun-exposed areas of adults. These lesions are premalignant **and may develop into squamous cell carcinoma. Bowen's disease or squamous cell carcinoma in** situ is a solitary, well-demarcated plaque. When Bowen's disease occurs on the glans penis, it is called **erythroplasia of Queyrat.**
- Bowen's disease and erythroplasia of Queyrat may both lead to a fungating and ulcerating squamous cell carcinoma. **Seborrheic keratosis** is the most common benign epithelial tumor. **Basal cell carcinoma** (BCC) is the most common type of skin cancer. It is invasive and aggressive but rarely metastasizes.
- These lesions are usually round, firm, glistening (pearly), and shiny. Histologically, basal cell carcinomas have **palisading nuclei.** Superficial spreading **melanomas** (SSMs) have five cardinal features: **A**symmetry, **B**order that is irregular, **C**olor that is mottled and haphazard, **D**iameter that is large, and **E**nlargement/**E**levation (**ABCDE**).

Ans. 171: (d) 1-a,b,c,d; 2-e,f; 3-g,h
Ref: Read the text below
Sol:

- The area between **the pleural sacs—the mediastinum—**is divided anatomically into the anterior mediastinum, middle **mediastinum, and posterior mediastinum.**
- The most common masses found in the **anterior mediastinum** are the **four Ts** **T**hymomas, **T**eratomas, **T**hyroid masses, and para**T**hyroid masses. Lymphomas may also be found in the anterior mediastinum.
- Masses in the **middle mediastinum** include enlarged **lymph nodes, lymphomas, vascular masses, pleuropericardial cysts, and bronchogenic cysts.**
- The **posterior mediastinum** is the likely area for neurogenic tumors, lymphomas, pheochromocytomas, myelomas, meningoceles, **meningomyeloceles, gastroenteric cysts, and diverticula**

Ans. 172: (d) 1-i; 2-a; 3-c; 4-e; 5-h
Ref: Read the text below.
Sol:

- Patients with **AIDS are at risk for numerous CNS infections, but** have an increased frequency of only two tumor types: **lymphoma and Kaposi's sarcoma.**
- **KS may metastasize to the CNS, but lymphoma is routinely primary to the CNS. This** tumor may produce blindness through direct invasion of the optic nerve. Medulloblastomas are one of the most common CNS tumors of childhood. They typically develop in the cerebellum, causing ataxia.
- Astrocytomas may also occur in children infratentorially**, primarily in the cerebellum and brainstem. In either location, hydrocephalus may develop because of obstruction at the level of the fourth ventricle. The astrocytoma that develops in** the cerebellum is usually cystic. Medulloblastomas are invariably infratentorial, at least initially.
- They may extend supratentorially or become disseminated supratentorially through seeding of cells carried in the CSF. Ependymomas, **another common tumor type in children, are derived from the lining of the ventricles and also carry the risk of hydrocephalus and seeding throughout the CNS.**
- **The neurofibromatoses are a pair of hereditary** neurocutaneous syndromes that result in a variety of congenital and later-occurring abnormalities and neoplasms affecting the skin, nervous system, and other **organs. Neurofibromatosis (NF) type 1, also called peripheral NF, is characterized by café au lait spots, which are light to dark brown spots found on the skin; multiple cutaneous and subcutaneous tumors; bone cysts; sphenoid bone dysgenesis; precocious puberty; pheochromoc**ytoma; syringomyelia; glial nodules; cortical dysgenesis; and macrocephaly. Optic nerve tumors are a particularly worrisome complication, and may produce blindness **in children.**
- **Schwannomas usually develop on the vestibular division of cranial nerve VIII and are pathologically derived from Schwann cells rather** than nerve tissue, and

are therefore more appropriately called vestibular schwannomas than acoustic neuromas, the traditional name. Although this is not the **division of the nerve that carries information from the cochlea, the cochlear division is crushed as the tumor expands.**

- **This type of tumor is especially likely with neurofibromatosis** type 2, a hereditary disorder characterized by a variety of tumors in the skin and nervous system. Pineocytomas are histologically benign lesions affecting the region of the pineal gland. They arise from the parenchymal cells of the pineal gland.
- This **patient's symptoms and signs constitute Parinaud syndrome, which may include loss of vertical gaze, loss of pupillary light reflex, lid retraction, and convergenceretraction nystagmus**, in which the eyes appear to jerk back into the orbit on attempted upgaze. This syndrome occurs in lesions due to involvement of the dorsal midbrain in the region of the superior colliculus.
- Other tumors appearing in the pineal region that can produce a **similar clinical picture include germ cell tumors (germinomas), teratomas, and gliomas. Malignant** pineal tumors, or pineoblastomas, may also occur, and are similar histologically to medulloblastomas.

Ans. 173: (c) 1-a; 2-g; 3-e
Ref: Read the text below
Sol:

- The patient has a **left colon cancer. In order to resect the tumor with a margin** of 3-5 cm on its proximal and distal ends as well as to remove the **draining lymph node basin, a left hemicolectomy should be performed.**
- A Dukes C tumor is one that extends through the bowel wall and involves adjacent lymph nodes. In a study of 1166 patients with stage B and C colon cancer, the National Surgical Adjuvant Breast and Bowel Project (NSABP) **reported an improved survival in patients randomized to receive adjuvant chemotherapy compared with no further treatment after resection.**
- Adjuvant radiation therapy has only been useful in preventing local recurrence in rectal cancers with positive surgical margins. The **liver is the most common site of bloodborne metastases from primary colorectal cancers.**
- **In a subgroup of patients, the liver may be the only** site of disease. Overall, surgical resection is associated with a 25–30% 5-year survival rate.

Ans. 174: (b) Chronic blood loss
Ref: Read the text below
Sol:

- The **lab values for hemotocrit and hemoglobin** indicate that this women has anemia. Her MCV value of 70 is **consistent with a microcytic anemia. The most common microcytic anemia is iron deficiency anemia.**
- **Chronic blood loss through the GI tract is the most common cause of iron deficiency** anemia in men and post menopausal women. An acquired hemolytic anemia likely would present with additional symptoms on physical exam, including signs of jaundice, dark urine upon standing and splenomegaly.
- Also, the **history does not suggest a cause for hemolysis**. Beta-thalassmia minor is a mild microcytic anemia. In the majority of cases, Beta-thalassemia minor is asymptomatic, and many affected people are unaware of the disorder.
- **This is an inherited anemia that would not present late in life with increasing shortness of breath. Folic acid deficiency and pernicious anemia** leading to Vitamin B_{12} deficiency are both types of macrocytic and megaloblastic anemia.
- The **MCV value** would be elevated above 96 micrometer^3 and these types of anemia are less common than iron deficiency anemia.

Ans. 175: (a) All require emergent intervention
Ref: Read the text below
Sol:

- **Lunate and perilunate** dislocations generally result from forced dorsiflexion and impact on the outstretched hand.
- These injuries generally require a significant amount of force to disrupt the intrinsic and extrinsic ligaments of the midcarpal region. The amount of force needed to produce these injuries **frequently results in associated fractures of the carpal bones in an arc around the lunate. Clinically, the patients have a significant amount of swelling but may lack an obvious gross deformity.**
- **Radiographs reveal a disruption in the linear arrangement** of the distal radius, the lunate, and the capitate. If the lunate bone retains contact with the radius on radiographs, the injury is classified as a perilunate dislocation. If the lunate is completely displaced off the radius and no longer articulates with the capitate as well, the injury is termed a lunate dislocation.
- **All patients with these injuries require emergency orthopedic consultation**. Open reduction and internal fixation are required for unstable, open, or irreducible injuries. Closed reduction and long arm splint immobilization may be appropriate if the injury is reducible, but some orthopedists prefer to operate on all perilunate and lunate dislocations.
- **Because the lunate is dislocated in a volar direction into** the carpal tunnel, median nerve

compression is sometimes an associated complication of these injuries. Early degenerative arthritis, malunion, nonunion, **and avascular necrosis are also possible complications if associated carpal fractures have occurred.**

Ans. 176: (b) Retinal detachment
Ref: Read the text below
Sol:
Sudden painless **loss of vision**
Cataract surgery 2 years back
IOP = 10 mm Hg

- History of **RD in other eye.**
- This history is **enough to diagnose retinal detachment.**
- History of diabetes is to confuse u guys, such questions are to be expected in AIIMS and PGI exams. They are not difficult but require a better **understanding of subject and thoughtful reasoning.**
- **Predisposing factors to RD are mainly 3:**
- **Trauma, myopia and post surgery** commonly cataract surgery.
- **IOP is commonly low in RD** due to mismatch between aqueous production and drainage.
- **Sympathetic Ophthalmia** occurs in eye after trauma to other eye. It's a hypersensitivity due to antibody production against uveal tissue Ag.
- History of RD in one eye increases the chances of RD in other eye by 30% this is very imp history to be noted.
- **Diabetes: Who said diabetics** cant have RD!
- Vitreous hmm and macular edema cant **be ruled out in this case but the ans is quite clear here with other components of history.**

Ans. 177: (b) Progressive
Ref: Read the text below
Sol:

- It's a non-**progressive disorder. Its commonly unilateral**. Anterior surface is normal.
- Vision is minimally affected **since the main refractive component is anterior surface of cornea.**
- Lens is normal.
- Compare **with anterior keratoconus, which is progressive in nature.**

Ans. 178: (a) Both A and R are true and R is correct explanation of A
Ref: Read the text below
Sol:
Hyperacute rejection

- Occurs within minutes to hours (due to preformed antibodies).
- **Morphology:** Rejected kidney becomes cyanotic, mottled and flaccid. May excrete a few drops of bloody urine.
- **Microscopy:** Endothelial injury with fibrin platelet thrombi. Neutrophilic infiltrate in arteriole, glomeruli, capillaries. Fibrinoid necrosis in arterial wall and a/c cortical necrosis.

Ans. 179: (c) A is true but R is false
Ref: Read the text below
Sol:

- A large right mass developing in a 60 year old postmenopausal woman, **must be considered a n ovarian malignancy unless proven otherwise.**
- **This is not only the diagnosis to be excluded, but also the most likely diagnosis.** Endometrial **carcinoma usually presents with postmenopausal** bleeding but usually does not have a adnexal mass, although the uterus may itself be enlarged.
- Follicular cyst are very rare after the menopause, a benign ovarian tumor is less common at this age and a degeneration fibroid **would be unusual, especially as the pelvic examination was normal 3 years previously.**

Ans. 180: (b) Both A and R are true and R is not correct explanation of A
Ref: Read the text below
Sol:

- **Microtubules are made up of two** globular protein subunits; α and β-tubulin.The α and β subunits form heterodimers, **which aggregate to form long tubes made** up of stacked rings, with each ring usually **containing 13 subunits.**
- Because of their constant assembly and disassembly**, microtubules are a dynamic portion of the cell skeleton.**
- Microtubule assembly is prevented by **colchicines and vinblastine. The anticancer** drug paclitaxel (Taxol) binds to microtubules and makes them so stable **that organelles cannot move. Mitotizc spindles cannot form and the cell dies.**

QUESTIONS

1. **Most common type of tracheoesophageal fistula likely results from:**
   a. Failure of the buccopharyngeal membrane to rupture.
   b. Failure of the tracheoesophageal ridges to fuse
   c. Incomplete formation of the septum secundum
   d. Incomplete recanalization of the larynx

2. **A woman comes to the physician for a prenatal visit. Examination reveals that her uterus is considerably larger than her gestational age would predict. An ultrasound examination is ordered and reveals that she has polyhydramnios. Which of the following congenital defects of the fetus would be most likely to be associated with this abnormality?**
   a. Atrial septal defect b. Esophageal atresia
   c. Lung hypoplasia d. Meckel diverticulum

3. **A 22-year-old patient is unable to unlock the knee joint to permit flexion of the leg. Which of the following muscles is most likely damaged?**
   a. Rectus femoris b. Semimembranosus
   c. Popliteus d. Gastrocnemius

4. **This variation is a result of abnormal development of which of the following structures?**
   a. Allantoic duct b. Metanephric duct
   c. Mesonephric tubules d. Ureteric bud

5. **Posterior glenohumeral instability is diagnosed by:**
   a. Crank test b. Fulcrum
   c. Jerk test d. Sulcus

6. **A 27-year-old pianist with a known carpal tunnel syndrome experiences difficulty in finger movements. Which of the following intrinsic muscles of her hand is paralyzed?**
   a. Palmar interossei and adductor pollicis
   b. Dorsal interossei and lateral two lumbricals
   c. Lateral two lumbricals and opponens pollicis
   d. Abductor pollicis brevis and palmar interossei

7. **A 23-year-old woman who receives a deep cut to her ring finger by a kitchen knife is unable to move the metacarpophalangeal joint. Which of the following pairs of nerves was damaged?**
   a. Median and ulnar
   b. Radial and median
   c. Musculocutaneous and ulnar
   d. Ulnar and radial

8. **A newborn baby is observed to be cyanotic immediately after birth. Diagnostic studies, including an ultrasound reveal that the baby has persistent truncus arteriosus. Which of the following additional defects is this baby most likely to have?**
   a. Dextrocardia
   b. Membranous ventricular septal defect
   c. Secundum-type atrial septal defect
   d. Tetralogy of Fallot

9. **Occlusion of the anterior descending branch of left coronary artery will lead to infarction of which area?**
   a. Anterior wall of left ventricle
   b. Posterior part of the interventricular septum
   c. Lateral part of the heart
   d. Inferior surface of the right ventricle

10. **On examination following surgical removal of a firm nodular cancer swelling in the right breast and exploration of the right axilla, a patient is found to have a winged scapula. This occurred due to injury to the:**
   a. Subscapular muscle
   b. Coracoid process of scapula
   c. Long thoracic nerve
   d. Circumflex scapular artery

11. **A 47-year-old woman develops accelerated hypertension (blood pressure 210/105 mm Hg) but no clinical symptoms except frequent headaches. Which of the following findings are most likely?**

On examination of the fundii (See Fig.)

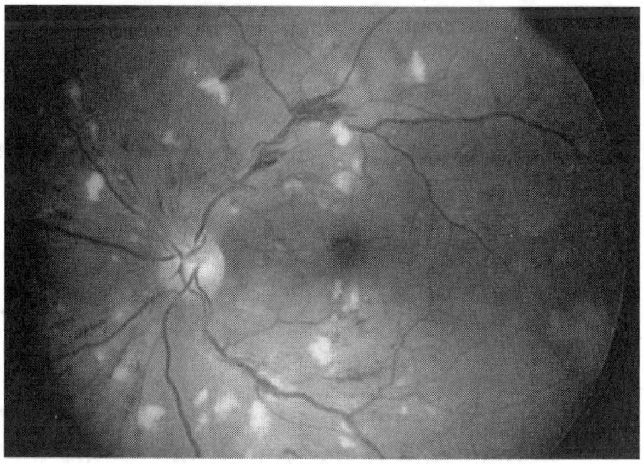

a. Retinitis obliterans
b. Cotton-wool spots
c. Retinal detachment
d. Optic atrophy

12. Fundus of the stomach is supplied by:
a. Left gastric artery
b. Right gastric artery
c. Short gastric artery
d. Right gastro-epiploic artery

13. Injury to the lower division of facial nerve during surgery will most likely result in:
a. Inability to furrow the brow (to frown) on the same side
b. Numbness over the angle and mental region of the jaw on the same side
c. Weakness in losing the eye on the same side
d. Weakness of the lower lip on the same side

14. The porto-systemic anastomoses involve the following veins of the portal group *except*:
a. Inferior rectal veins
b. Left gastric vein
c. Superior rectal vein
d. Paraumbilical veins

15. Coeliac plexus is present:
a. Anterior lateral and around the aorta
b. Posterior medial and around the aorta
c. Anterior medial to lumbar symp chain
d. Posterior lateral to lumbar symp chain

16. About prostatic urethra all are true *except*:
a. Trapezoid in cross section
b. Verumomentum is present in posterior wall
c. Opening of prostatic ducts lies in posterior wall
d. Relation of urethral crest in posterior wall

17. Middle superior alveolar nerve is a branch of :
a. Palatine branch of maxillary
b. Nasal branch of maxillary
c. Infraorbital nerve
d. Mandibular nerve

18. After an amniocentesis, a 29-year-old woman who is carrying twins learns that one fetus has XY chromosomes and the other has XX chromosomes. At 37 weeks' gestation, the woman deliver two healthy babies. Which of the following structures is likely to be present in the baby with the XY chromosomes but not in the one with XX chromosomes?
a. Bulbospongiosus muscle
b. Bulbourethral gland
c. Corpus cavernosum
d. Membranous urethra

19. A 32-year-old man complains of progressive, severe, generalized headaches that began 3 months ago, are worse in the mornings, and lately have been accompanied by projectile vomiting. He has also lost his upper gaze, and on physical examination the upper part of the sclera is visible above the downward looking, irises. Which of the following is the most likely diagnosis?
a. Nelson syndrome
b. Pituitary apoplexy
c. Posterior fossa tumor
d. Tumor in the area of the pineal gland

20. A patient with external haemorrhoids develops pain while passing stools. Nerve mediating this pain is:
a. Hypogastric nerve
b. Pudendal nerve
c. Splanchnic visceral nerve
d. Sympathetic plexus

21. Each of the following statements about Romano-Ward syndrome is true, *except*:
a. It is a heterogeneous disorder involving mutations in different ion channels
b. It is inherited as an autosomal recessive disorder
c. It is associated with sudden cardiac death in young patients
d. It is not associated with congenital deafness

22. **All of the following features are seen in neurons from dorsal root ganglia, *except*:**
   a. They have centrally located nuclei
   b. They are derived from neural crest cells
   c. They are multipolar
   d. They contain lipofuscin granules

23. **Hyponatremia has no effect on the resting membrane potential because:**
   a. The cell membrane is impermeable to Na+
   b. ECF Na+ concentration is high
   c. Intracellular K+ concentration is high
   d. Equilibrium potential for Na+ is + 60 mV

24. **The FRC is defined as the combination of:**
   a. Tidal volume and residual volume
   b. Tidal volume and expiratory reserve volume
   c. Inspiratory reserve volume and tidal volume
   d. Residual volume and expiratory reserve volume

25. **Parietal cells in the stomach secrete a protein crucial for the absorption of vitamin B_{12} by the ileum. What is this protein?**
   a. Intrinsic factor
   b. Gastrin
   c. Somatostatin
   d. Cholecystokinin (CCK)

26. **Gastric acid secretion is stimulated during several phases associated with the ingestion and digestion of a meal. Which phase is associated with the bulk of acid secretion?**
   a. Cephalic
   b. Esophageal
   c. Gastric
   d. Intestinal

27. **Which of the following would not favor the unloading of oxygen from hemoglobin in tissues?**
   a. Increase in P50
   b. Increase in tissue pH
   c. Increase in 2,3-DPG levels
   d. Increase in tissue PCO_2

28. **Hypoxemia is dependent on all *except*:**
   a. PcO_2 b. FiO_2
   c. Hb level d. Altitude

29. **Active transport occurs in:**
   a. Movement of sodium ions across the cell membrane
   b. Glucose absorption from the gut
   c. Potassium excretion in the distal convoluted tubule
   d. All of the above

30. **In the Wallerian degeneration of a peripheral nerve:**
   a. The axons regenerate at 1 cm/day
   b. Occurs in distal portion of the broken axons leaving empty tubule
   c. Is a feature of neuropraxia
   d. All of the above

31. **The metabolic function of parathormone includes all these *except*:**
   a. Mobilizes calcium from bone
   b. Decreases renal tubular reabsorption of calcium
   c. Promotes renal production of 1,25 hydroxy cholecalciferol
   d. Lowers serum phosphate level

32. **A patient with untreated diabetes mellitus is admitted to the hospital for treatment. Laboratory findings include a blood pH below 7.2. Which of the following is likely to directly result from this level of acidemia?**
   a. Arteriolar constriction
   b. Decreased catabolism
   c. Hyperkalemia
   d. Hypoventilation

33. **The change of which of the following substances is most commonly monitored as indicator for the efficiency of blood glucose control?**
   a. Hemoglobin A1c (HbA1c)
   b. Lipoprotein
   c. Modified albumin
   d. Myoinositol

34. **Vasopressin receptor wrong pair:**
   a. V1 - vascular receptor

b. V2 - distal nephron

c. V3 - pituitary

d. V4 - CNS

35. Which one of the following statements about aldosterone is correct?

a. It produces its effect by activating cAMP

b. It produces its effect by increasing distal tubular permeability to sodium

c. It causes an increased reabsorption of hydrogen ion

d. It has its main effect on the proximal tubule

36. The syndrome of inappropriate antidiuretic hormone secretion (SIADH) is caused by the excess release of ADH. SIADH will cause an increase in:

a. Concentration of plasma sodium

b. Intracellular volume

c. Urinary flow

d. Plasma oncotic pressure

37. A saccular aneurysm in the abdominal aorta is more likely to rupture than one in the normal aorta because:

a. More tension is exerted on the wall of the aneurysm

b. There is less pressure in the aneurysm

c. There is less turbulence in the aneurysm

d. There is more tension exerted on and less turbulence in the aneurysm

38. Hartnup's disease is an inherited autosomal recessive disorder involving the malabsorption of amino acids, particularly tryptophan, by the small intestine. Feeding dipeptides and tripeptides containing tryptophan to patients with this disease improves their clinical condition because:

a. Dipeptides and tripeptides, unlike free amino acids, can be taken up passively by enterocytes in the small intestine

b. Peptides, unlike free amino acids, can be taken up by defective amino acid transporters

c. Dipeptides and tripeptides use transporters that are different from the defective amino acid transporters

d. The presence of dipeptides and tripeptides in the intestinal lumen enhances the uptake of amino acids by the transporters

39. In dislocation of the jaw, displacement of the articular disk beyond the articular tubercle of the temporomandibular joint results from spasm or excessive contraction of which of the following muscles:

a. Buccinator

b. Lateral pterygoid

c. Medial pterygoid

d. Masseter

40. Calcium enters the cardiac cell during:

a. Rapid upstroke of the action potential

b. Down slope of the action potential

c. Plateau phase of the action potential

d. Slow diastolic depolarization (phase 4) of the action potential

41. Which of the following statements about diffuse esophageal spasm is true?

a. Chest pain due to esophageal spasm is readily differentiated from angina pectoris of cardiac origin

b. Bouts of esophageal obstruction and regurgitation of food are characteristic

c. During manometric assessment, unless the patient is having pain there may be no detectable multiphasic, high-amplitude, simultaneous esophageal contractions

d. The treatment of choice is a long esophagomyotomy from the aortic arch to the esophagogastric junction

42. Refsum's disease is a rare neurological disorder caused by:

a. Accumulation of glutamic acid

b. Accumulation of glycine

c. Accumulation or phytanic acid

d. Accumulation of phenylalanine

43. Which one of the following pairs of lipids and related compounds exhibit opposite biological activities?

a. 5-HPETE and leukotriene D4

b. Cholic acid and lithocholic acid

c. Thromboxane A2 and prostocyclin (PG12)

d. Acetone and beta-hydroxybutyrate

44. The cost in high-energy phosphate bonds for the formation of 1 mole of glucose from pyruvate is:

a. 8 moles of ATP
b. 6 moles of ATP
c. 4 moles of ATP
d. 2 moles of ATP

45. Which of the statements best characterize glucose ?

a. It usually exits in furanose form
b. It is a ketose
c. It forms part of the disaccharide sucrose
d. It is oxidized to form sorbitol

46. Factor III, or thromboplastin, of the blood-clotting scheme:

a. Directly activates prothrombin
b. Activates the intrinsic pathway
c. Activates the extrinsic pathway
d. Directly activates the common pathway

47. A polymorphism is best defined as:

a. Cosegregation of alleles
b. One phenotype, multiple genotypes
c. One locus, multiple abnormal alleles
d. One locus, multiple normal alleles

48. The synthesis of 3-hydroxy-3-methylglutaryl CoA can occur:

a. Only in mitochondria of all mammalian tissues
b. Only in the cytosol of all mammalian tissues
c. Only in the endoplasmic reticulum of all mammalian tissues
d. In both the cytosol and mitochondria

49. Which of the following would rule out hyperuricemia in a patient?

a. Lesch-Nyhan syndrome
b. Xanthine oxidase hyperactivity
c. Carbamoyl phosphate synthase deficiency
d. Purine overproduction secondary to Von Gierke's disease

50. Which one of the following contributes nitrogen atoms to both purine and pyrimidine rings?

a. Aspartate
b. Carbamoyl phosphate
c. Carbon dioxide
d. Glutamine

51. If a completely radioactive double-stranded DNA molecule undergoes two rounds of replication in a solution free of radioactive label, what is the radioactivity status of the resulting four double-stranded DNA molecules?

a. Half should contain no radioactivity
b. All should contain radioactivity
c. Half should contain radioactivity in both strands
d. One should contain radioactivity in both strands

52. Following ultraviolet damage of DNA in skin:

a. A specific excinuclease detects damaged areas
b. Purine dimers are formed
c. Both strands are cleaved
d. Endonuclease removes the strand

53. Inhibitor of ADP transport in and ATP out of mitochondria is:

a. Atractyloside
b. Oligomycin
c. Rotenone
d. Cyanide

54. Which of the following binds to acetyl CoA and condenses with OAA inhibiting citric acid cycle?

a. Arsenic
b. Fluoroacetate
c. Malonate
d. Fumarate

55. A 32 years old man is starving for the last 2 days. Which of the following enzymes will be activated in his body?

a. Glucokinase
b. Pyrovate dehydrogenase
c. Glycogen phosphorylase
d. Glucose 6 phosphatase

56. Which of the following statement regarding rothera's test is untrue?

a. Detects acetone
b. Brown colour is positive

c. May be used in diabetes mellitus patients to detect complications
d. Sodium nitoprusside is required

57. Alkaptonurea is characterized by:
a. Increased urinary homocystine
b. Increased conjugated bilirubin
c. Increased serum phenylalanine
d. Excessive homogentisic acid in urine

58. Microsatellite sequence:
a. Can determine paternity
b. Consists of 10-15 base pair sequence
c. Is irreproducible
d. Are neutral regions of DNA

59. Which of the following enzymes catalyze reactions in the biosynthesis of both catecholamines and indoleamines (serotonin)?
a. Dopamine beta-hydroxylase
b. Phenyl ethanolamine N-methyl transferase
c. Aromatic amino acid decarboxylase
d. Tryptophan hydroxylase

60. Which of the following statements about protein structure is correct ?
a. The extended beta-configuration is not found in globular proteins
b. The stability of the alpha helix is mainly due to hydrophobic interactions
c. Globular proteins tend to fold into configurations that keep hydrophobic side chains in the interior of the molecule
d. The primary structure of a peptide does not influence the formation of native three dimensional configurations

61. A 32-year-old woman presents with a history of fever, headache and is on sodium valproate. She receives a loading dose of intravenous phenytoin and a lumbar puncture is performed. A diagnosis of tuberculous meningitis is made. She is commenced on quadruple antituberculous therapy and makes a good recovery. She attends the outpatients clinic two months later, when she informs you that she is three weeks' pregnant. Which one of the following drugs would be safe to continue?
a. Phenytoin b. Isoniazid
c. Isotretinion d. Alcohol

62. All the following products contain a local anaesthetic *except*:
a. Dequacaine b. Merocaine
c. Burneze d. Anthisan

63. A 25-year-old man is brought in by ambulance to the Accident and Emergency Department with a Glasgow Coma Scale score of 13/15. It is suspected that he took a drug overdose 12 hours previously but he is unable to remember what he took. For which one of the following is a specific antidote not available?
a. Ferrous sulphate b. Cyanide
c. Amitriptyline d. Paracetamol

64. Which of the following opioid agonists is only administered by the parenteral route?
a. Morphine b. Codeine
c. Fentanyl d. Methadone

65. Inhibitors of serotonin (5-HT) uptake such as paroxetine interact significantly with which of the following drugs?
a. Chlorpromazine b. Tranylcypromine
c. Halothane d. Benztropine

66. Which of the following inhalation anesthetics is most likely to produce hepatotoxicity?
a. Isoflurane b. Enflurane
c. Methoxyflurane d. Halothane

67. A 70-year-old man has stable, well controlled atrial fibrillation and has been on digoxin for several years. He presents with nausea, vomiting and confusion. His serum digoxin level is raised. Which one of the following is most likely to exacerbate this problem?
a. Thyrotoxic heart failure
b. Left ventricular failure
c. Spironolactone
d. None

68. Drug having greater activity than ciprofloxacin against pneumococci is:
a. Nalidixic acid b. Norfloxacin
c. Levofloxacin d. Ofloxacin

69. Which one of the following drugs is most likely to cause gynaecomastia?
a. Diazepam b. Methysergide
c. Metoclopramide d. Climetidine

70. Which one of the following is a known cause of galactorrhoea?

a. Cannabis b. Phenothiazine
c. Alcohol d. Digoxin

71. Which one of the following statements about ergotamine is true?

a. It is chemically related to methysergide
b. It is a powerful vasodilator
c. It is an alpha-adrenoceptor blocker
d. It is safe for use in pregnancy

72. Which of the following products is not indicated for the management of peptic ulceration?

a. Zantac b. Gaviscon
c. Nexium d. Buscopan

73. Which one of the following agents can be used without caution in renal failure?

a. Magnesium trisilicate mixture
b. Amphotericin
c. Diazepam
d. Vancomycin

74. Ethambutol causes:

a. Retrobulbar neuritis b. Deafness
c. Red urine d. Peripheral neuritis

75 Pyridoxine deficiency can cause all *except*:

a. Convulsion in infants
b. Anemia
c. Peripheral neuritis
d. Growth retardation

76. Rubella is also known as:

a. The brown measles
b. The German measles
c. The 7-day measles
d. Roseola

77. At which stage of syphilis is the patient likely to have condylomata lata?

a. Primary syphilis b. Secondary syphilis
c. Latent syphilis d. Tertiary syphilis

78. Pulmonary KS is commonly mistakenly diagnosed as:

a. CMV pneumonia
b. Lymphoma
c. Pneumocystis carinii pneumonia
d. Pneumococcus

79. After initial exposure to cytomegalovirus (CMV), a normal host will:

a. Completely eradicate the virus
b. Continue to produce CMV IgM
c. Encapsulate the virus is selected lymph tissue
d. Recover but continue to harbor live virus

80. Which of the following is an appropriate treatment for Giardia lamblia?

a. Chloroquine
b. Metronidazole (Flagyl)
c. Amoxicillin
d. Praziquantel

81. Which of the following best describes signs of elevating intracranial pressure?

a. Mental status changes, vomiting and papilledema
b. Ataxia, positive Kernig's sign and scalp tenderness with palpation
c. Nuchal rigidity, fever and vomiting
d. Fever, forgetfulness and nausea

82. A patient with a suspected brain abscess should undergo a search for:

a. A secondary source of infection located in the middle ear
b. A potential secondary source of infection from a possibly infected tooth
c. Adequate views of the mastoids and sinuses
d. An EEG study

83. Which of the following is false about Cl. perfringes?

a. Food poisoning strains produce heat resistant spores
b. Show positive naegler reaction
c. Most important toxin is hyaluronidase
d. Most common cause gas gangrene

84. All can cause candidiasis *except:*

a. DM b. HTN
c. Ca breast d. Pregnancy

85. Amoebiasis is not transmitted through:

a. Vertical transmission b. Fecooral
c. Cockroach d. Oral

86. Genetic reassortment is found in:

a. Hepadna virus b. Parvo virus
c. Rota virus d. Astro virus

87. Which of the following statement is true regarding ascaris lumbricoides?

a. A lumbricoides is transmitted sexually

b. A lumbricoides is diagnosed by seeing cysts in a muscle biopsy

c. A lumbricoides can cause pneumonia

d. The intermediate hosts of A lumbricoides are dogs and cats

88. Which of the following are the most common fatal complications of measles?

a. Fever and bacterial pneumonia

b. Hepatitis and giant cell pneumonia

c. Meningitis and respiratory complications

d. SSPE and immunodeficiency

89. The etiologic agent of granuloma inguinale is:

a. Haemophilus ducreyi

b. Leishmania donovani

c. Calymmatobacterium granulomatis

d. Leptospira canicola

90. A 16-year-old boy from a rural area presents with two highly inflammatory lesions in the bearded area of his face. Skin scrapings from lesion margins mounted in potassium hydroxide demonstrate the presence of true hyphae and arthroconidia. Which drug or combination is most appropriate?

a. Amoxicillin

b. Amoxicillin and clavulanate

c. Amphotericin B

d. An imidazole such as itraconazole

91. Which of the following is not a cause of acute pancreatitis?

a. Hyperlipidemia b. Ethanol

c. Steroids d. Hypotension

92. A 59-year-old man complains of periorbital edema and gradually increasing ankle swelling. Blood pressure is 120/80 mm Hg. Urinalysis shows a 4+ proteinuria but no cells or casts. Serum albumin is moderately decreased but blood urea nitrogen (BUN) and creatinine are normal. Most likely diagnosis:

a. Acute proliferative glomerulonephritis

b. Diabetic nephropathy

c. IgA nephropathy

d. Membranous glomerulopathy

93. A 74-year-old woman with left heart failure develops pulmonary edema. This accumula-tion of fluid is best explained by which of the following mechanisms?

a. Decreased hydrostatic pressure

b. Decreased lymphatic drainage

c. Decreased oncotic pressure

d. Increased hydrostatic pressure

94. Which of the following is not directly related with Alzheimer's disease?

a. Senile plaques b. Diabetes mellitus

c. Tangles d. Dementia

95. Lipid can be stained in frozen sample by:

a. Oil red O b. Muciramine

c. PAS d. Giemsa

96. Lynch syndrome involves carcinoma of:

a. Breast, ovary, endometrium

b. Breast, ovary, colon

c. Breast, endometrium, colon

d. Colon, endometrium, ovary

97. Which of the following is not directly related with Horner's syndrome?

a. Miosis b. Malaise

c. Ptosis d. Anhidrosis

98. Which of the following is not directly related with Goodpasture's syndrome?

a. Hematuria

b. Paleness

c. Adrenal hypertrophy

d. Hemoptysis

99. Histological examination of the affected vertebral bone in a woman suffering from senile, or postmenopausal, osteoporosis would be?

a. Disorganized interconnecting trabeculae of woven bone rimmed by osteoblasts

b. Thickened, irregular trabeculae with prominent cement lines

c. Thinning of the cortical and trabecular bone

d. Widened osteoid seams of peripheral trabeculae

100. A 28-year-old woman complains of a chronic productive cough with blood-tinged sputum, night sweats, low-grade fever over the past 6 weeks. Chest X-ray reveals a cavitary lesion in the left upper lobe and a calcified left hilar lymph node. Biopsy of the left upper lobe mass will reveals:

a. Amorphous eosinophilic material surrounded by epithelioid cells and T-lymphocytes

b. Disorganized pleomorphic and hyperchromatic cells with rare mitotic figures

c. Numerous neutrophils and necrotic debris surrounded by a fibrous capsule

d. Scattered macrophages interspersed with regenerating alveolar cells and sparse collagen deposition

101. The Wilson's disease gene (ATP7B) has been mapped to:

a. Chromosome 11 b. Chromosome 13

c. Chromosome 17 d. Chromosome 21

102. Which of the following is not associated with Wilson's disease?

a. Asterixs b. Basal ganglia

c. Cirrhosis d. Pancreatitis

103. Which of the following is not associated with Reye's syndrome?

a. Coma b. Hyperglycemia

c. Influenza B d. Fatty liver tissue

104. Presenilin 1 (PSEN1) is related with:

a. Chromosome 11 b. Chromosome 14

c. Chromosome 19 d. Chromosome 21

105. Which of the following is not directly related with Hashimoto's thyroiditis?

a. Hypothyroidism

b. Slow onset

c. Neuropathy

d. Autoimmune disease

106. Witness in a trial who testifies for the opposing party or a witness who offers adverse testimony to the calling party during examination is:

a. Medical witness b. Expert witness

c. Hostile witness d. Atheist witness

107. Maximum death in mushroom poisoning is caused by:

a. Amanita phalloides

b. Amanita crustuliniforme

c. Amanita muscarina

d. None

108. Cephalic index is useful for determination of:

a. Age b. Sex

c. Race d. Religion

109. Delirium is seen in all of the following *except*:

a. Dhatura b. Lead

c. Nux vomika d. Opioid

110. Untrue statement regarding about somatic death is:

a. Cooling of the body

b. Cessation of spontaneous respiration

c. Cessation of circulation

d. Flat isoelectric EEG

111. Rigor mortis is resisted by:

a. Cold stiffness

b. Heat stiffness

c. Tetanus

d. Strychnine poisoning

112. Which of the following snake is neurotoxic:

a. Sea snake b. Russel viper

c. Elapids d. Pit viper

113. Brush burn are also known as:

a. Electrical injury b. Graze abrasion

c. Chemical injury d. None

114. Order of exhumation of body is given by:

a. Doctor

b. Police

c. District Magistrate

d. Chief Medical Officer

115. Topical mitomycin C is used to aid the following treatment:

a. Endoscopic treatment of angiofibroma
b. Treatment of laryngotracheal stenosis
c. Skull base osteomyelitis
d. Sturge-Weber syndrome

116. Microwick and microcatheter sustained release devices are used in:

a. Drooling of saliva
b. Frey's syndrome
c. Conrol of epistaxis
d. Delivering drug to the round membrane

117. A 72-year-old man is having difficulty hearing. He is being tested with a tuning fork. If he has disease of the middle ear, sound transmitted strictly by air conduction will be perceived as:

a. Louder than that transmitted by bone conduction
b. Quieter than that transmitted by bone conduction
c. Lower-pitched than that transmitted by bone conduction
d. Higher-pitched than that transmitted by bone conduction

118. A 58-year-old man complains of an enlarged, pitted nose and a facial rash that "flushes" in response to drinking hot liquids or alcohol. The rash is on both cheeks, and it is red and flushed in appearance, with some telangiectasia and small papules. Which of the following is the most likely diagnosis? (See Fig.):

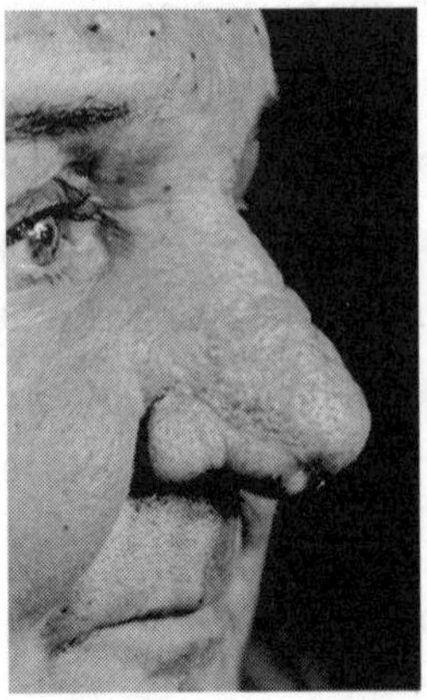

a. Acne vulgaris
b. Pemphigus
c. Rosacea
d. Psoriasis

119. The most common predisposing risk factor for otitis media in children is:

a. Allergies
b. Day-care attendance
c. Adenoidal hypertrophy
d. Upper respiratory infections

120. The most common biological cause of spontaneous rupture of the tympanic membrane in children is:

a. Beta lactamase-producing strains of Haemophilus influenza
b. Moraxella (Branhamella) catarrhalis
c. Group A beta-hemolytic streptococcus
d. Respiratory syncytial viruses

121. The paranasal sinuses most prone to osteomyelitis are:

a. Sphenoid b. Maxillary
c. Ethmoid d. Frontal

122. Which of the following could be considered as an extracranial complication of mastoiditis?

a. Labyrinthitis b. Meningitis
c. Brain abscess d. All of the above

123. In the physical assessment of a child with possible otitis media, the most predictive sign is:

a. Decreased motility of the tympanic membrane
b. The presence of pus in the ear canal
c. Tragal tenderness
d. Fever

124. In the surgical procedure known as Lasik, the shape of the cornea may be flattened. This will result in which of the following?

a. Decreased refraction of light by the cornea
b. A decreased amount of light entering through the cornea
c. Conversion of the cornea from a "stationary" to an "adjustable" form of refraction
d. Maintenance of the lens in a more flattened state

125. Retina receives its blood supply from all of following *except*:

a. Posterior ciliary artery
b. Central retinal artery
c. Retinal arteries
d. Plexus of Zinn and Haller arteries

126. **Typically bilateral inferior lens subluxation of the lens is seen in:**
a. Marfan's syndrome
b. Homocystinuria
c. Hyperlusinaemia
d. Ocular trauma

127. **Which of the following is the drug of choice for treatment of corneal ulcers caused by filamentous fungi?**
a. Itraconazole b. Natamycin
c. Nystatin d. Fluconazole

128. **In which of the following uveitic conditions is it contraindicated to put in an intraocular lens after cataract surgery?**
a. Fuch's heterochromic cyclitis
b. Psoriatic arthritis
c. Juvenile rheumatoid arthritis
d. Reiter's syndrome

129. **A white reflex on examination of the optic fundus of an infant is most suggestive of which of the following?**
a. Retinoblastoma
b. Retinocerebellar angioma
c. Choroidal angioma
d. Primary congenital glaucoma

130. **Enzyme deficient in gyrate atrophy is:**
a. Ornithine ketoacid transaminase
b. Phenylalanine hydroxylase
c. Tyrosinase
d. Propionyl CoA carboxylase

131. **Shaffer's sign is seen in:**
a. Lens dislocation
b. Anterior uveitis
c. Retinal detachment
d. Open angle glaucoma

132. **Lallo, 25-year-old man, presented with history of pain redness and watering of left eye for last 1 day. There is also intolerance to light. Most probable diagnosis is:**
a. Keratitis
b. Acute anterior uveitis
c. Acute posterior uveitis
d. Epidemic kerato conjunctivitis

133. **Kaplan Meire test is used for:**
a. Survival b. Incidence
c. Prevalence d. Frequency

134. **Incidence is derived from:**
a. Cross sectional b. Case and control
c. Prospective study d. Retrospective study

135. **All are true about cluster sampling *except*?**
a. Sample size based on hypothesis
b. Rapid assessment
c. Samples provide equal type of various clusters
d. Easy

136. **False + is more with screening test with?**
a. Decreased prevalence
b. Increased prevalence
c. Increased sensitivity
d. Decreased specificity

137. **Fish is a poor source of:**
a. Fe b. Iodine
c. Phosphorus d. Vitamin A

138. **Seventh disability is defined in part of Article of Disabilities Act of 1955 includes:**
a. Drug addiction b. Disability by accident
c. Mental illness d. Neurological illness

139. **Lepromin test is best for:**
a. Prognosis b. Diagnosis
c. Treatment d. Epidemiological investigations

140. **According to the WHO classification of obesity, 'Obese class 1' have body mass index of :**
a. 25.0 - 29.9 b. 30.0 - 34.9
c. 35.0 -39.9 d. 40.0

141. **You find that the specific disease that you are studying is very rare in your patient population. You are interested in determining which risk factors may contribute to the development of this disease. Which study design would be the most appropriate to further pursue this question?**
a. Case-control study
b. Cohort study
c. Prospective, randomized-controlled trial
d. Cross-sectional study

142. Which of the following is a commonly used mechanism for reducing medical errors in hospitals?

a. Confidential peer review

b. National hospital accreditation

c. Departmental grand rounds

d. Random drug testing

143. The Integrated Management of Childhood Illness (IMNCI) clinical guidelines target children less than:

a. 1 year old b. 2 years old

c. 3 years old d. 5 years old

144. Grass-roots functionaries primarily for Integrated Child Development Services Scheme (ICDS) are:

a. Anganwadi workers (AWW) and multipurpose worker

b. Multipurpose worker and Anganwadi helpers (AWH)

c. Multipurpose worker and school teachers

d. Anganwadi workers (AWW) and Anganwadi helpers (AWH)

145. Which statement about varicella is not true?

a. Varicella is highly contagious

b. Varicella is a notifiable disease in all states

c. Most adults are immune to varicella

d. Airborne transmission of varicella can occur

146. A male patient with hepatitis C is receiving interferon/ ribavirin combination therapy, and his viral load is reevaluated after 3 months of therapy. The viral load is reduced by 2 logs, but has still not normalized. Which of the following is the best next step?

a. Discontinue all therapy

b. Increase the dose of ribavirin

c. Continue with therapy and recheck viral load after 6 months of therapy

d. Discontinue the ribavirin and continue patient on long-term, low-dose interferon

147. All of the following purified protein derivative (PPD) test results are considered positive *except*:

a. 5 mm diameter induration in a 25-year-old homosexual man who uses intravenous drugs,HIV status unknown

b. 5 mm diameter induration in a 55-year-old patient with type I diabetes mellitus

c. 10 mm diameter induration in a 65-year-old nursing home patient

d. 10 mm diameter induration in a 45-year-old patient who has had a gastrectomy

148. All of the following prophylactic regimens are acceptable after meningococcus exposure in a 40-year-old man *except*:

a. Benzathine penicillin, 4 million units intramuscularly in a single dose

b. Rifampin, 600 mg orally twice a day for 2 days

c. Ceftriaxone, 250 mg intramuscularly in a single dose

d. Ciprofloxacin, 500 mg orally in a single dose

149. A recently discovered treatment for prostate cancer extends the lifespan but does not prevent the disease or lead to its cure. In this scenario, which of the following statements about prostate cancer is true?

a. Incidence will increase

b. Prevalence will increase

c. Incidence will decrease

d. Prevalence will decrease

150. In probability and statistics, the standard deviation is a measure of the dispersion of a collection of values. It is defined as the:

a. Root-mean-square (RMS) deviation of the values from their mean, or as the square root of the variance

b. Root-mean-square (RMS) deviation of the values from their mean, or as the square of the variance

c. Root-mean-square (RMS) deviation of the values from their median, or as the square of the variance

d. None

151. Plastic wrapper of used syringes is discarded in:

a. Red bag b. Black bag

c. Yellow bag d. Blue bag

152. Shortest incubation period is seen in:

a. Hepatitis A b. HBV

c. Rubella d. Influenza

153. Signs and symptoms of hyperlipidemia include:

a. Xanthomas

b. Abdominal pain

c. Pale creamy blood samples

d. All of the above

154. The risk of sudden death is increased in all the following *except*:

a. Smokers

b. Left ventricular hypertrophy

c. Paroxysmal atrial fibrillation

d. Left ventricular systolic dysfunction

155. Risk factors for the development of coronary atherosclerosis include all the following *except*:

a. Postmenopausal state

b. Hypertension

c. Elevated LDL cholesterol

d. Elevated HDL cholesterol

156. Stress echocardiograms demonstrate ischemia by:

a. Inducing mitral regurgitation

b. Inducing transient ventricular wall motion abnormalities

c. Demonstrating permanent ventricular wall motion abnormalities

d. Inducing right atrial diastolic collapse

157. Recommended first-line treatment for femoral vein deep venous thrombosis (DVT) is:

a. Urokinase b. Heparin

c. Warfarin (Coumadin) d. Aspirin

158. Management of infectious mononucleosis includes:

a. Instructing the patient to avoid contact sports or strenuous exercise

b. Symptomatic treatment of fever and pharyngitis

c. Penicillin or erythromycin for treatment of bacterial pharyngitis

d. All of the above

159. All the following are risk factors for developing cholangiocarcinoma *except:*

a. Choledochal cyst

b. Cholelithiasis

c. Liver flukes

d. Sclerosing cholangitis

160. The differential diagnosis of an isolated unconjugated (indirect) hyperbilirubinemia is limited. In a patient with isolated unconjuga-ted hyperbilirubinemia, which of these historic findings would be unlikely?

a. Calcium bilirubinate gallstones

b. Cryoglobulinemia

c. History of gout

d. Spherocytosis

161. An abnormal D-xylose test is suggestive of:

a. Pancreatic insufficiency

b. Hepatic insufficiency

c. A mucosal abnormality of proximal small intestine

d. Colonic disease

162. The treatment of herpes simplex viral encephalitis includes:

a. Zidovudine b. Acyclovir

c. Didanosine d. Symptomatic treatment only

163. The drug found to be beneficial in amyotrophic lateral sclerosis is:

a. Riluzole b. Methylprednisolone

c. Hydroxyurea d. None of the above

164. Drugs useful in the treatment of acute gouty arthritis include:

a. Allopurinol b. Colchicine

c. Probenecid d. Sulfinpyrazone

165. The single test that confirms the diagnosis of autoimmune hemolytic anemia is:

a. Coombs' test

b. Reticulocyte count

c. Peripheral smear

d. Hemoglobin electrophoresis

166. The most common manifestations in Takayasu's arteritis are related to occlusion of:

a. Abdominal aorta b. Renal arteries

c. Subclavian arteries d. Pulmonary arteries

167. All these conditions are autosomal dominant disorder *except*:

a. Marfan's syndrome

b. Hunter syndrome

c. Osteogenesis imperfecta

d. Achondroplasia

168. Which of the following statements regarding pancreatic cancer is true?

a. Five-year survival is ~5%

b. Most cases present with locally confined disease amenable to a surgical cure

c. Pancreatic adenocarcinomas occur most frequently in the pancreatic tail

d. The median age of diagnosis is 49 years

169. An 80-year-old man with Type II diabetes and hypertension presents with increasing dyspnea. He appears short of breath, blood pressure is 170/95 mm Hg, pulse 100/min and regular. The JVP is at 7 cm; there is a loud second heart sound and a systolic ejection murmur at the right sternal border, which does not radiate. The lungs have bibasilar crakles upto the scapula. The CXR has bilateral infiltrates and vascular redistribution. His echocardiogram reports aortic sclerosis, concentric left ventricular hypertrophy (LVH), and normal ejection fraction. Which of the following is the most likely mechanism for this condition? (See Fig.)

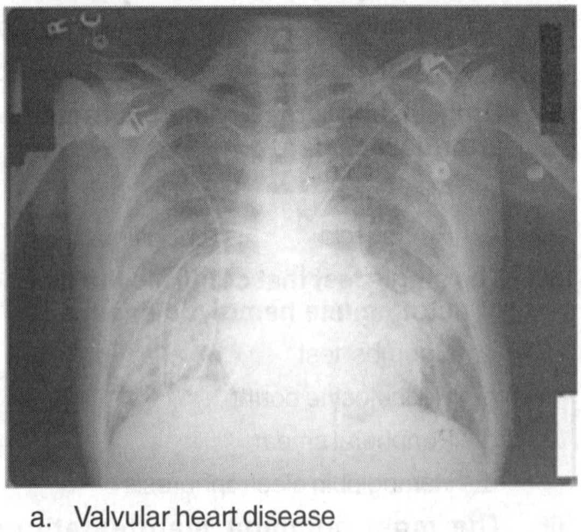

a. Valvular heart disease

b. Diastolic dysfunction

c. Systolic dysfunction

d. Hibernating myocardium

170. Complication of infectious mononucleosis include:

a. Hematologic b. Neurologic

c. Hepatic d. All of the above

171. A man 25 years old presents with renal failure. His maternal uncle died of renal failure 10 years ago. On slit lamp examination, keratoconus is present. Diagnosis is:

a. ADPKD

b. ARPKD

c. Alports syndrome

d. Denysh-Drash syndrome

172. A 35-year-old lady presents with chronic backache. On X-ray she had a D12 collapse. But intervertebral disc space is maintained. All are possible *except:*

a. Multiple myeloma b. Osteoporosis

c. Metastasis d. Tuberculosis

173. All are true about starting of β-blocker therapy in a case of heart disease *except:*

a. They should be started with optimum doses

b. They should be gradually incresed over weeks

c. Special precautions should be taken in cases of NYHA class III and IV

d. Carvedilol and metoprolol are the preferred drugs

174. A patient present with waxy flexibility, negativitism and rigidity. Diagnosis is:

a. Catatonic schizophrenia

b. Paranoid schizophrenia

c. Hebephrenic schizophrenia

d. Simple schizophrenia

175. Chandu, at age 32 presents with abdominal pain and vomiting. He also complains of some psychiatric symptoms and visual hallucina-tions. Most likely diagnosis is:

a. Intermittent porphyria

b. Hypothyroidism

c. Hyperthyroidism

d. Hysteria

176. A 37-year-old woman who was diagnosed with AIDS 3 years earlier is unable to work, is physically debilitated, and requests her physician to provide her with medications with which to take her own life. The most common emotional disorder that results in such requests by patients is:

a. Schizophrenic disorder
b. Factitious disorder
c. Major depressive disorder
d. Borderline personality disorder

177. Ability to filter unpleasant memories is called:

a. Dissociation b. Repression
c. Suppression d. Isolation

178. "Exclamation mark" hair are seen in:

a. Tinea capitis b. Alopecia areata
c. Trichotillomania d. Lichen planus pilaris

179. Wickham's striae is seen in:

a. Lichen nitidus b. Psoriasis
c. Pityriasis rosea d. Lichen planus

180. Herald patch is seen in:

a. Pityriasis vesicolor b. Pityriasis alba
c. Pityriasis rosea d. Pityriasis rubra pilaris

181. Darier's sign is seen in:

a. Darier's disease
b. Urticaria pigmentosa
c. Pemphigus vulgaris
d. Lichen planus

182. Advantages of crystalloid solution over colloid in fluid resuscitation include all of the following *except*:

a. Cost b. Availability
c. Retrievability d. Edema

183. A-22-year-old woman complains of palpitations and has a regular heartbeat at a rate of 170/min, with a blood pressure of 110/70 mm Hg. The rate abruptly changes to 75/min after applying carotid sinus pressure. Which of the following is the most likely diagnosis? (See Fig.)

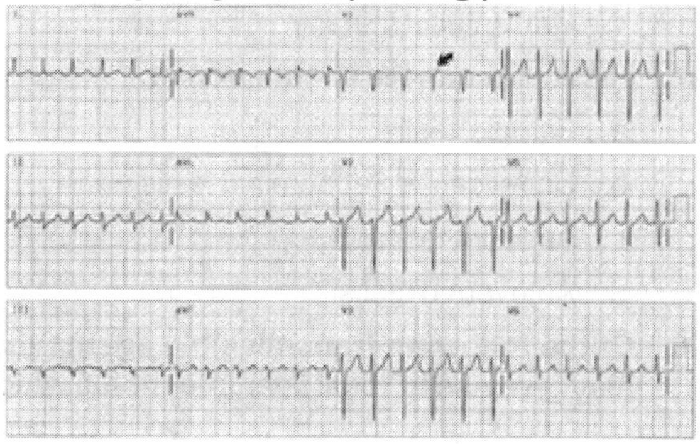

a. Paroxysmal atrial fibrillation
b. Paroxysmal atrial flutter
c. Paroxysmal supraventricular tachycardia (PSVT)
d. Paroxysmal ventricular tachycardia

184. Which of the following statements about Schatzki's ring is correct?

a. The ring represents a panmural fibrotic stricture resulting from gastroesophageal reflux
b. Dysphagia occurs when the ring diameter is 13 mm or less
c. The ring occurs within 1 to 2 cm of the squamocolumnar epithelial junction
d. Schatzki's ring indicates reflux esophagitis

185. Which of the following suggests unresectability of a left upper lobe lung cancer?

a. Hemoptysis
b. Pneumonia
c. Malignant pleural effusion
d. A cough specimen with positive sputum cytology

186. Paralytic ileus is seen in all of the following *except*:

a. Spinal cord injury b. Hypocalcemia
c. Hypermagnesemia d. Uremia

187. Management of pulmonary complications of tuberculosis refractory to antibiotic management include each of the following *except*:

a. Decortication
b. Chest wall reconstruction
c. Hyperbaric oxygen therapy
d. Bronchoscopic brush biopsy and lavage

188. One method of pre-operative therapy that has been helpful in facilitating liver resection for tumor has been:

a. Pre-operative external beam radiation
b. Arteriographic vascular occlusion
c. Portal venous thrombosis
d. Intensive cancer chemotherapy with leucovorin rescue

189. The presence of a non-malignant mid- or upper esophageal stricture always indicates the presence of:

a. Alkaline reflux esophagitis
b. Barrett's esophagus
c. Idiopathic reflux disease
d. Meditational fibrosis

190. A 50-year-old patient has undergone truncal vagotomy and antrectomy with Billroth II Reconstruction two years ago. The patient now complains of recurrent postprandial pain, nausea and vomiting. Endoscopic examina-tion reveals bile in the stomach; endoscopic biopsies demonstrate histologic evidence of moderately severe gastritis. No other endoscopic abnormalities are noted. appropriate therapy could include:

a. Octreotide administration
b. Total gastrectomy
c. Conversion of Billroth II gastrojejunostomy to Billroth I gastroduodenostomy
d. Conversion of Billroth II gastrojejunostomy to Roux-en-Y gastrojejunostomy

191. Staples may safely be placed during laparoscopic hernia repair in each of the following structures *except*:

a. Cooper's ligament
b. Tissues superior to the lateral iliopubic tract
c. The transversus abdominis aponeurotic arch
d. Tissues inferior to the lateral iliopubic tract

192. A 50-year-old male with a 2 years history of duodenal ulceration develops sudden, severe epigastric pain 4 hours prior to evaluation. Physical examination reveals T 101° F, pulse 80, BP 125/90, diminished bowel sounds, and abdominal muscular rigidity. An upright chest X-ray reveals pneumoperitoneum. At laparotomy, an anterior perforation in the first portion of the duodenum is observed. Optimal treatment would include:

a. Omental patch of the perforation followed by truncal vagotomy and antrectomy after 8 weeks
b. Omental patch of the perforation followed by truncal vagotomy and pyloroplasty after 8 weeks
c. Omental patch of the perforation followed by chronic cimetidine administration
d. Omental patch of the perforation plus proximal gastric vagotomy

193. Which of the following is most reliable for confirming the occurrence of a significant esophageal caustic injury?

a. History of the event
b. Physical examination of the patient
c. Barium esophagraphy
d. Endoscopy

194. Indications for surgical reconstruction of the esophagus include all of the following *except*:

a. Continuing requirement for frequent dilation of an extensive esophageal stricture for a minimum of 2 years
b. Failure or refusal of the patient to comply with a treatment regimen of regular dilation
c. Development of a fistula between the esophagus and tracheobronchial tree
d. Iatrogenic perforation of the esophagus during attempted dilation

195. First-line therapy for routine peptic duodenal ulcer disease includes:

a. Vagotomy and antrectomy
b. Upper endoscopy and biopsy to rule out tumor
c. Evaluation for Helicobacter pylori
d. Serum gastrin determination

196. Appropriate management of severe vomiting associated with gastric outlet obstruction from peptic ulcer disease includes all of the following *except*:

a. Intravenous hydration
b. Nutritional assessment; upper endoscopy to rule out malignancy
c. Intravenous H_2 antagonist
d. Oral antacid therapy

197. Testicular cancer is common in:

a. Ectopic testis
b. Undescended abdominal testis
c. Atrophic testis
d. Anteverted testis

198. Of the following transmissible agents that may give rise to focal liver infections, which

may cause an anaphylactic response if the contents are spilled in the event of resection or rupture?

a. Entamoeba histolytica
b. Staphylococcus aureus
c. Clonorchis sinensis
d. Echinococcus granulosus

199. Each of the following conditions is an indication for splenectomy *except*:

a. Thrombocytopenia
b. Traumatic splenic laceration in a child with minimum blood loss
c. A splenic artery aneurysm within the splenic pulp
d. Splenic abscess

200. Which of the following tumor cell types has the worst prognosis in the thyroid gland?

a. Lymphoma
b. Anaplastic carcinoma
c. Medullary carcinoma
d. Papillary carcinoma

201. A 22-year-old man has symptoms of low back pain and stiffness. After several months of mild symptoms, he notes more severe stiffness at night and hip pain. On physical examination, there is paravertebral muscle tenderness and limited flexion of the lumbar spine. Fig. shows an X-ray of the lumbar spine. Which of the following is the most likely diagnosis?

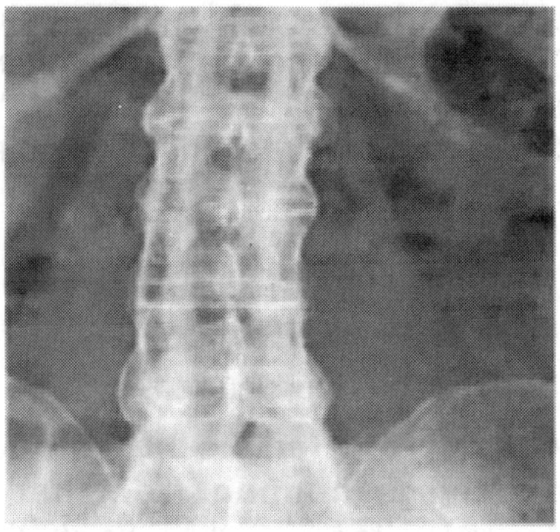

a. Reiter's syndrome
b. Marfan's syndrome
c. Ankylosing spondylitis (AS)
d. RA

202. Most common cause of neonatal intestinal obstruction:

a. Duodena atresia
b. Jejunal atresia
c. Necrotizing enterocolitis
d. Meconium ileus

203. Hill-Sachs lesion is seen in:

a. Recurrent dislocation of elbow
b. Recurrent dislocation of patella
c. Recurrent dislocation of hip
d. Recurrent dislocation of shoulder

204. Most serious complication of fracture of a long bone is:

a. Fat embolism
b. Pulmonary embolism
c. Deep vein thrombosis
d. Associated joint injuries

205. Bone commonly fractured in facial injuries is:

a. Nasal bones
b. Nasoethmoid bone
c. Zygomatic bone
d. Mandible

206. Investigation of choice for Zenker's diverticulum is:

a. Barium swallow
b. Endoscopy
c. Esophageal manometry
d. CT

207. All correlates with USG findings of pyloric stenosis *except*:

a. Accurate–95%
b. High gastric residue
c. Segment length >16 mm
d. Thickness > 4 mm

208. Which of following is least useful for diagnosing spondylolisthesis?

a. MRI
b. CT scan
c. X-ray lumbar spine-lateral view
d. X-ray lumbar spine-AP view

209. Characteristics of epidural anesthesia include all *except:*

a. A decreased risk for postdural puncture headache

b. A higher incidence of systemic hypotension
c. Ability to produce a segmental sensory block
d. A catheter can be placed in the epidural space

210. Basic anesthetic monitoring include(s):

a. Measuring the concentration of oxygen in patient breathing system by oxygen analyzer
b. All patients receiving anesthesia shall have continuous ECG display
c. Temperature monitoring to be done when clinically significant changes in body temperature are intended, anticipated or suspected
d. All of the above

211. All the undermentioned are true with respected of either anesthesia *except:*

a. It is flammable
b. Use of either is associated with quick induction time
c. There will be a delayed emergence from anesthesia
d. Use of the either is associated with a high incidence of nausea and vomiting

212. The most important maneuver in preserving renal function in septic shock is:

a. Intravenous infusion of furosemide
b. Infusion of dopamine at a rate of 1-3 g/kg/min
c. Rapid restoration of the circulating volume
d. Proper antibiosis against the offending organism

213. In the management of a child with ARDS and respiratory failure, all of the following measures are important *except*:

a. Normalize blood gases
b. Use permissive hypercapnia
c. Accept PaO_2 measurements of 60-80 mm Hg
d. Reduce airway pressures to prevent barotrauma and volutrauma

214. A pediatrician is examining a young infant and notes that the infant symmetrically abducts and extends his extremities after a loud noise and then begins to cry. This reflex is known as which of the following?

a. Asymmetric tonic neck reflex (ATNR)
b. Parachute reflex
c. Moro reflex
d. Hand-grasp reflex (grasping reflex)

215. In Burkitt's lymphoma, there is increased expression of a hybrid protein with an amino-terminus similar to immunoglobulin (Ig) heavy chain and an unknown carboxyterminus. Which of the following best explains this phenomenon?

a. Chromosome translocation that brings together an Ig heavy chain with an oncogene
b. Chromosome duplication involving a segment with an oncogene
c. Chromosome translocation involving a segment with Ig heavy chains
d. Chromosome deletion removing an oncogene

216. A young man with hypercholesterolemia is rushed to the hospital with crushing chest pain radiating to his left arm and a probable heart attack. Which of the following treatments should be considered?

a. A platelet transfusion
b. Heparin infusion
c. Fibrinogen infusion
d. Tissue plasminogen activator infusion

217. A 10-year-old child had an upper respiratory infection 5 days ago and was given aspirin for fever. She now presents with fever, protracted vomiting, and lethargy. Physical examination reveals mild hepatomegaly. Total bilirubin, serum transaminases, and serum ammonia are increased. Which of the following is the most likely diagnosis?

a. Hepatitis A virus (HAV)
b. Drug-induced hepatitis
c. Reye's syndrome
d. Infectious mononucleosis

218. A 4-day-old female has blood-tinged discharge coming from her vagina. According to the mother, the child has been afebrile and is feeding and sleeping well. At this point, the physician should do which of the following?

a. Draw a hematocrit (Hct)
b. Notify the child protective services

c. Reassure the mother that this is normal
d. Obtain a urinalysis

219. A mentally retarded 15-year-old boy is found to have macro-orchidism and large, prominent ears. The most likely diagnosis is:

a. Acromegaly
b. Hypothyroidism
c. Trisomy 21
d. Fragile X syndrome

220. A 5-year-old boy develops a headache, cough, myalgia and a fever. He is given a decongestant and an aspirin for his symptoms with some relief. However, 4 days later, he is brought back by his parents because of persistent vomiting and irritability. On physical examination, he is found to be semicomatose, becoming combative on stimulation. Which of the following levels should be measured to aid in the diagnosis of this patient?

a. Serum ammonia level
b. Serum blood urea nitrogen level
c. Serum calcium level
d. Serum opiate level

221. What is the treatment of choice of unruptured tubal pregnancy with serum beta hCG titer of 200 IU/Ml?

a. Single dose of methotrexate
b. Variable doses of methotrexate
c. Expectant management
d. Laparoscopic salpingostomy

222. Which of the following DNA alterations play a role in gynecologic cancer?

a. Amplification
b. Point mutations
c. Rearrangements
d. All of the above

223. Which of the following tumor-associated antigens is specific for the associated gynecologic malignancy?

a. Squamous cell carcinoma (SCC) antigen for cervical cancer
b. Carcinoembryonic antigen (CEA) for endometrial cancer
c. β-hCG for ovarian germ cell tumor
d. None of the above

224. Endometrial cancer involving > 50% of myometrium, extending to vagina, no pelvic extension, no pre and para aortic lymph nodes. Peritoneal lavage was positive, staged as:

a. III a
b. III b
c. III c1
d. III c2

225. Shock just after normal delivery, due to:

a. Amniotic fluid embolism
b. PPH
c. Uterine inversion
d. Postpartum eclampsia

226. A 21-year-old woman complains of vaginal discharge that she states has a fishy odor. It is particularly noticeable following coitus. You examine her and find the pH is 5. The most likely diagnosis is:

a. Candida albicans
b. Bacterial vaginosis
c. Trichomonas vaginalis
d. Normal postcoital discharge

227. The most common site of metastasis of a gestational trophoblastic tumor is the:

a. Vagina
b. Lung
c. Liver
d. Brain

228. Of the following features, which one is highly prognostic in patient with stage II and III gestational trophoblastic disease (GTD)?

a. Race
b. Smoking history
c. The parity of the patient
d. Interval between the antecedent pregnancy and the occurrence of the GTD

229. All of the following are true about anencephaly *except*:

a. Facial presentation
b. Increased alpha-fetoprotein
c. Enlarged adrenal gland
d. Polyhydramnios

230. Neural tube defects in the newborn can be prevented by:

a. Giving folic acid to the mother in periconceptional period
b. Correcting iron deficiency anaemia in early pregnancy

c. Supplemental vitamin 'A' to the mother in periconceptional period
d. Vitamin B12 in early pregnancy for proper foetal central nervous system development

231. Patients with non-metastatic gestational trophoblastic tumors are most commonly treated with:
a. Hysterectomy
b. Primary combination chemotherapy
c. Single agent chemotherapy with either cisplatin or Taxol
d. Single agent chemotherapy with either methotrexate or actinomycin-D

232. When a patient has achieved remission with chemotherapy for a gestational trophoblastic tumor, she should be advised that in later pregnancies:
a. She should expect a higher risk of congenital malformations
b. She should expect a higher risk of cesarean section
c. She should expect a higher risk of spontaneous abortion
d. She should expect a generally normal reproductive outcome

233. A 28-year-old complains of a "cottage cheese" discharge that has not responded the over-the counter clotrimazole, which she self-administered. The most likely reasons for the condition is:
a. Vaginal injury
b. Hypersensitivity reaction
c. Colonization resistance
d. Autoimmune reaction

234. Which of the following human papilloma virus (HPV) types is most common in patients with invasive cervical cancer, CIN 3 and CIN 2 ?
a. HPV type 6
b. HPV type 11
c. HPV type 16
d. HPV type 18

235. Which one of the following causes the greatest risk of ectopic pregnancy?
a. Pelvic inflammatory disease
b. Intrauterine contraceptive devices' use
c. Previous ectopic pregnancy
d. Previous medical termination of pregnancy

236. Poor prognostic factors in the management of cancer cervix are the following *except*:
a. Young age
b. Well-differentiated squamous cell carcionoma
c. Hydroureter
d. Adenocarcinoma

237. Which one of the following drugs not used in endometriosis?
a. Danazol
b. Progestins
c. GnRH agonists
d. Misoprostol

238. What is the most common ovarian tumour to undergo torsion?
a. Mucinous cystadenoma
b. Serous cystadenoma
c. Dermoid
d. Brenner tumour

239. Which one of the following is not a correct statement regarding the use of condom?
a. Air should be squeezed out of the tip
b. It should be tested by inflating
c. It should be unrolled on erect penis
d. K-Y jelly may be used for lubrication

240. The Mirena prevents the pregnancy primarily by:
a. Suppressing ovulation
b. Making endometrium unreceptive
c. Making cervical mucus thick
d. Making inflammatory changes within endometrium

EXPLANATIONS

Ans 1: (b) Failure of the tracheoesophageal ridges to fuse
Ref: Read the text below
Sol:

- The **tracheoesophageal ridges are two longitudinal ridges the separate the respiratory diverticulum from the foregut.**
- Eventually, they fuse to form a septum separating the esophagus (dorsal) from the trachea (ventral) **and lung buds, maintaining a communication only rostrally at the pharynx.**
- **Incomplete formation of the tracheoesophageal** septum (by fusion of ridges) results in the most common type of tracheoesophageal fistula, whereby the proximal part of the esophagus ends as a blind sac (esophageal atresia), while the distal part is connected to the trachea by a narrow **canal just above the bifurcation. This defect occurs in approximately 1 in 2500 births.**

Ans-2: (b) esophageal atresia
Ref: Read the text below
Sol:

- **Polyhydramnios is the presence of excess amniotic fluid. Because** amniotic fluid is normally swallowed by the fetus, esophageal atresia, an obstruction of the esophagus that prevents the fetus from **swallowing the amniotic fluid, an excess of fluid is retained in the amniotic cavity.**
- An atrial septal defect is a common acyanotic heart **defect. This defect has no relationship to abnormalities in amniotic fluid volume.**

Ans 3: (c) Popliteus
Ref: Read the text below
Sol:

- The **popliteus muscle** rotates the femur laterally (unlocks the knee) or rotates the tibia medially, **depending on which bone is fixed.**
- This **action results in unlocking of the knee joint** to initiate flexion of the leg at the joint. The rectus femoris flexes **the thigh and extends the knee**.
- The **gastrocnemius flexes** the knee and plantar flexes the foot. The semimembranosus extends the thigh **and flexes and rotates the leg medially.**
- The **biceps femoris** extends the thigh and flexes and rotates the leg laterally.

Ans 4: (d) Ureteric bud
Ref: Read the text below
Sol:

- The **ureteric bud forms the ureter, renal pelvis, major and minor ca**lyces, and collecting tubules of the kidney.
- The **ureteric bud is an outgrowth of the mesonephric duct** that grows toward the metanephric blastema and induces the metanephric blastema to develop into the nephrons of the kidney.
- The **caudal end of the mesonephric duct** become incorporated into the trigone of the urinary bladder Thus, the **ureteric bud drains urine from the filtration portion of the kidney into the bladder.**

Ans 5: (c) Jerk test
Ref: Turek's Orthopaedics: Principles and Their Application, 6th EditionP.388
Rockwood fracture in adults 5th ed
Sol:
GLENOHUMERAL INSTABILITY

- **Glenohumeral instability is a common problem** encountered by the orthopaedic surgeon, particularly in young, active individuals.
- **Jerk Test** For the jerk test the patient sits with the arm internally rotated and flexed forward to 90 degrees. The examiner grasps the elbow and axial loads the humerus in a proximal direction. While axial loading of the humerus is maintained, the arm is moved horizontally across the body. In many patients with recurrent posterior instability this test will produce a sudden jerk when the humeral head **slides off the back of the glenoid. When the arm is returned to the original position of 90 degrees of abduction, a second jerk may be observed—that of the humeral head returning to the glenoid**.

- **Push–Pull Test** For the push–pull test the patient lies supine with the shoulder off the edge of the table. The arm is in 90 degrees of abduction and 30 degrees of flexon.Standing next to the patient's hip, the examiner pulls up on the wrist with one hand while pushing down on the proximal humerus with the other. The shoulders of normal, relaxed patients often will allow 50% posterior translation on this test. Greater degrees of translation, apprehension, or reproduction of the **patient's symptoms suggest pathologic posterior instability. This test should be performed on both sides to compare the degrees of translation and the patient's response.**

Ans-6: (c) Lateral two lumbricals and opponens pollicis
Ref: Read the text below
Sol:

- The **median nerve innervates** the abductor pollicis brevis, opponens pollicis, and two **lateral lumbricals.**
- The **ulnar nerve innervates all interossei (palmar and dorsal), the adductor pollicis**, and the two medial lumbricals.

Ans-7: (d) Ulnar and radial
Ref: Read the text below
Sol:

- The **metacarpophalangeal joint of the ring finger is flexed by the lumbrical, palmar, and dorsal interosseous** muscles, which are innervated by the ulnar nerve. The extensor digitorum, which is innervated by the **radial nerve, extends this joint.**
- The musculocutaneous and axillary nerves do not supply muscles of the hand. The **median nerve supplies the lateral two lumbricals,**which can flex metacarpophalangeal joints of the index and middle fingers.

Ans-8: (b) Membranous ventricular septal defect
Ref: Read the text below
Sol :

- **Persistent truncus arteriosus** results from failure of the aorticopulmonary septum to form. **Normally, the aorticopulmonary septum divides** the truncus arteriosus into the ascending aorta and the pulmonary trunk.
- The **aorticopulmonary septum also contributes to** the formation of the membranous portion of the interventricular septum. When the aorticopulmonary septum does not **form, the truncus arteriosus persists rather than being divided, and the membranous interventricular septum is incomplete.**
- **Because neural crest cells contribute to** the formation of the aorticopulmonary septum, it is believed that this defect may result from a defect in migration of neural crest cells.

Ans-9: (a) Anterior wall of left ventricle
Ref: Read the text below
Sol:
The following is a description of the frequencies of critical narrowing and thrombosis of each of the 3 main arterial trunks and the corresponding sites of myocardial lesions:

- **Left anterior descending coronary artery** (40-50%, most common) - Lesions in anterior wall of left ventricle near apex and anterior 2/3 of interventricular septum.
- **Right coronary artery** (30-40%) - Lesions in inferior or posterior wall of left ventricle, posterior 1/3 of interventricular septum, and posterior right ventricular free wall in some cases.
- **Left circumflex coronary artery** (15-20%) - Lesions in lateral wall of left ventricle

Ans-10: (c) Long thoracic nerve
Ref: Read the text below
Sol:

- In the **normal individual, the pull of the serratus anterior** muscle keeps the medial border against the thoracic wall. However, when there is injury to the long thoracic nerve which supplies the serratus anterior muscle, **there is winging of scapula, which is excessive prominence of the medial border of the scapula.**
- Actions of the serratus anterior muscle are:

1. It **pulls the scapula forwards** around the chest wall to protect the upper limb, as in pushing and punching actions
2. It rotates the scapula **so that the glenoid cavity is turned upwards, which allows abduction of the arm above 90 degree.**

In **paralysis of the serratus anterior muscle, when movements** like pushing, punching and raising arm above 90 degree is attempted, winging of scapula occurs.

- Long Thoracic **nerve is also known as "Nerve of Bell".**
- Serratus anterior muscle arises by eight **digitations from the upper eight ribs.**

Ans-11: (b) Cotton wool spots
Ref: Read the text below
Sol:

- Cotton wool spots, hemorrhage, **and papilledema are common. Fibrinoid necrosis occurs on the arterioles of many organs.**
- **Earlier manifestations of arteriosclerosis** include thickening of the vessel wall.
- This is manifested by **obscuring of the venous column at arterial crossings.**

Ans-12: (c) Short gastric artery
Ref: Read the text below
Sol:

- The **lesser curvature of the stomach** is supplied by the right gastric artery inferiorly, and theleft gastric artery superiorly, **which also supplies the cardiac region.**
- The greater curvature is supplied by the **right gastroepiploic artery inferiorly and the left gastroepiploic arterysuperiorly.**
- The fundus of the stomach, and also the upper portion of the **greater curvature, is supplied by the short gastric artery.**

Ans-13: (d) Weakness of the lower lip on the same side
Ref: Read the text below
Sol :

- The motor **component (special visceral efferent) of the faci**al nerve (CN VII) exits the skull via the stylomastoid foramen, passes lateral to the styloid process, and then enters the parotid gland. Within the gland, two divisions can usually be identified (upper and lower), which in turn give off five named branches that **innervate the muscles of the face.**
- **The upper division gives rise to the temporal and zygomatic branches, which collectively innervate the frontalis, corrugators, and orbicularis oculi muscles.**
- The lower division gives off the buccal, mandibular, and cervical branches.
- The largest, the buccal, **innervates the muscles attaching to the upper lip, including the orbicularis oris and the levators, as well as the buccinators and the muscles of the nose.**

Ans-14: (a) Inferior rectal veins
Ref: Read the text below
Sol:

	SITE	PORTAL VESSEL	SYSTEMIC VESSELS
1.	Umbilicus	Paraumbilical veins	Superficial veins of abdominal wall
2.	Lower third of esophagus	Esophageal branches of left gastric vein	Esophageal veins draining the middle third into azygos vein
3.	Anal canal	Superior rectal veins	Middle and inferior rectal veins
4.	Bare area of liver	Hepatic venules	Phrenic and intercostal veins
5.	Posterior abdominal wall	Veins of retroperitoneal organs (duodenum, ascending and descending colon)	Retroperitoneal veins of the posterior abdominal wall
6.	Liver (if ductus venosus persists)	Left branch of portal vein	Inferior vena cava

Ans-15: (a) Anterior lateral and around the aorta
Ref: GRAY'S ANATOMY 40TH 1045
Sol:
COELIAC PLEXUS

- The **coeliac plexus is the largest major autonomic plexus, sited** at the level of the twelfth thoracic and first lumbar vertebrae.
- It is a dense network uniting two **large coeliac ganglia and surrounds the coeliac artery and the root of the superior mesenteric artery.**
- It is **posterior to the stomach and lesser sac, anterior** to the crura of the diaphragm and the commencement of the abdominal aorta, and lies between the suprarenal glands.
- The plexus and ganglia are **joined by greater and lesser splanchnic nerves and branches from the vagus and phrenic nerves.**
- **The plexus extends as numerous secondary** plexuses along adjacent arteries.
- The **coeliac ganglia** are irregular masses on each side of the coeliac trunk adjacent to the suprarenal glands.
- They lie **anterior to the crura of the diaphragm.**
- The **right ganglion** is posterior to the inferior vena cava, the left ganglion posterior to the origin of the splenic artery.
- The **ipsilateral greater splanchnic nerve joins** the upper part of each ganglion.
- The lower part of each ganglion forms a distinct subdivision usually termed the aorticorenal ganglion.
- This **receives the ipsilateral lesser splanchnic nerve and gives origin to the majority of the renal plexus.**
- It most commonly lies anterior to the origin of the renal artery.
- The coeliac plexus is connected to **or gives rise to the phrenic, splenic, hepatic, superior mesenteric, suprarenal, renal and gonadal plexuses.**

Ans-16: (a) Trapezoid in cross section
Ref: GRAY'S 40th ed., 1295
Sol:

- The **male urethra is18-20 cm long and extends from the internal** orifice in the urinary bladder to the external opening, or meatus, at **the end of the penis. It may be considered in two parts .**
- The relatively long anterior urethra (16 cm long) lies within the perineum (proximally) and the penis (distally) **surrounded by the corpus spongiosum and is functionally a conduit.**
- The relatively short **posterior urethra (4 cm) lies in the pelvis proximal to** the corpus spongiosum and is acted upon by the urogenital sphincter mechanisms and also acts as a conduit.
- The anterior urethra is subdivided into a proximal component, the bulbar urethra, which is surrounded by the **bulbospongiosus and is entirely within the perineum, and a pendulous or penile component, which continues on to the tip of the penis.**
- The posterior urethra is divided into preprostatic, prostatic, and membranous segments.
- In the flaccid penis, the urethra as a whole presents a double curve.
- **Except during the passage of fluid along** it, the urethral canal is a mere slit: in transverse section, the slit is transversely arched in the prostatic **part, in the preprostatic and membranous portions it is stellate, in the bulbar and penile portions it is transverse, while at the external orifice it is sagittal**

MEMBRANOUS PART

- The **membranous part of the urethra is the shortest (c.1.5 cm), least dilatable and**, with the exception of the external orifice, the narrowest, section of the urethra.

PREPROSTATIC PART

- The preprostatic urethra is c.1-1.5 cm in length, extending almost vertically from the bladder neck to the superior aspect of the verumontanum.

PROSTATIC PART

- The **prostatic urethra is c.3-4 cm in length and tunnels** through the substance of the prostate closer to the anterior than **the posterior surface of the gland.**
- The **urethra turns anteriorly as it passes** through the prostate making an angle of 35.
- Throughout most of its length the posterior wall possesses a midline ridge, the urethral crest, which projects into the **lumen causing it to appear crescentic in transverse section.**

- **On each side of the crest** there is a shallow depression, termed the prostatic sinus, the floor of which is perforated by the orifices of c.15-20 prostatic ducts.
- An elevation, the verumontanum (colliculus seminalis), at about the middle of the length of the urethral crest, contains the slit-**like orifice of the prostatic utricle.**
- **On both sides of, or just within, this orifice are the two small openings of the ejaculatory ducts.**
- The prostatic utricle is a cul-de-sac c.6 mm long, which runs upwards and backwards in the substance of the prostate behind its median lobe.
- Its walls are composed of fibrous tissue, **muscular fibres and mucous membrane; the latter is pitted by the openings of numerous small glands.**

Ans-17: (c) Infraorbital nerve
Ref: Gray's 40th 699
Sol:
MAXILLARY NERVE

- The maxillary nerve is a sensory division of the trigeminal nerve.
- Most of the branches from **the maxillary nerve arise in the pterygopalatine fossa.**
- It gives rise to the zygomatic and infraorbital nerves that pass into the orbit through the inferior orbital fissure and two others that pass through the **pterygopalatine ganglion without synapsing and are distributed to the nose, palate and pharynx.**

Zygomatic nerve

- The zygomatic nerve is located close to the base of the lateral wall of the orbit. It soon divides into two branches, the zygo-maticotemporal and **the zygomaticofacial nerves, which run for only a short distance in the orbit before passing onto the face through the lateral wall of the orbit.**
- They may either enter separate canals within the zygomatic bone or the zygomatic nerve itself may enter the bone before dividing.
- The zygomaticotemporal nerve exits the zygomatic bone **on its medial surface, and pierces the temporal fascia to supply the skin over the temple.**
- It also gives a branch to the lacrimal nerve which may carry parasympathetic fibres to the **lacrimal gland .**

Infraorbital nerve

- The infraorbital nerve initially lies in the infraorbital groove on the floor of the orbit.
- The infraorbital nerve supplies the skin of the lower **eyelid, possibly the conjunctiva, and skin over the upper jaw, and also provides the middle and anterior** superior alveolar nerves.

Ans-18: (b) Bulbourethral gland
Ref: Read the text below
Sol :

- The **bulbourethral glands are paired structures** located within the deep perineal pouch, embedded within the sphincter urethrae. Their ducts pass to the spongy urethra. The homologous female structures are the greater vestibular (Barthlin's) glands, **which are located in the superficial perineal pouch.**
- The bulbospongiosus muscles lie superficial to the bulb of the penis in males and to the bulbs of the vestibule in females.
- The corpora cavernosa are paired **structures, portion of the cavernous erectile tissue, that form a large portion of the penile shaft in males and of the body of the clitoris in females.**

Ans-19: (d) Tumor in the area of the pineal gland
Ref: Read the text below
Sol :

- The first **lines of the question clearly suggest a brain tumor.** The additional ocular findings (loss of upper gaze and "sunset eyes" – the upper part of the sclera is visible above the downward-**looking irises) locate it to the pineal gland area.**
- **The frontal lobe when pressed on by tumors** produces changes in social behavior and olfactory and visual deficits.
- Nelson syndrome occurs in people who have had bilateral adrenalectomies performed for Cushing disease **secondary to a nonresected pituitary microadenoma. The symptom is that of pressure on the chiasma (hemianopsia)**

Ans-20: (b) Pudendal nerve
Ref: Read the text below
Sol:

- **External haemorrhoids occur below the pectinate** line and are very painful. This region is supplied by Inferior Rectal nerve (S2, S3, **S4), a somatic nerve, which in turn is a branch of the pudendal nerve.**
- In **contrast, the anal canal above the pectinate line is supplied by Sympathetic** (Inferior Hypogastric plexus, L1 and L2) and Parasympathetic (**Pelvic Splanchnic, S2, S3, S4)**
- **They carry pain fibres from the internal haemorrhoids.**

Ans 21: (b) It is inherited as an autosomal recessive disorder
Ref: Read the text below
Sol

- Romano-Ward **syndrome is a heterogeneous disorder associated with** prolonged QT interval and recurrent syncope, cardiac arrest, or **sudden death.**
- It is inherited in an autosomal dominant pattern and several mutations involving sodium and potassium channels have been recognized. Jervell and Lange-**Nielsen syndrome is inherited in an autosomal recessive pattern.**
- It is associated with prolonged QT interval, history of recurrent **syncope or sudden death, and congenital neural deafness.**
- The Romano-Ward syndrome is more frequent than the **Jervell and Lange-Nielsen syndrome.**

Ans-22: (c) They are multipolar
Ref: Read the text below
Sol:

- They have centrally located nuclei as in the picture
- The dorsal root ganglia develop in the embryo from neural crest cells.
- These neurons are of the pseudo-unipolar type, meaning they have an axon with two branches that act as a single axon, often referred to as a distal process and a proximal process.

Ans-23: (d) Equillibrium potential for Na+ is + 60 mV.
Ref.: Ganong's Physiology, 23rd edn. Pg. 8.
Sol :

- The **gradient present on an ion due to the difference** in its intracellular and extracellular concentration is called concentration **gradient whereas the gradient present due to the charge on an ion is called electrical gradient.**
- **The membrane potential at which the equilibrium** exists is called as equllibrium potential.
- In case of Na+ the extracellular concentration is much higher compared to the intracellular concentration, and the electrical gradient is also towards the inside (the RMP is normally -70 mV and the equilibrium **potential for Na+ is – 60 mV), so any alteration of the concentration of Na+ would affect the RMP.**

Ans-24: (d) Residual volume and expiratory reserve volume.
Ref.: Harrison's, 17th edn. Pg. 1587.
Sol :

- Functional **residual capacity is the volume of air** in the lungs at the end of a normal exhalation. It is a combination of residual volume and expiratory reserve volume.
- FRC = ERV + RV = **1100 + 1200 = 2300 ml**

Ans-25: (a) Intrinsic factor
Ref: Read the text below
Sol:

- **Intrinsic factor is critical** for the absorption of vitamin B12 by the ileum.
- None of the other **substances is secreted by parietal cells.**
- Gastrin, somatostatin, and CCK are secreted by **specialized GI endocrine cells, whereas chylomicrons are produced by enterocytes.**

Ans-26: (c) Gastric
Ref: Read the text below
Sol:

- Although the **cephalic and intestinal phases stimulate** gastric secretion, the gastric phase is,by **far, the most important.**

Ans-27: (b) Increase in tissue pH
Ref: Read the text below
Sol:
All will favor the unloading of oxygen from hemoglobin except a rise in pH.

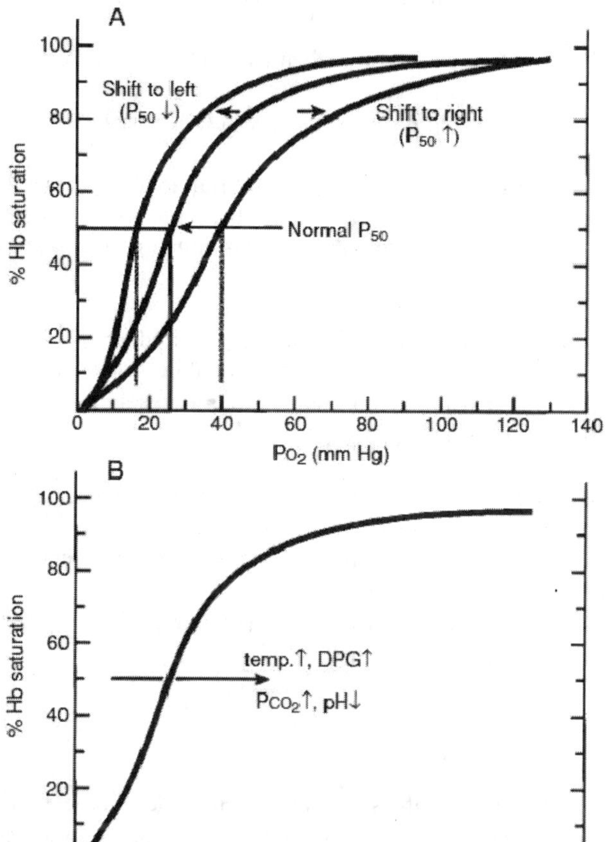

Hemoglobin (Hb) binding affinity for O2. A, A shift in the oxyhemoglobin equilibrium curve affects the P50. **B,** An increase in temperature, $[H^+]$, or arterial PCO2 causes a rightward shift of the oxyhemoglobin equilibrium curve. A P50 increase indicates that binding affinity for oxygen decreases, which favors the unloading of O2 from Hb at the tissue level. An increase in red cell levels of 2,3-diphosphoglycerate (DPG) will also shift the curve to the right. The increase in DPG occurs with hypoxemic conditions.

Ans-28: (c) Hb level
Ref: Harrison's principle of internal medicine 17th ed pg 229
Sol:
Hypoxia or tissue hypoxia refers to the unavailability of adequate oxygen to the cells to maintain aerobic metabolism. It is used to denote deficiency of oxygen supply at the tissue level. Depending on the mechanism of occurrence there are four types of hypoxia is of four- hypoxic hypoxia, histotoxic hypoxia, anemic hypoxia and stagnant hypoxiat.
Hypoxemia, on the other hand, is reduced blood PO_2 less than 80 mms of Hg.

Respiratory Hypoxemia

- When hypoxia occurs consequent to respiratory failure, Pa_{O2} declines, and when respiratory failure is persistent, the hemoglobin-oxygen ($Hb\text{-}O_2$) dissociation curve is displaced to the right, with greater quantities of O_2 released at any level of tissue P_{O2}.
- Arterial hypoxemia, i.e., a reduction of O_2 saturation of arterial blood (Sa_{O2}), and consequent cyanosis are likely to be more marked when such depression of Pa_{O2} results from pulmonary disease than when the depression occurs as the result of a decline in the fraction of oxygen in inspired air (FI_{O2}).
- In this latter situation, Pa_{CO2} falls secondary to anoxia-induced hyperventilation and the $Hb\text{-}O_2$ dissociation curve is displaced to the left, limiting the decline in Sa_{O2} at any level of Pa_{O2}.
- The most common cause of respiratory hypoxia is ventilation-perfusion mismatch resulting from perfusion of poorly ventilated alveoli.
- Respiratory hypoxemia may also be caused by hypoventilation, and it is then associated with an elevation of Pa_{CO2}
- These two forms of respiratory hypoxia are usually correctable by inspiring 100% O_2 for several minutes (i.e., FI_{O2} of 100%)
- A third cause is shunting of blood across the lung from the pulmonary arterial to the venous bed (intrapulmonary right-to-left shunting) by perfusion of nonventilated portions of the lung, as in pulmonary atelectasis or through pulmonary arteriovenous connections. The low Pa_{O2} in this situation is correctable only in part by an FI_{O2} of 100%.

Hypoxemia Secondary to High Altitude

- As one ascends rapidly to 3000 m (~10,000 ft), the reduction of the O_2 content of inspired air (FI_{O2}) leads to a decrease in alveolar P_{O2} to about 60 mmHg, and a condition termed high-altitude illness develops.
- At higher altitudes, arterial saturation declines rapidly and symptoms become more serious; and at 5000 m, unacclimatized individuals usually cease to be able to function normally

Anemic Hypoxia

- A reduction in hemoglobin concentration of the blood is attended by a corresponding decline in the O_2-carrying capacity of the blood.
- Although the **Pa_{O2} is normal in anemic hypoxia**, the absolute quantity of O_2 transported per unit volume of blood is diminished i.e., the oxygen content of the blood is reduced.
- As the anemic blood passes through the capillaries and the usual quantity of O_2 is removed from it, the P_{O2} and saturation in the venous blood decline to a greater degree than normal.

Ans-29: (d) All of above
Ref: Read the text below
Sol:

- The **sodium ion pump is responsible** for the active transport of the sodium ions across the cell membrane.
- **Glucose absorption from the gut, potassium excretion** in the distal convoluted tubule and water reabsorption from the collecting **ducts are other examples of active transport.**
- Water reabsorption from the proximal convoluted tubule occurs **due to the concentration gradient.**

Ans-30: (b) Occurs in distal portion of the broken axons leaving empty tubule
Ref.: Essential orthopedics, Maheswari, - 50
Sol :

- Nerve **degeneration : The part of neuron distal** to the point of injury undergoes secondary or Wallerian degeneration. Wallerian degeneration is a feature of axonotmesis and neurotmesis.
- The **rate of recovery of axon is 1 mm/day.**
- **Neuropraxia is a physiological disruption of conduction** in the nerve fiber; no structural changes occur. Recovery occurs spontaneously within a few weeks and is complete.

Ans-31: (b) Decreases renal tubular reabsorption of calcium
Ref.: KD **Tripathi, 6th edn. Pg. 327-28.**
Sol :

Functions of parathormone

- Increases resorption of calcium from bone.
- Increases calcium reabsorption in the distal tubule of the nephrons.
- It also promotes phosphate excretion and thus lowers serum phosphate level.
- It activates I-alpha hydroxylase and enhances the formation of calcitriol (active form of vitamin D) in the kidney.

Ans 32: (c) Hyperkalemia
Ref.: Read the text below
Sol :

- **Acidemia is the presence of excess H□□ ions** in blood, which tends to create a rise in the extracellular potassium concentration.
- The rule of thumb for an **inorganic acid** that causes the acidity is that a decrease in pH of **0.1 unit leads to a rise in plasma potassium of 0.6 milliequivalents per liter.**
- The effect of an **organic acid is a lot less**. The mechanism responsible for the relationship between pH and extracellular potassium concentration is not completely understood.
- One effect is that the intracellular acidosis **inhibits K □□influx by reducing the activity of the Na-K-pump.**
- An exchange of extracellular **H □□for intracellular K□□ might also contribute.**

Ans 33: (a) Hemoglobin A1c (HbA1c)
Ref.: Read the text below
Sol :

- The **hallmark of poorly controlled diabetes mellitus** is elevated blood glucose, which causes **unphysiological glycosylation of proteins.**
- An important long-term measure of blood glucose control in patients with diabetes mellitus is to monitor the modification of hemoglobin A to form glycated hemoglobins. HbA1c is the major subfraction, **and determination of HbA1c is usually achieved by ion-exchange or gel electrophoresis.**
- The **level of glycated hemoglobins** in the blood is directly related to the average blood glucose levels over the life span of the hemoglobin in the circulation. Since the half-life of red blood cells is **about 120 days, a single determination of glycated hemoglobin reflects the average blood glucose level during the preceding 8–12 weeks.**
- **Lipoprotein (a) is a lipoprotein particle** implicated in atherosclerosis and thrombosis. Albumin is the most abundant plasma protein, but is not significantly affected by glycosylation.
- **Myoinositol is a signaling molecule the decrease** in response of which to elevated sorbitol has been suggested as a complication of diabetes.
- **Sorbitol** is another sugar derivative, unrelated to HbA1c that is believed important in causing other diabetic complications such as cataracts and peripheral neuropathy.

Ans-34: (d) V_4 – CNS
Ref: Ganong 23rd edi pg 666
Sol:

- **V_1 or V_{1A} receptors are** found on the vascular smooth muscle- mediates vasoconstriction. V_{1A} receptors are also found in the liver- cause glycogenolysis and in the area postrema of the brain where vasopressin acts to cause a decrease in cardiac output.

- **V_2 receptors** are found on the apical or luminal membrane of the P cells of the collecting duct of the kidney. ADH acting via the V_2 receptors causes insertion of water channels- acquaporin 2, thereby increasing the water reabsorption.

- V_3 **receptors (or V_{1B} receptors) are found on the anterior pituitary, where they mediate increased secretion of ADH**

Ans-35: (b) It produces its effect by increasing distal tubular permeability to sodium
Ref: Read the text below
Sol:

- **Aldosterone binds to an intracellular receptor** that causes an increased synthesis of a variety of proteins, including K+ **and Na+ ion channels and Na+-K+-ATPase, which together act to increase Na+ reabsorption and K+ secretion by the tubular cells of the distal nephron.**
- **H+ secretion is also enhanced by aldosterone**.
- Aldosterone secretion is stimulated by a decrease in blood volume (through the renin-angiotensin system) and by **increased plasma K+ concentrations**.
- High blood pressure, if it has any effect on aldosterone, **will cause a decrease in its secretion.**

Ans-36: (b) Intracellular volume
Ref: Read the text below
Sol:

- The **increased secretion of antidiuretic hormone (ADH)** increases the permeability of the distal nephron to water and therefore **increases the reabsorption of water from the kidney.**
- The excessive reabsorption of water dilutes the extracellular fluid, producing a decrease in plasma **sodium, osmolarity, and oncotic pressure.**
- The decreased extracellular osmolarity causes water to flow from the extracellular fluid compartment into the intracellular fluid **compartment, increasing intracellular volume.**
- Because more water is being reabsorbed, less is excreted and urinary flow is decreased

Ans-37: (a) More tension is exerted on the wall of the aneurysm
Ref: Read the text below
Sol:

- **Tension in the wall of a vessel** represents a force which, if large enough, will cause the wall to rupture.
- In blood vessels,the source is the pressure inside the **vessel,but the magnitude of wall tension also depends upon the radius of the vessel.**
- The relationship is: **T : P X r**. At a given pressure, the greater the vessel readius the greater the wall tension.
- Thus, because an aneurysm had a greater radius, it will have **a greater wall tension and is more likely to rupture than the surrounding normal aorta.**

Ans 38: (c) Dipeptides and tripeptides use transporters that are different from the defective amino acid transporters.
Ref: Read the text below
Sol

- **Amino acids, as well as dipeptides and tripeptides**, use different brush border transporters for their uptake.
- **Dipeptides and tripeptides** are not taken up passively by any part of the GI tract

Ans 39: (b) Lateral pterygoid.
Ref.: Read the text below
Sol

- **The temporalis, masseter, and medial and lateral pterygoid muscles** attach to the mandible and are the major muscles involved in movements of the jaw.
- The **buccinator muscle**, which controls the contents of the mouth during mastication, is innervated by the seventh cranial nerve and constitutes the chief muscle of facial expression.
- The **lateral pterygoid muscles**, acting bilaterally, protract the jaw and, acting unilaterally, rotate the jaw during chewing.
- Because the fibers of the **superior head of the lateral pterygoid muscle insert onto the anterior aspect of the articular disk of the temporomandibular** joint as well as onto the head of the mandible, spasm of this muscle, such as in a yawn, can result in dislocation of the mandible by pulling the disk anterior to the articular tubercle. Reduction is accomplished by pushing the mandible downward and back, so that the head of the mandible reenters the mandibular fossa.
- **The temporalis, medial pterygoid, and masseter muscles primarily elevate the jaw in molar occlusion**.

Ans-40: (c) Plateau phase of the action potential
Ref.: Harrison-1370
Sol :

- During **the plateau of the action potential** (phase 2), there is a slow inward current through L-**type Ca^{2+} channels in the sarcolemma.**
- The depolarizing current not only extends across the surface of the cell but penetrates deeply **into the cell by way of the ramifying T tubular system. The absolute quantity of Ca2+ that crosses** the sarcolemma and T system is relatively small and itself appears to be insufficient to bring about full activation of the contractile apparatus.
- However, this Ca2+ **current triggers the release of much larger quantities of Ca2+ from the SR, a process termed Ca2+**- induced Ca2+ release. The latter is a major determinant of intracytoplasmic [Ca2+] and therefore of myocardial contractility.

Ans 41: (c) During manometric assessment, unless the patient is having pain there may be no detectable multiphasic, high-amplitude, simultaneous esophageal contractions.
Ref.: Read the text below
Sol:

- **The chest pain of diffuse esophageal spasm is often indistinguishable from that of angina pectoris of cardiac origin.**
- Many patients undergo **cardiac catheterization to rule out coronary artery disease**. Patients may experience slow emptying of the esophagus, but obstructive symptoms and regurgitation of food are unusual.
- **Psychiatric disorders (depression, psychosomatic complaints, and anxiety) have been documented** in more than 80% of patients with esophageal contraction abnormalities. The classic manometric criteria of diffuse esophageal spasm are simultaneous, multiphasic, repetitive, high-amplitude contractions occurring after a **swallow and spontaneously. These changes may not be detected if manometry is performed when the patient is having no pain.**
- As the cause of esophageal spasm is unknown, treatment is far from ideal. Conservative management—avoidance of "trigger" foods **and drinks, psychiatric counseling, treatment of reflux, esophageal dilatations, use of histamine H 2 blockers, anti-spasmodics, and smooth muscle relaxants—should always be attempted first.**
- **Esophagomyotomy provides** no lasting relief of esophageal spasm for as many as 50% of patients and should be used only in a minority of these patients.

Ans-42: (c) Accumulation or phytanic acid
Ref.: Harrison's, - 2664.
Sol :

- **Refsum's disease is due to** accumulation of phytanic acid due to deficiency of enzyme phytanic acid hydroxylase.
- It is **an autosomal recessive condition characte**rized by mixed motor and sensory neuropathy, palpable nerves, ataxia, **retinitis pigmentosa, night blin**dness, sensorineural deafness, elevated CSF protein, and age of onset before 20 years.
- Histopathologically **severe onion bulb formation is seen.**

Ans-43: (c) Thromboxane A2 and prostocyclin (PG12)
Ref.: Lippincott's Biochemistry 2nd edn. Pg. 186.
Sol :

Thromboxane A_2	**Prostacyclin**
Produced primarily by platelets	Produced primarily by endothelium of vessels
Promotes platelet aggregation	Inhibits platelet aggregation
Decreases formation of cAMP	Increases formation of cAMP
Vasoconstriction	Vasodilatation
Mobilizes intracellular calcium	
Contraction of smooth muscle	

Ans-44: (b) 6 moles of ATP
Ref.: Vasudevan Biochemistry - 95.
Sol :

- **Energy requirement for gluconeogenesis**

▪ Six ATP's are required to generate one glucose molecule from pyruvate
o 2 molecules of pyruvate → oxaloacetate = 2 ATP
o 2 molecules of oxaloacetate →phosphoenolpyruvate (2 GTP) = 2 ATP
o 2 molecules of 3 phosphoglycerate → 1-3 bisphosphoglycerate = 2 ATP
▪ Total = 6 ATP.

Ans-45: (c) It forms part of the disaccharide sucrose
Ref.: Lippincott's Biochemistry, 2nd edn. Pg. 120, 130.
Sol :

- **Glucose is reduced** by aldose reductase to form sorbitol
- **Glucose is a monosaccharide (hexose)**. It has an aldehyde group (CHO) and hence is an aldose (aldohexose).
- Fructose **is a ketohexose.**
- Glucose exists in **biologic systems as a pyranose ring.**
- Sucrose **consists of glucose + fructose.**

Ans-46: (c) Activates the extrinsic pathway
Ref: Read the text below
Sol:

- **Factor III activates** the extrinsic pathway.
- Factor III **is also known as thromboplastin** or tissue factor.

Ans 47 : (d) One locus, multiple normal alleles
Ref: Read the text below
Sol:

- **Polymorphic loci** have multiple alleles because of DNA sequence variation, **including one or more with frequencies greater than 1%.**
- This higher frequency and benign connotation differentiate polymorphic loci **from those that harbor multiple disease-causing alleles.**
- The **DNA sequence changes** may alter restriction sites [producing restriction fragment length polymorphisms (RFLPs)], change the numbers of repeated segments [producing **variable numbers of tandem repeats (VNTRs)], or alter the genetic code (producing variant proteins, or protein polymorphisms).**
- **Polymorphisms may cosegregate** (be inherited together) with disease alleles, allowing diagnosis by linkage analysis or estimates of risk through allele association (a.k.a. linkage disequilibrium, as with **certain HLA alleles and diabetes mellitus).**
- **Different mutant alleles may cause indistinguishable phenotypes (allelic heterogeneity), as may mutations at different loci (genetic heterogeneity).**

Ans 48 : (d) In both the cytosol and mitochondria
Ref. Read the text below
Sol:

- The **synthesis of 3-hydroxy-3- methylglutaryl** CoA requires the condensation of **three acetyl CoA groups.**
- The two enzymatic steps involved are the first two steps of cholesterol synthesis and ketone **body synthesis. While cholesterol synthesis occurs in the cytosol of** most mammalian tissues, ketone body synthesis can only occur in the mitochondria of liver cells.
- **Not only are cholesterol synthesis** and ketone body synthesis separated by **compartmentalizetion, they are separated by metabolic needs.**

- **Cholesterol synthesis** is an anabolic pathway that takes place when acetyl CoA production from excess dietary precursors is possible.
- In contrast, ketone body production by the liver occurs when acetyl CoA levels from β oxidation are high. This catabolic **situation exists during fasting, starvation, and uncontrolled diabetes.**

Ans 49 : (c Carbamoyl phosphate synthase deficiency
Ref: Read the text below
Sol:

- **Carbamoyl phosphate (CAP) synthase I** is found in mitochondrial matrix and is the first step in urea synthesis, condensing CO2 and $NH4^+$. **Hyperammonemia occurs when CAP is deficient.**
- **CAP synthase II forms CAP** as the first step in pyrimidine synthesis. Its complete deficiency would probably be a lethal mutation.
- When its activity is decreased, purine catabolism to uric acid is decreased, decreasing the possibility of hyperuricemia. In contrast, gout, **Lesch-Nyhan syndrome,high xanthine oxidase activity, and von Gierke's disease [glycogen storage disease type Ia (232200)] all lead to increased urate production and excretion.**

Ans 50 : (a) Aspartate
Ref: Read the text below
Sol:

- During **purine ring biosynthesis**, the amino acid glycine is completely **incorporated to provide C4, C5, and N7.**
- Glutamine contributes **N3 and N9, aspartate provides N1,** and derivatives of tetrahydrofolate furnish **C2 and C8.** Carbon dioxide is the **source of C6.**
- In pyrimidine ring synthesis, **C2 and N3** are derived from carbamoyl phosphate, while **N1, C4, C5, and C6** come from aspartate.

Ans 51: (a) Half should contain no radioactivity
Ref: Read the text below
Sol:

- The **replication of double-stranded DNA is semiconservative**, meaning that each strand separates and serves as a template for synthesis of a new complementary strand.
- The **first round of replication of a labeled DNA helix** in a cold (unlabeled) solution will yield two daughter double-stranded molecules, **each with one labeled and one unlabeled strand.**
- The second round of replication will yield four double-stranded DNA molecules.
- Two of these will have one original labeled strand and one unlabeled strand; the **other two will have two unlabeled strands and contain no radioactivity**.

Ans 52: (a) A specific excinuclease detects damaged areas
Ref: Read the text below
Sol:

- **Ultraviolet irradiation** causes thymine dimers to form in DNA. Replication is inhibited in cells until the pyrimidine dimmers are removed. **Removal of the damaged areas occurs in two ways.**
- The process can be simply reversed by a photoreactivating enzyme that cleaves **the dimers and yields the original bases. Blue light is required for this.**
- **Alternatively, the dimer is removed**. A UV-specific excinuclease nicks the dimer on its 5'side. DNA polymerase I replicates the damaged sequence,while the damaged sequence swings out.
- **Finally, the damaged piece is hydrolyzed by the 5□ to 3□ exonuclease activity of the DNA polymerase** I. DNA ligase then joins the new piece to the original DNA at the cleavage site.

Ans-53: (a) Atractyloside
Ref: Read the text below
Sol:

- A highly toxic glycoside isolated from Atractylis gummifera and other thistles.

- It inhibits **mitochondrial translocase i.e.inhibition of ADP/ATP translocation in inner mitochondria**. Its inhibitory action blocks oxidative phosphorylation of adenosine nucleotides through mitochondrial membranes.

INHIBITORS OF ETC

- Complex I (NADH DEHYDROGENASE)-
  - a.Amytal(barbiturate) b.Piercidin A c.Rotenone
- Complex II(SUCCINATE DEHYDROGENASE)-
  - a. Atpenins b. Malonate c. Carboxin d. TTFA e. HQ NITRIC OXIDE
- Complex III(CYT C REDUCTASE)-
  - a. Antimycin b. myxothiazol c. stigmatellin
- Complex IV (cyt. c reductase)-
  - a. cyanide b. azide c. sulfide d. co

Ans-54: (b) Fluoroacetate
Ref: Read the text below
Sol:
Fluoroacetate binds to CO A and forms fluoroacetyl coa. This fluoroacetyl coa condenses with oxaloacetate to form fluorocitrate which inhibits krebs cycle.
Inhibitors krebs cycle-

Enzyme	Inhibitor
1. Aconitase	- Fluoroacetate
2. Alpha ketoglutarate dehydrogenase	- Arsenate
3. Succinate dehydrogenase	- Malonate

Ans-55: (c) Glycogen phosphorylase
Ref: Read the text below
Sol:

- When the body **begins to starve it needs to break down its glycogen reserves** in order **to neurish the body so Glycogen phosphorylase will be activated**

Ans-56: (b) Brown colour is positive
Ref: Read the text below
Sol:

- **Rotheras test is a method of testing** urine for the presence of acetone or acetoacetic acid: a sign of diabetes mellitus.
- Strong ammonia is **added to a sample of urine saturated with ammonium** sulphate crystals and containing a small quantity of **sodium nitroprusside.**
- A purple colour confirms the presence of **acetone or acetoacetic acid.**

Ans. 57: (d) Excessive homogentisic acid in urine
Ref: Read the text below
Sol:

- **Alkaptonuria (black urine disease or alcaptonuria**) is a rare inherited genetic disorder of phenylalanine and tyrosine metabolism.
- This is an autosomal**recessive condition that is due to a defect in the enzyme homogentisate 1,2-dioxygenase**, which participates in the degradation oftyrosine.
- As a result, a toxic **tyrosine byproduct called homogentisic acid (or alkapton**) accumulates in the blood and is excreted in urine in large amounts (hence -uria).
- Excessive homogentisic acid causes damage to cartilage **(ochronosis, leading to osteoarthritis) and heart valves as well as precipitating as kidney stones**.

Ans. 58: (a) Can determine paternity
Ref: Read the text below
Sol:
Can determine paternity

- **Microsatellites, Simple Sequence Repeats (SSRs), or tandem repeats,** are repeating sequences of 1-6 base pairs of DNA.
- Microsatellites can be amplified for identification by the polymerase chain reaction (PCR) process, using the unique **sequences of flanking regions as primers so they can be reproduced.**
- As there are often many alleles present at a microsatellite locus,genotypes within pedigrees are often fully **informative, in that the progenitor of a particular allele can often be identified. In this way, microsatellites** are ideal for determining paternity, population genetic studies **and recombination mapping.**
- **Microsatellites owe their variability to an increased rate of mutation compared to other neutral regions of DNA.**

Ans. 59: (c) Aromatic amino acid decarboxylase
Ref.: Lippincott's Biochemistry - 266-67
Sol :

- In synthesis **of catecholamines, dopa is** decarboxylated to dopamine (dopa-decarboxylase). Catecholamines are **derived from tyrosine.**
- In synthesis of serotonin, 5-hydroxytryptophan is **decarboxylated to serotonin (decarboxylase). Serotonin is derived from tryptophan.**

Ans-60: (c) Globular proteins tend to fold into configurations that keep hydrophobic side chains in the interior of the molecule
Ref.: Lippincott's Biochemistry
Sol :

- The structure of **globular protein in aqueous solution** is compact, with a high density of the atoms in the core of the molecule. **Hydrophobic side chains are buried in the** interior whereas, hydrophilic groups are generally found on the surface of the molecule.
- The stability **of the alpha helix is mainly due to hydrogen bonding.**
- In globular proteins, alpha helices and beta strands are present.
- The primary structure of a polypeptide chain **determines its tertiary structure (three dimensional structures).**

Ans 61: (b) Isoniazid.
Ref: Read the text below
Sol:

- **Phenytoin** causes **cleft palate, microcephaly and mental retardation**, and screening is advised.
- **Retinoids** may cause hydrocephalus and neural tube defects. Alcohol in high concentrations causes the fetal alcohol syndrome.
- **Sodium valproate may cause neural tube defects.**

Ans 62: (d) Anthisan.
Ref: Read the text below
Sol:

- **Anthisan** contains mepyramine, an antihistamine**. Dequacaine** contains benzocaine and dequalinium, Merocaine contains benzocaine and cetylpyridinium, Burneze contains benzocaine, and **Proctosedyl** contains cinchocaine and hydrocortisone.

Ans 63: (c) Amitriptyline.
Ref: Read the text below
Sol:

- The antidote for **iron poisoning is desferrioxamine**; for **paracetamol it is** N-acetylcysteine or methionine; for morphine or other opiates it is naloxone, an oral opiate antagonist; **and for cyanide it is sodium thiosulphate or cobalt edetate.**

Ans 64: (c) Fentanyl.
Ref: Read the text below

Sol:

- **Fentanyl is a chemical relative of meperidine** that is nearly 100 times more potent than morphine.
- The **duration of action**, usually between 30 and 60 min after parenteral administration, is shorter than that of meperidine.
- **Fentanyl citrate** is only available for parenteral administration intramuscularly and intravenously.
- **Transbuccal ("lollipop") and transdermal patches avoid firstpass metabolism of fentanyl.**

Ans 65: (b) Tranylcypromine.
Ref: Read the text below
Sol:

- Fatalities have been reported when **fluoxetine and MAO inhibitors (MAOIs)** such as **tranylcypromine have been given simultaneously.**
- The **MAOIs** should be stopped at least two weeks before the administration of **fluoxetine or paroxetine.**
- The mechanism of this interaction is under **investigation.**

Ans 66: (d) Halothane.
Ref: Read the text below
Sol:

- **Halothane is a substituted alkane general anesthetic.**
- It undergoes **significant metabolism** in humans with about 20% of the absorbed dose recovered as metabolites.
- **Halothane can cause postoperative jaundice and hepatic necrosis with repeated administration in rare instances.**

Ans 67: (b) Left ventricular failure
Ref: Read the text below
Sol:

- **Digoxin toxicity** is depends on the plasma concentration of the drug and on the myocardial **sensitivity to it (often increased in heart failure).**
- **Toxicity** is more likely in the presence of hypokalamia, so diuretic therapy given with digoxin should either be potassium-sparing or given with potassium supplements.
- **Digoxin toxicity** is exacerbated by hypercalcaemia, verapamil, Beta-blockers, **amiodarone and quinidine.**

Ans 68: (c) Levofloxacin.
Ref: Read the text below
Sol:

- Both **levofloxacin and ciprofloxacin** are quinolones.
- **Levofloxacin** has greater activity against **pneumococci than ciprofloxacin.**

Ans 69: (d) Climetidine .
Ref: Read the text below
Sol:

- Other drugs associated with **gynaecomastia include tricyclic antidepressants, cytotoxic agents, phenothiazines, spironolactone, diethylstilbestrol (stilboestrol), digoxin and methyldopa.**
- **Methysergide** may cause retroperitoneal fibrosis.

Ans 70: (b) Phenothiazine.
Ref: Read the text below
Sol:

- Other drugs associated with **galactorrhoea include cimetidine, metoclopramide, L-dopa, oestrogens and benzodiazepines.**
- **Cannabis, alcohol, digoxin and spironolactone** are all known causes of gynaecomastia.

Ans 71: (a) It is chemically related to methysergid.
Ref: Read the text below

Sol:

- **Ergotamine is a powerful Alpha-adrenoreceptor blocker. Side effects include abdominal pain and vomiting.**
- **Repeated administration of high doses** may cause ergotism with gangrene and confusion. It is licensed for use in the treatment of migraine in patients who do not have any contraindications.
- It causes post-**partum contraction of the uterus. Pleural and peritoneal fibrosis may occur, as with methysergide.**

Ans 72: (d) Buscopan.
Ref: Read the text below
Sol:

- **Buscopan contains hyoscine**, which is a quaternary ammonium compound having antimuscarinic activity. It is indicated for symptomatic relief of gastrointestinal or genitourinary disorders characterised by smooth muscle spasm.
- **Zantac contains ranitidine**, which is an H2-receptor antagonist that promotes healing of peptic ulcers by reducing gastric output as a result of histamine H2-receptor blockade.
- **Nexium contains esomeprazole and Pariet contains rabeprazole**, both of which are proton pump inhibitors. The **proton pump inhibitors** inhibit gastric acid output by blocking the hydrogen–potassium–adenosine **triphosphatase enzyme system of the gastric parietal cells.**

Ans 73: (c) Diazepam.
Ref: Read the text below
Sol:
The following drugs should be avoided in renal failure:

- Antimicrobial drugs (amphotericin B, tetracyclines, nitrofurantoin).
- Aspirin and NSAIDs.
- Lithium.
- Narcotic analgesics.
- Potassium-sparing diuretics.

The following drugs should have their dose reduced when used in renal failure:

- Antimicrobials.
- Cardiac Drugs.
- Insulin.
- Chlorpropramide.
- H2¬-antagonists.

Ans-74: (a) Retrobulbar neuritis
Ref: Read **the text below**
Sol :
Ethambutol (commonly abbreviated **EMB** or simply **E**) is a bacteriostatic antimycobacterial drug prescribed to treat tuberculosis.
It is usually given in combination with other tuberculosis drugs, such as isoniazid, rifampicin and pyrazinamide.
It is sold under the trade names **Myambutol** and **Servambutol**.
Adverse effects

- Optic neuritis.[2] Hence contraindicated in children below 6 yrs of age.
- Red-green color blindness
- Peripheral neuropathy
- Arthralgia
- Hyperuricaemia
- Vertical nystagmus
- Milk skin reaction

Ans-75: (d) Growth retardation
Ref: Read the text below
Sol :
Pyridoxine deficiency

- Symptoms **include epithelial changes**
- Severe deficiency can lead to peripheral neuropathy, abnormal EEG, personality changes including **depression and confusion.**
- **In infants, diarrhea, seizures** and anemia has been reported.
- Microcytic, hypochromic anemia is due to diminished hemoglobin synthesis, as this is required in Hb synthesis.

Ans-76: (b) The German measles
Ref: Read the text below.
Sol:

- **Rubella is commonly known as the German measles** or the 3-day measles. It has also been called the easy measles, since the symptoms are quite mild.
- After an incubation period of 14–**21 days, German measles causes symptoms that are similar to the flu.**
- The primary symptom of rubella virus infection is the appearance of a rash (exanthem) on the face which spreads to the trunk and limbs and usually fades after three days (**that is why it is often referred to as three-day measles). The facial rash usually clears as it spreads to other parts of the body.**
- Other symptoms include **low grade fever, swollen glands (sub occipital & posterior cervical lymphadenopathy), joint pains, headache and conjunctivitis.**
- **The swollen glands or lymph nodes** can persist for up to a week and the fever rarely rises above 38 °C (100.4 °F).
- The rash of German measles is typically pink or light red. The rash causes itching and often lasts for about three days. The rash disappears after a few days with no staining or peeling of the skin.
- When the rash clears up, the patient may notice that his skin sheds in very small flakes wherever the rash **covered it. Forchheimer's sign occurs in 20% of cases, and is characterized by small, red papules on the area of the soft palate.**

Ans-77: (b) Secondary syphilis
Ref: Read the text below.
Sol:

- **Condylomata lata** or **condyloma latum**, is a cutaneous condition characterized by wart like lesions on the genitals.
- They are generally **symptoms of the secondary phase of syphilis, caused by the spirochete, Treponema pallidum.**
- **Condylomata lata occurs in about one** third of patients and is characterized by painless, mucosal, warty erosions. They tend to develop in warm, moist sites of the genitals and perineum.
- These lesions hold a high **accumulation of spirochetes and are highly infectious.**
- Complete resolution of the lesions is spontaneous and occurs after a few days to many weeks where it is **either resolved completely or enters the tertiary phase, defined by a latent state**

Ans-78: (c) Pneumocystis carinii pneumonia
Ref: Read the text below.
Sol:

- **Kaposi's sarcoma** in the lung is fairly uncommon, but must be kept in mind whenever a **patient who is HIV+ presents with dyspnea.**
- KS commonly causes pleural effusions, but may appear without effusions.
- PCP remains the most common **respiratory disease in HIV disease; failure to** respond to PCP therapy should prompt to search for other diagnoses, among them KS.

Ans-79: (d) Recover but continue to harbor live virus
Ref: Read the text below.
Sol:

- **CMV remains in the body indefinitely, probably** in multiple tissue sites as a latent virus.
- The virus is not eradicated when a person becomes immune compromised, so the virus **is free to multiply and cause further disease.**

Ans-80: (b) Metronidazole (Flagyl)
Ref: Read the text below.
Sol:

- **Human infection is** conventionally treated with metronidazole, tinidazole or nitazoxanide. **Although Metronidazole is the current first-line therapy, it is mutagenic in bacteria and carcinogenic** in mice, so should be avoided during pregnancy.
- It has not directly been linked to causing cancer in humans, only in other mammals, therefore **appears safe. One of the most common alternative treatments is berberine sulfate (found in Oregon grape root, goldenseal, yellowroot, and various other plants).**
- **Berberine has been shown to have an antimicrobial** and an antipyretic effect.
- Berberine compounds cause uterine stimulation, and so should be avoided in pregnancy.
- Continuously high **dosing of berberine may lead to bradycardia and hypotension in some individuals**

Ans-81: (a) Mental status changes, vomiting, and papilledema
Ref: Read the text below.
Sol:

- **Changes in the mental status of a patient, vomiting, and** papilledema are sure signs of increasing intracranial pressure, and **need immediate evaluation as to the cause.**

Ans-82: (c) Adequate views of the mastoids and sinuses
Ref: Read the text below.
Sol:

- The source of the abscess is **most likely the mastoid or paranasal** sinuses, so adequate views of these structures **are vital in detecting a brain abscess.**

Ans-83: (c) Most important toxin is hyaluronidase .
Ref: Ananthanarayan and Paniker's textbook of microbiology 8th ed pg 252.
Sol:

- Four **major toxins produced by clostridia** species are alpha, beta, epsilon, iota.
- Tha **alpha toxin is produced by all strains of clostridia and most predominantly by type A strain**
- **This is the most important** toxin biologically and is responsible for profound toxaemia in gas gangrene

Resistance:

- Spores are destroyed by boiling within five minutes but those of food poisoning strains of type A and certain type C strains resists boiling for 1-3 hours

Nagler's reaction

- When cl.perfringes is grown on a medium containing 6% agar, 5% fildes' peptic digest of sheep blood and 20 % human serum, with the antitoxin spread on one half of the plate, colonies on the other half without **the antitoxin will be surrounded by a zone of opacity. There will be no opacity around the colonies on the other half of the plate with the anti toxin due to the specific neutralisation of alpha** toxin. This specific lecithinase effect is known as nagler's reaction

Ans-84: (b) HTN.
Ref: Harrison's principle of internal medicine 17th ed pg 1254.
Sol:

Candidiasis have identified the following predisposing factors or conditions:

a) Antibacterial agents,
b) Indwelling intravascular catheters,
c) Hyperalimentation fluids,
d) Indwelling urinary catheters,
e) Parenteral glucocorticoids,
f) Respirators, neutropenia,
g) Abdominal and thoracic surgery,

h) Cytotoxic chemotherapy, and
i) Immunosuppressive agents for organ transplantation.
j) Patients with severe burns, low-birth-weight neonates, and persons using illicit iv drugs are also susceptible. Hiv-infected patients with low cd4+ t cell counts and patients with diabetes are susceptible to mucocutaneous infection, which may eventually develop into the disseminated form when other predisposing factors are encountered.
k) Women who receive antibacterial agents may develop vaginal candidiasis.

Ans-85: (a) Vertical Transmission.
Ref: Harrison's principle of internal medicine 17th ed pg 1275.
Sol:
Mode of infection

- Fecal oral route: E. histolytica is acquired by ingestion of viable cysts from fecally **contaminated water, food, or hands. Food**-borne exposure is most prevalent and is particularly likely when food **handlers are shedding cysts or food is being grown with feces-contaminated soil, fertilizer, or water. Besides the drinking of contaminated water, less common means of transmission include oral and anal sexual practices and—in rare instances—direct rectal inoculation through** colonic irrigation devices. Motile trophozoites are released from cysts in the small intestine and, in most patients, remain as harmless commensals in the large bowel
- Sexual transmission
- **Vectors such as flies, cockroaches and rodents**

1. Boy with skin ulcer on leg. Culture reveals beta hemolysis, Bacitracin sensitive. Cultures from school children with sore throat some days back also revealed beta hemolysis. What is the similarity between both
   a) **C carbohydrate antigen is different**
   b) **M protein is same**

Ans-86: (c) Rota virus.
Ref: Harrison's principle of internal medicine 17th ed pg 1206.
Sol:

- **Rotaviruses are members of the family Reoviridae.**
- The viral genome consists of 11 segments of double-strand RNA that are enclosed in a triple-layered, nonenveloped, **icosahedral capsid 75 nm in diameter.**
- Viral protein 6 (VP6), the major structural protein, is the target of commercial immunoassays and determines the group specificity of rotaviruses.
- There are seven major groups of **rotavirus (A through G); human illness is caused primarily by group A and, to a much lesser extent, by groups B and C. Two outer-capsid proteins, VP7 (G-protein) and VP4 (P-protein)**, determine serotype specificity, induce neutralizing antibodies, and form the basis for binary classification of rotaviruses (G and P types).
- The **segmented genome of rotavirus allows genetic reassortment** (i.e., exchange of genome segments between viruses) during co-infection—a property that may play a role in viral evolution and has been **utilized in the development of reassortant animal-human rotavirus–based vaccines.**

Ans-87: (c) A lumbricoides can cause pneumonia.
Ref: Read the text below.
Sol:

- **Larval worms are carried via** the bloodstream to the alveoli of the lungs, where they may cause pneumonia.
- **Transmission is usually hand to mouth.**
- The diagnosis is made by seeing the **characteristic eggs in a stool sample.**
- **There is no intermediate host.**

Ans-88: (C) Meningitis and respiratory complications
Ref: Read the text below.

Sol:

- **Complications with measles are relatively** common, ranging from relatively mild and less serious diarrhea, to pneumonia and acute encephalitis (and rarely subacute sclerosing panencephalitis); **corneal ulceration leading to corneal scarring.**
- **Complications are usually more severe amongst** adults who catch the virus.
- The most common fatal complications of measles are **meningitis and respiratory complications, such as pneumonia.**

Ans-89: (c) Calymmatobacterium granulomatis
Ref: Read the text below
Sol :

- **Calymmatobacterium granulomatis** is the etiologic agent of granuloma inguinale.
- The other organisms are **responsible for diseases other than granuloma inguinale.**

Ans 90 : (d) An imidazole such as itraconazole.
Ref– Read the text below
Sol:

- This patient has a **fungal infection requiring an oral antifungal, such as an imidazole, griseofulvin, or terbinafine**

Ans 91 : (d) Hypotension
Ref:Read the text below
Sol:
Acute Pancreatitis
Most common causes

- I - idiopathic. Thought to be hypertensive sphincter or microlithiasis.
- G - gallstone. Gallstones that travel down the common bile duct and which subsequently get stuck in the Ampulla of Vater can cause obstruction in the outflow of pancreatic juices from the pancreas into the duodenum. The backflow of these digestive juices causes lysis(dissolving) of pancreatic cells and subsequent pancreatitis.
- E - ethanol (alcohol)
- T - trauma
- S - steroids
- M - mumps (paramyxovirus) and other viruses (Epstein-Barr virus, Cytomegalovirus)
- A - autoimmune disease (Polyarteritis nodosa, Systemic lupus erythematosus)
- S - scorpion sting (e.g. Tityus trinitatis), and also snake bites
- H - hypercalcemia, hyperlipidemia/hypertriglyceridemia and hypothermia
- E- ERCP (**E**ndoscopic **R**etrograde **C**holangio-**P**ancreatography - a procedure that combines endoscopy and fluoroscopy)
- D - drugs (- steroids & sulfonamides, azathioprine, NSAIDS, diuretics such as furosemide and thiazides, & didanosine) and duodenal ulcers

Ans 92: (d) Membranous glomerulopathy
Ref: Read the text below
Sol:

- This patient has **nephrotic syndrome as indicated by the edema, 4+ proteinuria, and hypoproteinemi**a and the most common cause of this syndrome in adults is membranous nephropathy.
- **Acute proliferative glomerulonephritis** produces a nephritic syndrome marked by a mild proteinuria, hematuria, azotemia, and hypertension.
- **Diabetic nephropathy does produce proteinuria** that is sometimes sufficient to cause nephrotic syndrome, but hypertension is often present along with some indication of chronic renal failure neither of which are seen in this case.
- **IgA nephropathy or Berger** disease is a cause of nephrotic syndrome but with hematuria often associated with an upper respiratory infection unlike the presentation in this case.
- Patients with lupus nephritis may present with either nephritic or nephritic syndrome, but certainly this is a much less common cause of nephrotic syndrome than membranous glomerulonephritis.

Ans 93 : (d) Increased hydrostatic pressure
Ref:Read the text below
Sol:

- In **left-sided heart failure**, poor chamber contractility results in impaired systolic outflow, creating an increase in **end diastolic volume and a corresponding increase in ventricular hydrostatic pressure.**
- **Impaired ventricular emptying** cause's stasis in the pulmonary circulation, resulting in a similar increase in volume and pressure in the microvasculature.
- Capillary congestion leads to widening of endothelial intercellular junctions, leakage of fluid into the **interstitium alveoli, and the formation of pulmonary edema.**

Ans 94 : (b) Diabetes mellitus
Ref:Read the text below
Sol:

- A study found that **deposition of amyloid plaques** does not correlate well with neuron loss. This observation **supports the tau hypothesis,** the idea that tau protein abnormalities initiate the disease cascade.
- In this model, **hyperphosphorylated tau begins to pair with other threads of tau.** Eventually, they form neurofibrillary tangles inside nerve cell bodies. When this occurs, the microtubules disintegrate, **collapsing the neuron's transport system.**
- This may result first in **malfunctions in biochemical communication between neurons and later in the death of the cells.**
- **Herpes simplex virus type 1** has also been proposed to play a causative role in people carrying the susceptible versions of the apoE gene

Ans 95 : (a) Oil red O
Ref:Read the text below
Sol:

- Other stains used Sudan black B

Ans 96 : (d) Colon, endometrium, ovary
Ref:Read the text below
Sol:

Syndrome	Histologic Type	Distribution of Polyps	Malignant Potential	Associated Lesions
Nonpolyposis syndrome (Lynch syndrome)	Large intestine (often proximal	Adenoma	Common	• Endometrial and ovarian tumors
Gardner's syndrome	Large and small intestines	Adenoma	Common	• Osteomas • Fibromas • Lipomas • Epidermoid cysts ampullary cancers • Congenital hypertrophy of retinal pigment epithelium
Familial adenomatous polyposis	Large intestine	Adenoma	Common	None
Peutz-Jeghers syndrome	Small and large intestines, stomach	Hamartoma	Rare	• Mucocutaneous pigmentation; • Tumors of the ovary, breast, • Pancreas, • Endometrium
Juvenile polyposis	Large and small Hamartoma, rarely Rareprogressing to adenomaintestines, stomach	Hamartoma, rarely progressing to adenoma	Rare	• Various congenital abnormalities

Ans 97 : (b) Malaise
Ref:Read the text below
Sol:

- **Signs found in all patients on affected side of face include; ptosis** (which is drooping of the upper eyelid from loss of sympathetic innervation to the superior tarsal muscle, also known as Müller'smuscle), upside-down ptosis (slight elevation of the lower lid), and miosis (constricted pupil), and anhidrosis (decreased sweating on the affected side of the face). dilation lag (slow response of **the pupil to light), Enophthalmos (the impression that the eye is sunk in) loss of ciliospinal reflex and bloods hot conjunctiva may occur depending on the site of lesion.**
- Sometimes there is **flushing of the face is on the affected side of the face** due to dilation of blood vessels under the skin.

Ans 98 : (c) Adrenal hypertrophy
Ref:Read the text below
Sol:

- **Goodpasture's syndrome** can cause to cough up blood or feel a burning sensation when urinating. But its first signs may be vague, such as fatigue, nausea, difficulty breathing, or paleness.
- These signs are followed by kidney involvement, represented first by small amounts of blood **in the urine, protein in the urine, and other clinical and laboratory findings**
- Lung symptoms may present as nothing more serious than a dry cough and minor breathlessness; and such mild symptoms may last for many years before more severe ones develop. **At its most serious, however, lung damage may cause severe impairment of oxygenation so that intensive care is required.**
- Deterioration between the two extremes may occur very rapidly, often at the same time as rapid deterioration occurs in the kidney. **The patient often does not seek medical attention until he or she begins coughing up blood (hemoptysis).**

Ans 99 : (d) Widened osteoid seams of peripheral trabeculae
Ref:Read the text below
Sol:

- **This woman is suffering from senile, or postmenopausal, osteoporosis**. In such patients, the calcium and phosphate levels will typically be within the reference range. The alkaline phosphatase will also usually be normal**, but may be increased following fractures.**
- **Microscopic examination of affected bones** will reveal loss of bone mass tending to affect horizontal more than vertical trabeculae. Disorganized interconnecting trabeculae of woven bone rimmed by osteoblasts describes the appearance of an osteoblastoma, a benign bone tumor that is **histologically very similar to and often described in conjunction with an osteoid osteoma.**
- A **characteristic difference between these two benign bone tumors** is that osteoid osteomas are very painful lesions (excess prostaglandin E production) that respond dramatically to aspirin, while osteoblastomas produce a dull, achy pain that does not respond to aspirin.
- Thickened, irregular trabeculae with prominent cement lines describe the morphology seen in Paget disease. **Widened osteoid seams of peripheral trabeculae** reflect the appearance of unmineralized osteoid found in osteomalacia. **Alkaline phosphatase levels are typically increased in osteomalacia (and rickets) and Paget disease**

Ans 100 : (a) Amorphous eosinophilic material surrounded by epithelioid cells and T-lymphocytes
Ref:Read the text below
Sol:

- This **clinical scenario describes secondary tuberculosis (TB).** Upon initial exposure to the bacillus, an individual develops primary TB, where M. **tuberculosis is phagocytosed by alveolar macrophages and transported to the hilar lymph nodes.**
- As **naive macrophages** are unable to kill the mycobacterium, bacteria multiply and lyse the host cell, at **which time they infect other macrophages.**
- **T-cell immunity develops** after a few weeks to control the initial infection. An epithelioid-cell granulomatous inflammation occurs at the site of original parenchymal infection, which, **upon**

healing,results in scar formation, at times with late calcification that may leave a residual lesion potentially visible on chest x-ray.

- This **parenchymal scar in association with an enlarged** (and possibly calcified) hilar lymph node is known as **the Ghon complex.**
- In approximately 90–95% **of immunocompetent individuals, complete healing occurs. Because M. tuberculosis** may persist within macrophages for many years, reactivation may occur, although the mechanisms responsible for keeping the bacilli dormant as well as those leading to reactivation are unknown.
- **Reactivation (or, on less frequent occasions, reinfection) of TB is known as secondary TB. Typical clinical symptoms include weight loss, low-grade fever, and drenching night sweats.**
- Reactivated TB has a predilection for the upper lung zones, presumably due to the greater availability of oxygen **in this area, which enhances multiplication of the aerobic bacilli.**

Ans 101 : (b) chromosome 13
Ref:Read the text below
Sol:

- The **Wilson's disease gene (ATP7B)** has been mapped to chromosome 13 (13q14.3) and is expressed primarily in the liver, kidney, and placenta. The gene codes for a P-type (cation transport enzyme) ATPase **that transports copper into bile and incorporates it into ceruloplasmin.**
- Mutations can be detected in 90% of patients. Most (60%) are homozygous for ATP7B mutations (two abnormal copies), and 30% have only one abnormal copy. 10% have no detectable mutation.
- Although **300 mutations of ATP7B have been described**, in most populations the cases of Wilson's disease are due to a small number of mutations specific for that population. For instance, in Western populations the H1069Q mutation (replacement of a histidine by a glutamine at position 1069 in the protein) **is present in 37-63% of cases, while in China this mutation is very uncommon and R778L (arginine to leucine at 778) is found more often.**
- Relatively little is known about the relative impact of various mutations, although the H1069Q mutation seems to **predict later onset and predominantly neurological problems, according to some studies.**

Ans 102 : (d) Pancreatitis
Ref:Read the text below
Sol:
WILSON'S DISEASE
Signs and symptoms
The main sites of copper accumulation are the liver and the brain, and consequently liver disease and neuropsychiatric symptoms are the main features that lead to diagnosis.
Liver disease
Liver disease may present as tiredness, increased bleeding tendency or confusion (due to hepatic encephalopathy) and portal hypertension. On examination, signs of chronic liver disease such as spider naevi (small distended blood vessels, usually on the chest) may be observed. Chronic active hepatitis has caused cirrhosis of the liver in most patients by the time they develop symptoms.
Neuropsychiatric symptoms
About half the patients with Wilson's have neurological or psychiatric problems. Most patients initially have mild cognitive deterioration and clumsiness, as well as changes in behavior. Specific neurological symptoms then follow, often in the form of parkinsonism (increased rigidity and slowing of routine movements) with or without a typical hand tremor, masked facial expressions, slurred speech, ataxia (lack of coordination) or dystonia (twisting and repetitive movements of part of the body). Seizures and migraine appear to be more common in Wilson's disease.

Ans 103 : (b) Hyperglycemia
Ref:Read the text below
Sol:

- **Reye's syndrome** is a potentially fatal disease that causes numerous detrimental effects to many organs, especially the brain and liver, as well as causing hypoglycemia.
- The **exact cause is unknown**, and while it has been associated with aspirin consumption by children with viral **illness, it also occurs in the absence of aspirin use.**

- The disease causes fatty liver with **minimal inflammation and severe encephalopathy (with** swelling of the brain). The liver may become slightly enlarged and firm, and there is a **change in the appearance of the kidneys. Jaundice is not usually present.**

Ans 104 : (b) chromosome 14
Ref:Read the text below
Sol:
Familial cases with a defined inheritance pattern account for about 10% of Alzheimer disease. Genetic defects in familial cases have been identified on 4 chromosomes (Blennow et al, 2006):

Chromosome	Gene
21	Amyloid Precursor Protein (APP)
19	Apolipoprotein E (ApoE)
14	Presenilin 1 (PSEN1)
1	Presenilin 2 (PSEN2)

Ans 105 : (c) Neuropathy
Ref:Read the text below
Sol:

- **Hashimoto's thyroiditis** or **chronic lymphocytic thyroiditis** is an autoimmune disease in which the thyroid gland is gradually destroyed by a variety of cell and antibody mediated immune processes.
- **Hashimoto's thyroiditis very often results in hypothyroidism with bouts of hyperthyroidism.**
- Physiologically, **antibodies against thyroid peroxidase and/or thyroglobulin** cause gradual destruction of follicles in the thyroid gland. Accordingly, the disease can be detected clinically by looking for these antibodies in the blood. It is also characterized by invasion of the thyroid tissue by leukocytes, mainly T-lymphocytes. It is associated with non-Hodgkin lymphoma.
- **Symptoms of Hashimoto's thyroiditis include weight gain**, depression, mania, sensitivity to cold, fatigue, panic attacks, bradycardia,tachycardia, high cholesterol, reactive hypoglycemia, constipation, migraines, **muscle weakness, cramps, memory loss, infertility and hair loss.**

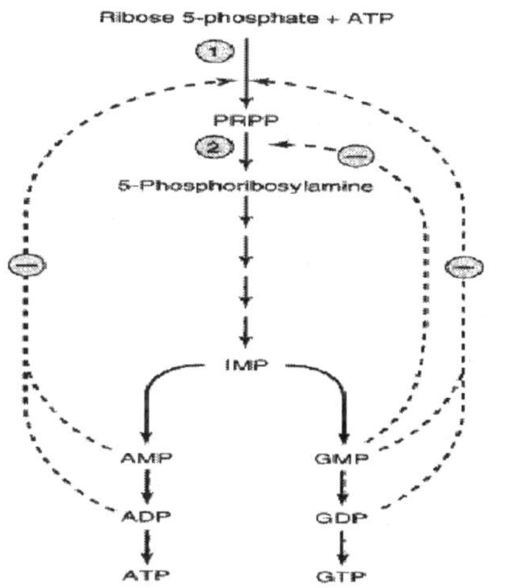

Control of the rate of de novo purine synthesis. Solid lines represent metabolite flow and dashed lines feedback inhibition by end products of the pathway.

Ans-106: (c) Hostile witness
Ref: Read the text below
Sol:

- A **hostile witness** is a witness in a trial who testifies for the opposing party or a witness who offers adverse testimony to the calling party during direct examination.
- **A witness called by the opposing party is presumed hostile.**
- A witness called by the **direct examiner can be declared hostile by a judge**, at the request of the examiner, when the witness' testimony is openly antagonistic or clearly prejudiced to the opposing party.
- **A party examining a hostile witness may question the witness as if in cross-examination, thus permitting the use of leading questions.** A hostile witness is sometimes known as an **adverse witness**.

Ans-107: (a) Amanita **Phylloides**
Ref: Read the text below
Sol:

- **Amanita phalloides** commonly known as the **death cap** is a poisonous basidiomycete fungus. In some cases, death cap has been accidentally introduced to new regions with the cultivation of non-native species of oak, chestnut, and pine.
- **Coincidentally, these toxic mushrooms** resemble several edible species (most notably the straw mushroom) commonly consumed by humans, increasing the risk of accidental poisoning.
- **A.phalloides is one of the most poisonous of all known toadstools. It has been involved in the majority of human deaths from mushroom poisoning.**
- The principal toxic constituent is α-amanitin, which damages the liver and kidneys, often **fatally. No antidote is known.**

Ans 108: - (c) Race
Ref- Parikh---67
Sol:

$$\textbf{Cephalic index} = \frac{\text{Maximum breadth of skull}}{\text{Maximum length of skull}} \times 100$$

Cephalic index is useful for determination of Race

Ans 109: - (3) Nax vomika
Ref- Parikh---904
Sol:
The deliriant poisons are:

a) Dhatura
b) Atropa belladonna
c) Hyoscyamus nigar
d) Cannabis indica
e) Cocaine
f) Opiates.
g) Chronic lead poisoning

- **Nux-vomica is a spinal poison.**
- **The active principle of nux-vomica is strychnine.**

Ans 110: - (a) Cooling of the body.
Ref- Parikh---67
Sol:

- **Somatic death or clinical death** is the complete and irreversible cessation of the vital functions of brain, heart and lungs.
- In **somatic death through life ceases**, cell responds to chemical, thermal and electrical stimuli.
- **Cooling of body is the sign of cellular death**

The **signs of somatic death or immediate signs** of death are:

- Insensibility to touch, pain, temperature and loss of voluntary power.
- Cessation of circulation.
- Loss of E.C.G. rhythm.
- Loss of E.E.G. rhythm .
- Cessation of respiration.

Ans 111: - (d) Strychnine poisoning
Ref- Parikh---921
Sol:
Strychnine poisoning resists Rigor mortis

Ans 112: - (c) Elapids
Ref- Parikh---806
Sol:

SNAKE	TYPES OF POISONS
Elapids	Neurotoxin
Viper	Vasculotoxic
Sea snake	Myotoxic

Ans-113: (b) Graze Abrasion
Ref: Read the text below
Sol:

- An **abrasion is a superficial injury**, commonly known as a **'graze' or 'scratch'.**
- This **type of wound damages** only the epidermis (uppermost skin layer), and should not therefore bleed. However, abrasions do usually extend into the dermis causing slight bleeding.
- **Abrasions are commonly caused by a 'glancing' impact across the surface of the skin, but if the force is directed vertically down onto the skin surface it may be termed a 'crush' injury**.
- These wounds are seen where an object has struck the skin (e.g. a blow from a fist), or where the injured person has fallen onto a rough surface, such as road.

Ans-114: (c) District magistrate
Ref: Read the text below
Sol:

- The term **exhumation** is applied only when a proper inhumation (ritual burial of the body in a legal and legitimate fashion) was done in the first place.
- This **difference is not merely academic; it has important legal repercussions.**
- In India, while a **proper exhumation can only be done a magistrate under section 176 of Criminal Procedure Code (Cr.P.C.),** retrieval of an illegally buried body can be done even by the police under section 174 of Cr.P.C.

Ans-115: (b) Treatment of laryngotracheal stenosis.
Ref: Read the text below.
Sol:

- Studies in humans **report the utility of topical mitomycin C for severe subglottic tracheal stenosis that recur after different treatments (concentrations ranging from 0.4 mg/ml to 10 mg/ml).**

Ans-116: (d) Delivering drug to the round membrane.
Ref: Read the text below.
Sol:

- The wick absorbs medication (which can be administered by the patient at home) that has been applied to the external ear canal and delvers it to the RWM. The advantage of this system is that fitting the device is a very simple and minimally invasive procedure (only nominally **more invasive than tympanostomy tube placement) and can be removed without anesthesia. Long-term use is not advised, because the wick material may become adherent to the mucosa of the round window niche.**

Ans 117: (b) Quieter than that transmitted by bone conduction
Ref– Read the text below
Sol:

a. The **traditional test** for detecting conductive deafness is the Rinne test. The vibrating tuning **fork is applied to the mastoid process.**
b. When the patient can no longer hear the vibration of the fork, it is taken off the skull and moved to the **external auditory meatus**. With nerve deafness, acuity may be generally reduced, but **perception with air conduction will be superior to that with bone conduction. This will also be true in normal persons.**
c. With conductive hearing loss, the sound waves are transmitted more effectively to the cochlea directly through **the bones of the skull than through the air and along the pathway that starts at the external auditory meatus.**

Ans-118: (c) Rosacea
Ref:Read the text below
Sol:

- **Rhinophyma is a complication of rosacea. It can be** treated surgically by shaving off the excessive tissue with a scalpel, but **regrowth occurs in time.**
- There is very little evidence to support the association between **alcoholism and rhinophyma.**
- The other conditions do not cause flushing or blushing-type **appearance. Psoriasis and seborrheic dermatitis have lesions that have white dry scales.**

Ans-119: (d) Upper respiratory infections
Ref: Read **the text below**
Sol :

- Children average **6 to 9 upper respiratory infections per year** during the **first 6 years of life.**
- Upper respiratory **infections are the most common predisposing factor, followed closely by day-care attendance.**
- Allergies and adenoidal hypertrophy are less common factors.
- Tonsillar hypertrophy has little or no **relationship to otitis-prone children.**

Ans-120: (c) Group A beta-hemolytic streptococcus
Ref: Read the text below
Sol :

- Although **spontaneous rupture can occur with** any ear infection, regardless of the pathogen, group A beta-**hemolytic streptococcus (GABHS) has been** found to be the most common. Selecting an appropriate antibiotic that covers GABHS would be important if a **spontaneous perforation is present. Pseudomonas aeruginosa may be present in otitis exterma, and is a rare middle-ear pathogen.**

Ans-121: (d) Frontal
Ref: Read the text below
Sol :

- The frontal **sinuses statistically** are the ones most **commonly prone to osteomyelitis.**

Ans-122: (a) Labyrinthitis
Ref: Read the text below
Sol :

- Although **meningitis and brain abscess are** both potential complications of mastoiditis, they are intracranial, not extracranial.
- **Labyrinthitis is the only** extracranial complication listed.

Ans-123: (a) Decreased motility of the tympanic membrane
Ref: Read the text below
Sol :

- Decreased **motility of the tympanic membrane (TM)** assessed by the pneumatic otoscope, has been found to be more predictive than color changes in diagnosing acute **otitis media. Crying and fever can cause the TM to appear red.**
- Acute infections may also have an opacified, yellow appearance without redness. Tragal tenderness is a **sign commonly seen in otitis externa, not otitis media. The presence of pus in the ear canal is nospecific, and is not predicitive of a middle-ear source.**

Ans 124: - (a) Decreased refraction of light by the cornea
Ref- Read the text below
Sol:

- **LASIK has largely replaced radial, or refractive, keratotomy. Both methods can be used to decrease the refraction of light by the cornea.**
- **LASIK alters corneal (not lens) anatomy** to create a new shape that is more flattened in the center and higher at the periphery of the cornea. This occurs because intraocular pressure will cause a reshaping of the cornea due to induced weakness produced by the laser removal of tissue.
- The **purpose of the procedure is to reduce myopia to eliminate the need for corrective lenses.**
- The **reduction in curvature of the central portion** of the cornea results in decreased refractive power of the cornea.
- The **removal of tissue and the degree of correction** required is estimated by computer simulations.

Ans-125: (d) Plexus of Zinn and Haller arteries
Ref:Read the text below
Sol:

- The retina is placed **between two sets of arteries and veins—the ciliary vessels of the choroid and the branches of the central retinal vessels**. It depends on both circulations, neither alone being sufficient to maintain full visual activity in the retina.
- The main blood supply to the optic disc is from the ophthalmic and carotid arteries to the short posterior ciliary arteries (PCAs), **which supply the choroid and the circle of Zinn-Haller. The circle of Zinn-Haller is a doughnut-shaped vascular plexus that encircles the papilla and is part of the choroidal vascular bed**. It is the portion of the choroid that nourishes most of the orbital portion of the optic nerve.
- On their way to the globe, the PCAs give **off small branches extending through the dura matter and forming and anastomosing plexus with the pia matter. This pial plexus is also supplied by branches from the central retinal artery at its entrance to the optic nerve.**
- **Near the posterior wall of the globe, the PCAs** divide into about 10 to 20 small branches. Direct branches travel to the lamina, the choroid or the circle of Zinn-Haller. Solan Singh Hayreh suggested that the peripapillary **vascular supply is not evenly distributed around the optic disc and can vary significantly between individuals. Hayreh also reported that the medial and temporal quadrants are more often well perfused, while the superior and inferior quadrants have less arterial influx. These** areas with less perfusion may often behave as watershed indicator zones; optic nerve axons are more susceptible to ischemic insult in the hypo-perfuse areas at the inferior and superior disc margins.

Ans-126: (b) Homocystinuria.
Ref: Read the text below
Sol:

- **Systemic disorders associated with displacement of the lens include Marfan syndrome, homocystinuria, Weill-Marchesani syndrome, and sulfite oxidase deficiency**.
- **Ectopia lentis occurs in approximately 80% of patients** with Marfan syndrome, and in about 50% of patients the ectopia is evident by the age of 5 yr. In most cases the lens is displaced superiorly and temporally; it **is almost always bilateral and relatively symmetric.**
- **In homocystinuria the lens is usually displaced inferiorly and somewhat nasally.** It occurs early in life and is often evident by 5 yr of age.

- In Weill-Marchesani syndrome the **displacement of the lens is often downward and forward, and the lens tends to be small and round.**

Ans-127: (b) Natamycin.
Ref:Read the text below
Sol:

- **Natamycin is a tetraene polyene antibiotic** derived from Streptomyces natalensis. It possesses in vitro activity **against a variety of yeast and filamentous fungi, including Candida, Aspergillus, Cephalosporium,** Fusarium and Penicillium.
- The mechanism of action appears to be through binding of the molecule to the sterol moiety of the fungal cell **membrane. The polyenesterol complex alters the permeability of the membrane to produce depletion** of essential cellular constituents.
- Although the activity against fungi is dose-related, natamycin is predominantly fungicidal.
- Natamycin is not effective **in vitro against gram-positive or gram-negative bacteria. It is used to treat fungal keratitis.** It is especially effective against Aspergillus and Fusarium corneal
- Natamycin, also known as pimaricin, is a macrolide polyene antifungal drug.
- Topical administration **appears to produce effective concentrations of natamycin within the corneal stroma but not in intraocular fluid. Systemic absorption should not be expected following topical administration of NATACYN (natamycin ophthalmic suspension) 5%. As with other polyene** antibiotics, absorption from the gastrointestinal tract is very poor. Studies in rabbits receiving topical natamycin revealed no measurable compound in the aqueous humor or sera, but the sensitivity of the measurement was no greater than 2 mg/mL.

Ans-128: (c) Juvenile rheumatoid arthritis.
Ref:Read the text below
Sol:
Contraindications to **implantation of intraocular lenses (IOL) are as follows,:**

- The patient's desire not to have an implant;
- Axial myopia greater than 7 diopters;
- A poor result from an implant or cataract extraction alone in the first eye;
- A patient with only one eye with potentially good vision;
- **A relatively young patient;**
- Individuals with senile macular choroidal degeneration without dense cataracts in both eyes;
- Endothelial corneal dystrophy;
- Proliferative diabetic retinopathy and possibly significant background retinopathy;
- Uncontrolled glaucoma;
- Previous retinal detachment in either eye ;
- Congenital cataracts (particularly rubella cataracts) and cataracts associated with
- certain other ocular abnormalities (such as recurrent iritis, essential iris atrophy, or atopic dermatitis);
- Significant complications during the cataract extraction procedure

Since Juvenile Rheumatoid arthritis affects young patients, IOL is contraindicated

Ans-129: (a) Retinoblastoma
Ref:Read the text below
Sol:

- **Retinoblastoma causes a white reflex (leukocoria).** This is a life-threatening malignant tumor rarely seen in infants and children. **Leukocoria may also be due to a cataract.**
- **Retinocerebellar angiomatosis is part of a rare autosomal dominant disease (von Hippel-Lindau disease); patients present with nystagmus,** retinal detachment, cerebellar hemangioblastoma, intraabdominal cysts, and renal carcinoma.
- Choroidal angioma is found in Sturge-Weber **disease; patients present with congenital glaucoma, cloudiness of the cornea, and marked enlargement of the eye at birth (buphthalmos). Infants with Sturge-Weber disease may** also have facial angiomas

Ans-130: (a) Ornithine ketoacid transaminase
Ref:Read the text below
Sol:

- In **gyrate atrophy the blood ornithine is** grossly elevated, due to deficiency of ornithine ketoacid transaminase, which **converts ornithine towards glutamic acid.**
- It is a autosomal recessive disorder **with gene on chromosome 10**

Ans-131: (c) Retinal detachment
Ref:Read the text below
Sol:

- **Pigment cells in the anterior vitreous (Shafer's** sign) are known to be associated with retinal breaks. Sometimes termed **"tobacco dust," it can be very significant clues to a retinal break or detachment.**
- Hamilton **and Taylor found that 98% of patients in their clinical review with this sign had retinal detachments and 60% had** flat retinal holes.
- The source of the pigment **granules is not known though is suspected to arise from the retinal pigment epithelium (RPE).**
- **There are a large number of patients** with retinal detachments that are totally asymptomatic an simply checking the retrolental (Berger's Space) & anterior vitreous for cells is important.
- The failure to check for this **sign on a symptomatic patient could be considered gross negligence.**

Ans-132: (a) Keratitis
Ref:Read the text below
Sol:
The symptoms of pain, tearing, and photophobia are characteristically seen in corneal lesions
• In **acute anterior uveitis,** though pain & photophobia is seen but tearing is minimal.
• In **acute posterior uveitis** there is no pain, redness or photophobia. Symptoms typically include, floaters, loss of visual field or scotoma or decreased vision.
• **Epidemic Keratoconjunctivitis** is usually b/l, photophobia and corneal lesions appear 5-14 days after the onset of symptoms. Symptoms gradually appear in phases not in a single day as this patient has.

Ans 133: (a) Survival
Ref: biostatistics pg 116-120)
Sol:

Kaplan Meire curves are also known as survival curves

- There are **methodologic problems** that require the use of a different form of analysis, usually called **life table analysis or survival curve analysis.**
- Patients are usually **enrolled into the study over a protracted period of time**. There are always less no of patient at one point of time who can start trial at same time with long studies there are **drop out and we have no way what happened to them**. Another thing is patient die before the completion of study.
- What do we do with the withdrawals? Obviously, we can't determine length of survival from their data, because of the different survival and loss of substantial patients from study (due to drop out and death) so we have to discard lot of our data, withdrawals did provide useful information before they withdrew.

So we have two **methods for calculation of survival**:-

➢ **Actuarial method** for survival analysis, in which the status of the subjects is looked at after a fixed period of time (each month, or every 6 months, or every year, depending on the length of follow-up and how frequently the end points occur). Slight modification of the technique, called the **Kaplan-Meier (K-M) approach**.
➢ The **major difference between it and the actuarial method** is that calculating the probability of survival only at the fixed intervals, the K-M analysis calculates it only when an end point occurs. So it's possible that there may be 6 months between the first and second analyses but only 2 days between the second and third.

- The **K - M method is usually more efficient than the actuarial method when there are fewer than 50 subjects, but the differences between the results are quite minor for the most part.**

Ans 134: (c) Prospective study
Ref: Park- 74
Sol:

- **Incidence** – total no of new cases occurring in a defined population during specified period of time.
- **Cross-sectional studies** give an estimate of prevalence, while case-control is an example of retrospective study and both give an estimate of the relative risk, known as Odds ratio.
- **Incidence** – the no. of new cases occurring in a defined population during specified period of time.
- **Here period is usually one year**
- **Special incidence rates – Attack rate, sec attack rate, hospital admission ratio**

- **Incidence is derived during epidemiology study – Cohort study**

Ans 135: (a) Sample size based on hypothesis
Ref: Park -501,502
Sol:

- Choice a seems to be the **right answer as the sample size** is not based any hypothesis but then again option c is not clear.
- The clusters **are not equal in cluster sampling technique and the meaning of 'equal' is not mentioned as in what sense.** Still I would go with option a as the correct answer.

Ans 136: (d) Decreased specificity
Ref: Read the text below
Sol:

- Decreased specifity means increased number of false positives.
- Specifity is the ability of a test to correctly identify the true negatives out of all disease negatives.

Ans 137-C – Phosphorus
Ref: Read the text below
Sol:

- A **tricky question.** In fact, fish is a rich source of all the above mentioned nutrients. However it is exceptionally good source of **Iodine and Vitamin A.**
- Of the remaining two choices, **Phosphorus** seems to be the better answer as it is in same quantities in fish as **other meat products.**

Fish – Protein rich – (15-25%)
Rich in

- Unsaturated fatty acids
- Vit A – also remember fish oil – richest natural source of Vit A (retinol)
- Vit D

Ans 138: (c) Mental illness
Ref:http://www.indiatogether.org/health/opinions/jabidi2.htm,
http://www.hinduonnet.com/mag/2003/11/30/stories/2003113000240400.htm,
http://socialwelfare.delhigovt.nic.in/disabilityact.htm
Sol:
The **Persons with Disabilities (Equal Opportunities, Protection of Rights and Full Participation) Act** was passed by both the Houses of our Parliament in a single day in **December 1995**. The law was notified on 7th February 1996.
The Disability Act of 1995 defines 'disability' to mean

- Blindness;
- Low vision;
- Leprosy-cured;

- Hearing impairment;
- Locomotor disability;
- Mental retardation, and
- **Mental illness.**

- The **Disability Act of 1995** not only included mental illness under the definition of 'disability' but also mandates that its Central Coordination Committee (which has representation at the 'Secretary to the Government of India' level of the Health Ministry!) will: **(1)** review and coordinate the activities of all Governmental and Non-Governmental Organizations which are dealing with matters relating to persons with disabilities; **(2)** develop a national policy to address issues faced by persons with disabilities; **(3)** advise on the formulation of policies, programmes, legislations and projects with respect to disability.
- In a tragic incident at Erwadi in Tamilnadu during August 2001, 25 people, including 11 women, were charred to death. A devastating fire broke out at 5 a.m. in the thatched hostel housing them. Out of the 46 hostel inmates, 40 were chained to their beds.
- They kept screaming for help but no one came to their rescue. The 46 hostel inmates were mentally ill. The Erwadi tragedy of Aug 2001 attracted international attention. That it happened is indicative of a deep-rooted apathy towards people with mental illness.

Ans 139: (a) Prognosis
Ref: Park /19th ed. /page no. 271
Sol:

- **Lepromin test** – done intradermally, 0.1 ml of lepromin into the inner aspect of forearm of the individual examined on 48 hr and 21 days
- **Early reaction (Fernandez reaction)** – inflammation response disappear after 3-4 days, d/t soluble constituent of bacteria. **Diameter of red area is measured**
- **Late reaction (Mitsuda reaction)** – apparent in 7-10 days
- Test read at 21 days, it is d/t – type IV hypersensitivity
- **Diameter of nodule is measured**

Value of this test
Not a diagnostic test
Evaluation of the cell mediated immunity of leprosy patient [not general population]
Classification of the type of disease
Prognosis of the disease
Now coming to option (D) – epidemiological studies
Park 271 – writes – "probably the most important recent advance in the study of the epidemiology of leprosy is the development of sociological tests"
They have importance in
Detection of subclinical infection
Preclinical manifestation
Follow up efficacy of drug treatment
Includes:

- FLA – ABS [Fluorescence leprosy Ab absorption test]
- Monoclonal ab – ab competition test (SALT)
- Others – Radioimmunoassay, ELISA – PGL Ag based [phenolic glycolipid]

Ans 140: (b) 30.0 – 34.9
Ref– Read the text below
Sol:
According to the **WHO classification** following cut off points to define the obesity were used in this study.

BMI	Classification
< 18.5	Under weight
18.5 – 24.9	Normal weight
25.0 – 29.9	Pre-obese (overweight)

30.0 – 34.9	Obese class 1
35.0 -39.9	Obese class 2
> 40.0	Obese class 3

Ans 141:(a) Case-control study
Ref– Read the text below
Sol:

- A **case-control study** is very useful and efficient at studying **diseases that occur rarely.**
- In a case-**control study, persons** with a disease are identified and then information is determined by looking **back in time (i.e., retrospective review).**
- **Apopulation of those without the disease** (controls) is also defined and studied in the same way.
- The **prevalence of a risk factor in the cases and controls** can then be determined and compared.
- A **case-control study cannot prove cause and effect**, but it can be a powerful tool to determine risk factors that can generate hypotheses for further study.

Ans 142:(a) Confidential peer review
Ref– Read the text below
Sol:

- **Peer review, morbidity and mortality rounds**, shorter work weeks, and root cause analysis are all mechanisms to prevent future errors from fatigue, impaired system processes, and inadequate knowledge.
- **Frequently when medical errors occur,** the families want to know what is being done to prevent this from happening again.
- Although **the peer review process is confidential** and not subject to subpoena, it provides an effective mechanism to honestly evaluate our colleagues and enforce necessary discipline to improve patient safety.
- **Random drug testing is not a systemic solution.**

Ans 143: (d) 5 years old.
Ref– Read the text below
Sol:

Integrated Management of Childhood Illness (IMCI).

- During the mid-1990s, the **World Health Organization (WHO),** in collaboration with **UNICEF** and many other agencies, institutions and individuals, responded to this challenge by developing a strategy known as the **Integrated Management of Childhood Illness (IMCI).**
- This strategy has been adapted for **India as Integrated Management of Neonatal and Childhood Illness (IMNCI).**
- The IMNCI clinical guidelines target children **less than 5 years old** — the age group that bears the highest burden of deaths from common childhood diseases.
- The guidelines take an evidence-based, syndromic approach to case management that supports the rational, effective and affordable use of drugs and diagnostic tools

Ans 144: (d) Anganwadi workers (AWW) and Anganwadi helpers (AWH)
Ref– Read the text below
Sol:

- Universalisation of the **Integrated Child Development Services Scheme** (ICDS) will be achieved during the Tenth Plan in all the 5652 blocks of the country.
- **Anganwadi workers (AWW) and helpers (AWH)** who are the most visible grass-root **functionaries primarily for ICDS,** also play an important role in other development activities.
- To suitably compensate them and also to boost their morale, the honorarium of **AWW and AWH has been doubled.**

Ans 145: (b) Varicella is a notifiable disease in all states
Ref: Read the text below
Sol:

- **Varicella is a notifiable disease** in fewer states (less than 70%) than are measles, mumps, or rubella.

- This fact and **the fact that many cases of varicella are mild and never** come to medical attention contribute to the low **rate of reporting of varicella.**

Ans 146: (c) Continue with therapy and recheck viral load after 6 months of therapy
Ref: Read the text below
Sol:

- Continue with **therapy and recheck viral load after 6 months of therapy**. The 3-month viral response is a good predictor of sustained virologic response in **patients receiving monotherapy.**
- However, in the registration **trials for interferon/ribavirin therapy, a number of patients first became PCR negative between months three and six of therapy**, and later became sustained virologic **responders after a total of 12 months of therapy.**
- In these trials, all sustained responders to interferon **monotherapy were PCR negative by month three.**

Ans 147: (b) 5-mm diameter induration in a 55-year-old patient with type I diabetes mellitus
Ref: Read the text below
Sol:

- **5-mm diameter induration in a 55-year-old patient with types I diabetes** mellitus. The intravenous drug user is at **high risk for HIV.**
- With unknown **HIV status** he should be considered at high risk for developing active TB**; therefore, a 5-mm induration diameter is a positive PPD result.**
- The **diabetes patient and the gastrectomy patient** are considered to be in populations at increased risk; therefore, a **diameter of 10 mm or greater is considered to be a positive PPD result.**

The nursing home patient is in a high-**prevalence group; therefore, a diameter of 10 mm or greater is also a positive PPD result.**

Ans 148 : (a) Benzathine penicillin, 4 million units intramuscularly in a single dose
Ref:Read the text below
Sol:

- **Benzathine penicillin, 4 million units intramuscularly in a single dose**. Penicillin does not eradicate nasopharyngeal carriage and is not appropriate for meningococcal prophylaxis.
- **Rifampin 600 mg orally twice a day for 2 days, ceftriaxone 250 mg** intramuscularly in a single dose, and ciprofloxacin 500 mg orally in a single dose are all acceptable regimens **for eradication of meningococcal pharyngeal colonization in adults.**
- **Rifampin is the least expensive option** and has the most clinical experience, and thus is the first-line recommendation.

Ans 149: (b) Prevalence will increase
Ref– Read the text below
Sol:

- As the **length of survival from prostate cancer** increases because of the new treatment (**assuming the rate of new cases diagnosed remains unchanged**), the number of cases present at any point in time (**prevalence) increases, not decreases.**
- **Incidence, based on the number of new cases only, remains unchanged.**

Ans 150: (a) Root-mean-square (RMS) deviation of the values from their mean, or as the square root of the variance.
Ref– Read the text below
Sol:

Standard deviation

- In probability and statistics, the **standard deviation** is a measure of the dispersion of a collection of value

Ans 151: (b) Black bag
Ref: Read the text below
Sol:

- **Black bag** is used for collecting general waste i.e., paper, non-infectious plastics, cardboard boxes, and other dry waste **generated in hospital office or in the wards**

Colour coding and type of container for disposal of biomedical waste

Colour coding	Type of container	Waste category	Treatment option as schedule I
Yellow	Plastic Bag	Cat 1, 2, 3, 6	Incineration/deep burial
Red	Disinfected container/plastic bag	Cat 3, 6, 9	Autoclave/microwave chemical t/t
Blue/wt.	Plastic bag/puncture proof	Cat 4, 7	Destruction/shredding
Black	Plastic Bag	Cat 5, 9 & 10 (solid)	Disposal in secured land fide

The plastic bag for incineration does not contain. Chlorinated plastic

Ans 152: (d) Influenza
Ref: Park 19th ed. /page no.134
Sol:

Incubation period of various disease are

- Hep A – 20-30 days [15-45 days]
- Hep B – < 100 days [45-180 days]
- Rubella – 18 days [2-3 weeks]
- **Influenza – 18-72 hrs**
- Varicella/chickenpox – 14-16 days [7-21 days]
- Measles (Rubeola) – 10-14 days
- Mumps – 18 days [2-3 weeks]
- Dipheria – 2-6 days
- Pertussis – 7-14 days [Not more than 3 weeks]
- Meningococcal meningitis – 3-4 days [2-10 days]
- Cholera – few hrs – 5 days [commonly 1-2 days]
- Typhoid fever – 10-14 days [3-21 days]

Ans-153: (d) All of the above
Ref: Read the text below
Sol :

- Each **sign or symptom noted is an indication** of extreme elevations of either triglycerides **or cholesterol.**

Ans-154: (c) Paroxysmal atrial fibrillation
Ref: Read the text below
Sol :

- The **Framingham Study has demonstrated** key risk factors in sudden-death syndrome.
- In contrast, **paroxysmal atrial fibrillation increases risk of stroke.**

Ans-155 : (d) Elevated HDL cholesterol
Ref: Read the text below
Sol :

- **Epidemiologic studies have** defined risk factors in coronary atherosclerotic heart disease.
- Changes in diet and **cessation of smoking, in addition to modern medicinal therapy, are reducing disease risk.**

Ans-156: (b) Inducing transient ventricular wall motion abnormalities
Ref: Read the text below
Sol :

- Myocardial **ischemia can be provoked through several diagnostic modalities.**

- **These include exercise-induced** and pharmacologic-induced techniques.
- Exercise- or **dobutamine-induced ischemia can be diag**nosed by demonstration of transient ventricular wall **motion abnormalities on the echocardiogram.**

Ans-157: (b) Heparin
Ref: Read the text below
Sol :

- **Urokinase is more commonly used to** lyse arterial clots. Warfarin (Coumadin) may be used to initiate **treatment of calf vein DVTs and for** continued outpatient therapy for DVTs of larger or more proximal vessels.
- Aspirin may be effective adjuvant therapy **for thrombotic or embolic** arterial occlusive disease. Recommended treatment **for popliteal or iliofemoral DVT is intravenous heparin titrated to maintain** the APTT at 1.5 to 2 times normal.

Ans-158: (d) All of the above
Ref: Read the text below
Sol :

- Treatment of **uncomplicated infectious mononucleosis is supportive.** Warm saline gargle or topical anesthetic will relieve sore throat.
- Acetaminophen is used for fever. Superinfection by group A **beta-hemolytic streptococcus will require treatment with penicillin or erythromycin.**
- Amoxicillin or ampicillin should be avoided since they will cause a rash in persons with mononucleosis.
- Splenomegaly **is seen in 50 percent of patients. Strenuous activity or contact sports increase risk of rupture of the enlarged spleen.**

Ans 159: (b) Cholelithiasis
Ref – Read the text below
Sol

- **Cholangiocarcinoma occurs most commonly in the sixth** and seventh decades of life. Patients often present with symptoms and signs **of biliary obstruction, including right upper quadrant pain, jaundice, and cholangitis.**
- Unfortunately, most patients present with **unresectable disease, and 5-year survival is dismal. Diagnosis is often made by cholangiography.**
- Chronic infection with the liver flukes **Opisthorchis and Clonorchis confers an added risk** of cholangiocarcinoma. Similarly, exposure to toxic dyes in the automobile and rubber industries, primary sclerosing cholangitis, and congenital malformations of the **biliary tree such as choledochal cysts and Caroli disease predispose to the development of** cholangiocarcinoma.
- Cholelithiasis is **not clearly a predisposing factor.**

Ans 160: (b) Cryoglobulinemia
Ref – Read the text below
Sol

- Causes of **isolated unconjugated (indirect) hyperbilirubinemia include inherited (sickle** cell disease, spherocytosis, glucose-6-phosphate **dehydrogenase deficiency) and acquired (microangiopathic hemolytic anemia, paroxysmal nocturnal hemoglobinuria, immune hemolysis) hemolytic disorders, ineffective erythropoiesis (nutritional** deficiencies), inherited conditions (Gilbert's syndrome, Crigler-Najjar **types I and II), and drugs (probenecid, ribavirin, rifampicin).**
- Inherited hemolytic disorders with chronic hemolysis carry a high risk of developing calcium bilirubinate gallstones.
- Patients with hemolytic disorders that cause excessive heme production seldom have a serum bilirubin >5 mg/dL. Higher levels may occur during **acute hemolytic conditions (sickle cell crisis) or with concomitant renal or hepatocellular disease.**
- **Probenecid (used to treat gout) and rifampicin cause unconjugated hyperbilirubinemia** by diminishing hepatic uptake of bilirubin.

- Cryoglobulinemia is associated with hepatitis C infection which, if **present, is associated with a mild hepatocellular pattern of injury and an elevated direct bilirubin.**

Ans-161: (c) Hyponatremia
Ref: Harrison's, 17th edn. Pg 1878.
Sol:

- **Urinary D-Xylose Test for carbohydrate** absorption provides an assessment of proximal small-intestinal mucosal function.
- D-Xylose, a pentose, is **absorbed almost exclusively in the proximal small intestine.**
- The D-xylose test is **usually performed by giving 25 g D-xylose and collecting urine for 5 h.**
- An **abnormal test (<4.5 g excretion) primarily reflects the presence** of duodenal/jejuna mucosal disease.

Ans-162: (b) Acyclovir
Ref: Read the text below
Sol:

- There are **several antivirals that are effective for treating herpes including:** aciclovir (acyclovir), valaciclovir (valacyclovir), famciclovir, **and penciclovir.**
- **Aciclovir was the first discovered and is now available in generic.**

Ans-163: (a) Riluzole
Ref: Davidsons, 20th edn. Pg. 1223.
Sol:

- **Patterns of involvement in motor neuron** disease (amyotrophic lateral sclerosis) is of 3 types-progressive **muscular atrophy; progressive bulbar palsy; amyotrophic lateral sclerosis.**
- The **glutamate antagonist Riluzole 100 mg/day appears** to be modestly effective in prolonging survival/life expectancy in patients with motor neuron disease by about 2 months

Ans-164: (b) Colchicine
Ref: Harrison's-216.
Sol:

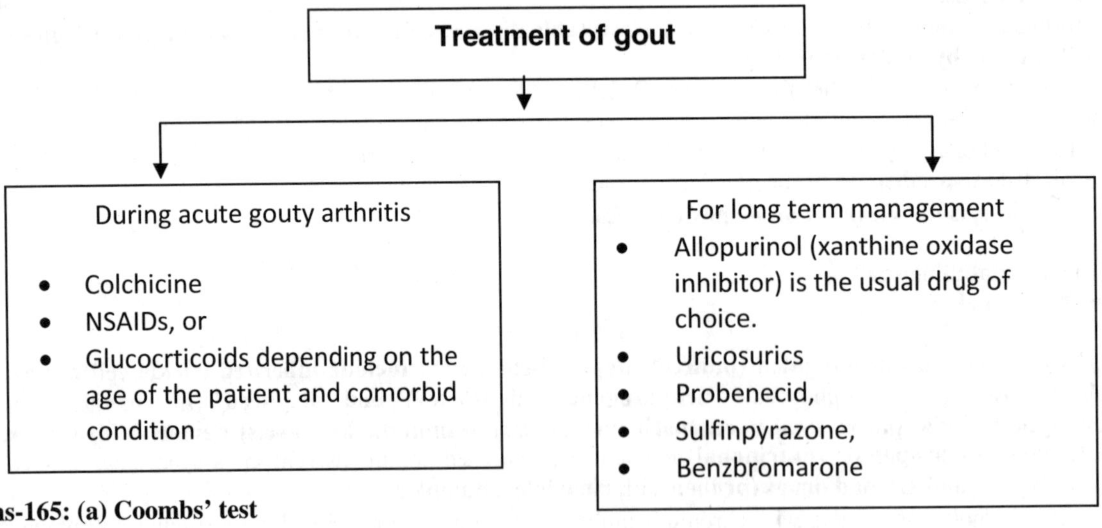

Ans-165: (a) Coombs' test

Ref: Harrison's, 17th -659
Sol:

- The **diagnostic test for Autoimmune Hemolytic Anemia (AIHA)** is the antiglobulin test worked out in 1945 by R R A. Coombs and known since by his name.
- The beauty of this test is that it directly detects the pathogenetic mediator of the disease, i.e. the **presence of antibody on the red cells themselves.**
- **When the test is positive, it clinches the diagnosis, when it is negative, the diagnosis is unlikely.**

Ans-166: (c) Subclavian arteries
Ref: Harrison's -Pg 2127, Table 319-6
Sol:

- Takayasu's **arteritis is an inflammatory and stenotic disease** of medium-and large-sized arteries characterized by a strong **predilection for the aortic arch and its branches.**
- For this reason, it is often referred to as the aortic arch syndrome. The most common artery affected is Subclavian artery **(93%) > Common carotid > Abdominal aorta > Renal arteries > Pulmonary artery (20%)**

Ans-167: (b) Hunter syndrome
Ref: Harrison's-2456
Sol:

- **Hunter disease (MPSII) is an X-linked disorder** due to deficiency in iduronate sulfatase; it has manifestations very **similar to MPS I,** including neurologic degeneration, but there is NO corneal clouding or **other eye disease.**

Ans 168: (a) Five-year survival is ~5%.
Ref – Read the text below
Sol

- Ductal **adenocarcinomas of the exocrine pancreas are the** most common type (>90%) of pancreatic neoplasm.
- The pancreatic head is the most common **site. The median age of diagnosis is 72 years, with the peak incidence between 65 and 85 years.**
- **The incidence is slightly higher in men than women** and in African Americans than Caucasians. Pancreatic carcinoma is uncommon **below the age of 50.**
- **These tumors are aggressive and usually present with locally inoperable disease with local and distal metastases.**
- The 5-year survival is only about 5%. It is the fourth leading cause of cancer death.
- Other less common types of pancreatic neoplasms **include islet cell tumors and neuroendocrine tumors.**

Ans-169: (b) Diastolic dysfunction
Ref:Read the text below
Sol:

- Diastolic dysfunction is an important cause **of heart failure in the elderly. It is commonly associated with a history of hypertension and diabetes.**
- Normal ejection fraction and aortic sclerosis rule out **either systolic or valvular heart disease as causes. In HOCM there is nonconcentric hypertrophy.**

Ans-170: (d) All of the above
Ref: Read the text below
Sol :

- **Complications of infectious mononucleosis** are rare but may be the major manifestation of the illness. Hematologic complications include hemolytic anemia, mild **thrombocytopenia in 50 percent of cases, and mild granulocytopenia.**
- **Severe hematiologic complications** can occur. Splenic rupture is rare. It is accompanied by abdominal pain and occurs in the second or third week of illness. Neurologic **complications may be the presenting manifestation of the illness. Most frequent** are cranial nerve palsies (especially Bell's palsy) and encephalitis.
- The majority of patients with neurologic complications recover spontaneously. Hepatitis is common. Almost 90 percent of patients will have elevated serum transaminases. Cardiac complications are uncommon but can occur. Airway obstruction can **occur from adenopathy. Pulmonary infiltrates may occur, especially in children.**

Ans-171: (c) Alports syndrome
Ref: Harrison internal medicine 17th ed pg 2469

Sol:

As per the history given this condition is **a X linked disease as no female affection has been shown**

In all these conditions only **X linked inheritance is seen in Alport syndrome**

- Classically, **patients with Alport's syndrome develop hematuria**, thinning and splitting of the GBMs, mild proteinuria (<1–2 g/24 h), and **chronic glomerulosclerosis, leading to renal failure in association with sensorineural deafness.**
- Some patients develop lenticonus of the anterior lens capsule and, rarely, mental retardation or leiomyomatosis. Approximately **85% of patients with Alport's syndrome** have an X-linked inheritance of mutations in the **alpha 5 (IV) collagen chain on chromosome Xq22–24.**
- **Female carriers have variable penetrance depending** on the type of mutation or the degree of mosaicism created by X inactivation. **Fifteen percent of patients have autosomal** recessive disease of the alpha3 (IV) or alpha4 (IV) chains on chromosome 2q35–37.
- Rarely, some kindred have an autosomal **dominant inheritance of dominant-negative mutations in alpha3 (IV) or alpha4 (IV) chains.**

Ans-172: (d) Tuberculosis

Ref: Campbell's Operative Orthopaedics, 11th ed

Sol:

About multiple myeloma

The median age at diagnosis is 68 years; it is uncommon under age 40

About tuberculosis

- **Spinal tubercular infections** account for one third to one half of the bone and joint infections. The **thoracolumbar spine is the most commonly infected area.**
- The incidence of infection **seems to increase with age, but males and females are almost equally infected**
- Early radiographic findings **include a subtle decrease in one or more disc spaces and localized osteopenia.**
- Later findings include **vertebral collapse, called "concertina collapse"**
- **Soft-tissue swelling** and its late calcification are highly predictable radiographic findings. CT scanning, with or without contrast, allows better evaluation of the pathological process and the degree of neural compromise.
- **MRI permits further delineation of the pathological process.**
- **Ga scanning was most useful in patients with disseminated tuberculosis.**

Ans-173: (a) They should be started with optimum doses

Ref: Coronary care manual. Peter L Thomson 2nd edition PG 244.

Sol:

- **Beta Blocker drug** in cardiac failure should be started with lowest possible dose and titrated slowly **with optimal dose and start low and go slow.**
- Rate of increase of dose depends on patient's **symptomatic response, BP, heart rate.**
- Patient may need to be advised that the response to beta blocker can **be delayed and three months may be needs to obtain benefit.**

Ans-174: (a) Catatonic Schizophrenia

Ref: Read the text below

Sol:

Catatonic schizophrenia is characterized by marked disturbance of motor behaviour in addition to the general features of schizophrenia. **The patient in question present with typical signs of retarded catatonia, and hence is catatonic schizophrenia.**

Certain characteristics catatonic sings often in our examinations include:

1. Mutism: absence of speech
2. Rigidity: Maintenance of Rigid posture against efforts to be moved
3. Posturism: Voluntary assumption of bizarre, inappropriate posture for long period of Time
4. Negativis: Motivates resistance to all commands and attempts to be moved

5. Echolalia: Repetition, echo or mimicking of phrases of words heard
6. Echopraxia: Repetition, echo or mimicking of actions observed

Ans-175: (a) intermittent, porphyria
Ref:Read the text below
Sol:

- Acute **intermittent porphyria is a neurovisceral** syndrome, and should be suspected whenever a patient presents with a **constellation of symptoms, suggestions involvement of both viscera and nervous system.**
- The patient in question is presenting with **symptomatology that is consistent with a diagnosis of acute intermittent porphyria.**

Ans-176: (c) Major depressive disorder
Ref: Read the text below
Sol:

- Many people who **request physician-assisted suicide have one of two conditions present: either a poorly controlled painful condition or severe depression.**
- If the painful condition is adequately treated or the **depression is brought under good medical control, the request for physician assistance in terminating** the situation is typically withdrawn.
- It is important to note that bringing these conditions under control requires the intervention of caregivers who are **specifically trained in the management of these two conditions; primary care physicians usually are not adequately trained to address these difficult presentations.**
- Patients who are diagnosed as bipolar disorder borderline personality disorder), and schizophrenic disorder often make suicide **attempts (and frequently complete those attempts), they do not generally ask their physician** for assistance in the suicide.
- Persons with factitious disorder are seeking **primary gain, often for dependency needs, and are seeking to enter the "sick role" not the "dead role.**

Ans-177: (b) Repression
Ref:Read the text below
Sol:
Repression may refer to:

- **Memory inhibition,** the ability to filter irrelevant memories from attempts to recall
- Political repression, the oppression or persecution of an individual or group for political reasons
- **Social repression**
- Psychological repression, the psychological act of excluding desires and impulses from one's **consciousness**
- Repression, a theoretical concept that **describes the act of creating a repressed memory that excludes a particular episode from consciousness and** the ability to recall it

Ans-178: (b) Alopecia areata
Ref.: Davidson's, 20th dn. Pg. 1278
Sol :

- Typical first symptoms of alopecia areata are small bald patches. **The underlying skin is unscarred and looks** superficially normal. These patches can take many shapes, but are most usually round or oval.
- Alopecia areata most often affects the scalp and beard, but may occur on any hair-bearing part of the body
- Different skin areas can exhibit hair loss and regrowth at the same time. The disease may also go into remission for a time, or permanently. **Common in children.**
- **The area of hair loss may tingle or be painful.**
- **The hair tends to fall out over a short period of time, with the loss commonly occurring more on one side of the scalp than the other.**
- Exclamation point hairs are often present. Exclamation point hairs are hairs that become narrower along the length of the strand **closer to the base, producing a characteristic "exclamation point" appearance.**
- **In the case of healthy hair, if you were to try to pull some out, at most a few should come out, and ripped hair should not be distributed evenly across the tugged portion of the scalp. In cases of alopecia areata hair will tend to pull out more easily along the edge of the patch where the follicles**

are already being attacked by the body's immune system than away from the patch where they are still healthy.

- Nails may have pitting or trachyonychia

Ans-179: (d) Lichen planus
Ref.: Harrison's, 17th edn. Pg. 316
Sol :

- **Wickham striae** are whitish lines visible in the papules of lichen planus and other dermatoses, typically the macroscopic appearance of the histologic phenomenon hypergranulosis, and named for Louis Frédéric Wi

Ans-180: (c) Pityriasis rosea
Ref.: Harrison's, 17th edn. Pg. 315
Sol :

- **Pityriasis rosea** (also known as **pityriasis rosea Gibert**[l]) is a skin rash. It is non-dangerous but may inflict substantial discomfort on some people.
- Classically, it begins with a single "herald patch" lesion, followed in 1 or 2 weeks by a generalized body rash lasting about 6 weeks

Ans-181: (b) Urticaria pigmentosa
Ref.: Harrison-333.
Sol :
Darier's sign is a change observed after stroking the skin of a person with systemic mastocytosis or urticaria pigmentosa.
In general, the skin becomes swollen, itchy and red. This is a result of compression of mast cells, which are **hyperactive in these diseases. These mast cells release inflammatory granules which contain histamine. It is the histamine which is responsible for the response seen after rubbing the skin.**

Ans:182: (d) Edema
Ref: Read the text below
Sol:

- **Crystalloid solution is readily available at 1/20th of the cost** of albumin, and has fewer associated pyrogenic reactions.
- It is also possible to retrieve infused **crystalloid through diuresis in patients with functioning kidneys.**
- It does cross permeable membranes to accumulate in "third space" components of extracellular fluid; whereas, **albumin has a longer circulating half life in patients tending toward congestive edema**.

Ans-183: (c) Paroxysmal supraventricular tachycardia (PSVT)
Ref:Read the text below
Sol:

- The patient most likely has **PSVT, since the tachycardia terminates after carotid sinus massage (CSM).**
- CSM increases vagal tone **(parasympathetic) which decreases AV nodal conduction and terminates AV node re-entry arrhythmias.**
- Sinus tachycardia differs from PSVT tachycardia in that it does not start or stop abruptly. In PSVT, the QRS is usually narrow **without clearly discernible P waves.**
- A wide QRS in PSVT can result from a preexisting bundle branch block, or a functional bundle branch block secondary to the tachycardia. This can make the **distinction from a ventricular arrhythmia quite difficult.**

Ans 184: (b) Dysphagia occurs when the ring diameter is 13 mm. or less.
Reference: Read the text below
Sol:

- **Schatzki's ring is seen radiographically as an annular weblike constriction at the esophagogastric junction in a patient with a sliding hiatalhernia.**

- It represents prominence of the **esophagogastric junction with slight submucosal fibrosis** but not true panmural fibrotic reflux stricture. Intermittent dysphagia may occur when the ring size is 20 mm. or less, but dysphagia is almost invariable when the **ring measures 13 mm. or less.**
- Schatzki's ring occurs precisely at the squamocolumnar epithelial junction. It is indicative of the presence of a hiatal hernia but not of gastroesophageal reflux or esop**hagitis.**
- **An asymptomatic**
- Schatzki's ring requires no therapy per se. Patients with refractory severe reflux symptoms after dilation therapy is candidates for **antireflux surgery.**

Ans-185: (c) Malignant pleural effusion
Ref: Read the text below
Sol :

- **Pneumonia, hemoptysis and clubbing are** all signs that may be related to benign pulmonary disease **as well as resectable malignancy,** and positive sputum cytology on cough specimen does not rule out resection for cure since is its presumed to originate **from the cancer already identified in the left upper lobe.**
- **If the cytology were from a catheter transbronchial** aspirant from the right lung, it would suggest bilateral disease making this patient with clubbing and pneumonia inoperable as well as suggesting a tumor that is nonresectable.
- The single contraindication to **operation planned for resection for cure is the** positive finding of a malignant pleural effusion, since this indicates that the cancer has spread beyond the confines of the lobe and **would not be cured even by left pneumonectomy.**

Ans-186: (c) Hypermagnesemia
Ref: Bailey - 1201
Sol :
Paralytic ileus (neurogenic ileus): Defined as failure of transmission of peristaltic wave secondary to neuromuscular failure
CAUSES

- **Peritonitis (MC)**
- **Reflex ileus** : Following fracture of spine or ribs, retroperitoneal hemorrhage.
- **Infection : Intra**-abdominal abscess, pneumonia, sepsis.
- **Metabolic** : Uremia, hypokemia are most common contributing factors, hyponatremia. Hypo and hypermagnesemia, hypothyroidism can also contribute.
- **Ischemia :** Mesenteric ischemia, myocardial infarction.
- **Postoperative** : Paralytic ileus should be considered only after 72 hrs. of operation.
- **Drugs :** Anticholinergics, opiates, calcium channel blockers, tricyclic antidepressants.

Ans-187: (c) Hyperbaric oxygen therapy
Ref: Read the text below
Sol :

- **Tuberculosis can result in local destruction of** affected lung with cavitation. If this cavitary destruction is large, if it is **multiple in one lobe, and if it is not** successfully drained intrabronchially through the assistance of bronchoscopic brush biopsy to enter the cavity **and lavage, lobectomy may be advised.**
- A **thickened pleura is likely**, particularly if a secondary bacterial infection and **empyema result which may require thorough drainage of the pleural** space and decortications of the encased lung in order to allow expansion.
- If that expansion is not possible with the lung coming up to chest wall, the chest wall is actually **collapsed down onto the lung, in a type of chest wall reconstruction called thoracoplasty.**
- Each of these surgical methods has **been used with success with management of complications of tuberculosis.**
- Hyperbaric oxygen is not **successful in managing these complications.**

Ans-188: (b) Arteriographic vascular occlusion
Ref: Read the text below
Sol :

- **Hepatoma is not a radiosensitive tumor and no** pre-operative utility would be expected from radiotherapy or intensive **cytotoxic chemotherapy, since it is alos highly unresponsive to drug therapy.**
- **Immunotherapy and nutritional** therapy might make a marginal difference in the host response to **operation, but are inadequate to make any marginal difference that would be worth a delay.**
- The one **technique listed that has been proven** effective in selective instances is **devascularization of the liver segment anticipated** to be resected, which gives a head-start on the regeneration of liver function in adjacent liver to be preserved.
- It is also suggested to decrease the **tumor neovascularity involved in the** tumor-bearing segment, but this is difficult to judge prospectively and impossible to control in comparative trials.
- Radiographic occlusion is nonetheless and **advocated for some selected pre-operative hepatoma management.**

Ans 189: (b) Barrett's esophagus.
Reference: Read the text below
Sol:

- **A stricture at or above the aortic arch is almost certainly situated above an esophagus lined at its lower end with columnar epithelium.**
- **Barrett's esophagus is suggested radiographically** when local esophagitis, ulcer, or stricture is at the limits of a normal-looking segment of esophagus under the stricture but above a herniated stomach.
- The **columnar-lined esophagus is not always associated with a high stricture; however Messiaen and Halpert documented strictures** in 80% of their Barrett's patients. These high strictures, when seen with alkaline reflux esophagitis, with idiopathic reflux disease, or in association with scleroderma, always suggest the presence of a columnar-lined esophagus.
- **Mediastinal fibrosis is a rare condition that can cause multilevel strictures on the esophagus.**

Ans 190: (d) Conversion of Billroth II gastrojejunostomy to Roux-en-Y gastrojejunostomy
Reference: Read the text below
Sol:

- **Symptoms related bile reflux gastritis occur transiently in 10% to 20% of patients after truncal vagotomy and resection or drainage.**
- Symptoms **persist in only 1% to** 2%. No completely satisfactory solution to bile reflux gastritis exists. Medicinal and dietary treatments have not been proven to be beneficial.
- Operative diversion of biliary secretions away from the gastric mucosa by construction of a **Roux-en-Y gastrojejunostomy with an intestinal limb of 50 to 60 cm has been widely reported.**
- The procedure eliminates bilious vomiting in nearly 100% of patients, but **pain persists in up to 30%, and 20% develop delayed gastric emptying as a result of the procedure.**

Ans 191: (d) Tissues inferior to the lateral iliopubic tract.
Reference: Read the text below
Sol:

- **Placement of staples inferior to (below) the lateral iliopubic tract** may result in injury to the **lateral femoral cutaneous nerve or the genitofemoral nerve.**
- Staples should also not be placed within the triangle of doom, owing to the risk of major vascular injury.

Ans 192: (d) Omental patch of the perforation plus proximal gastric vagotomy
Reference: Read the text below
Sol:

- Simple **omental patching of a perforation** in patients with chronic ulcer disease does not yield satisfactory long-term results.
- **Up to 80% of patients so treated develop recurrent ulceration and 10% develop secondary complications.**
- A definitive ulcer operation should be performed during the initial laparotomy if the following circumstances apply: **1) there has been no preoperative shock, 2) the perforation has been present for less than 48 hours, and 3) no life-threatening medical co-morbidity exists.**

- Omental patching of the perforation combined with proximal gastric vagotomy is a preferred approach because it combines safety, freedom from disabling **postoperative symptoms, and a low rate of recurrent ulceration.**

Ans 193: (d) Endoscopy.
Reference: Read the text below
Sol:

- In the absence of **physical or radiographic evidence of upper airway obstruction or esophagogastric perforation, the presence of a significant** caustic injury can be defined reliably only by direct visualization at the time of endoscopy.
- Although the history may shed light on the possibility of a burn and its severity, all too often the event goes unwitnessed or the **type and amount of ingested substance are not known with certainty.**
- The **identification of oropharyngeal burns clearly indicates the need for endoscopy, but as many as 70% of patients** with such lesions escape associated esophageal injury. Conversely, 10% to 30% of patients with no external evidence of burns have subsequently been confirmed by esophagoscopy to have sustained damage.
- In the absence of an identifiable perforation, a barium esophagogram can rarely be considered unequivocally diagnostic of acute injury, though such an injury may be suggested when the esophagus **appears atonic and dilated, rigid and persistently narrowed, or excessively irritable.**
- Because of the importance of early confirmation of the presence or absence of a significant esophageal burn as a guide to formulating appropriate treatment, esophagoscopy should be performed expeditiously as soon as sufficient **time has elapsed to allow gastric emptying and stabilization of the patient, preferably within the first 12 to 48 hours after ingestion.**

Ans 194: (a) Continuing requirement for frequent dilation of an extensive esophageal stricture for a minimum of 2 years.
Reference: Read the text below
Sol:

- **Development of a tracheobronchial fistula almost always necessitates some form of esophageal reconstruction because of the extensive damage usually associated with it.**
- Failure of the patient to cooperate effectively condemns to failure any attempt at restoring esophageal patency by **bougienage, because sporadic attempts at dilation do not allow** progressive lumen enlargement but, rather, invite additional injury because of the necessity for repeated instrumentation of a recurrent, tight stricture.
- The need for repeated dilation of extensive or multiple strictures over a period exceeding 6 months should prompt surgical reconstruction of the esophagus, especially in young children, for whom the **psychological and physical hazards are intensified by prolonged treatment. In such circumstances, a 2-year period of attempted bougienage is excessive**.
- Although iatrogenic perforation often signals the need for esophageal reconstruction, this misadventure should not be considered **an absolute indication but should be assessed in relation to (1) the extent and complexity of the stricture, (2) the potential for eventually achieving successful bougienage, and (3) the severity** of complications caused by the secondary injury.

Ans 195: (c) Evaluation for Helicobacter pylori.
Reference: Read the text below
Sol:

- **Vagotomy and antrectomy** is the definitive surgical therapy for peptic ulcer disease but should be applied only for complications of the disease or after refractory disease has been documented.
- Biopsy of routine peptic duodenal ulcer is not indicated to rule out malignancy except in special circumstances, **such as an endoscopic appearance typical of malignancy.**
- H. pylori are found in a large percentage of peptic ulcer patients, and treatment alters the rate of recurrence if therapy is directed toward reduction of H. pylori in addition to acid. Measurement of serum gastrin is recommended for patients **with resistant or persistent peptic ulcer disease for patients undergoing surgery for peptic ulcer disease.**

- **The Sippy diet has not been recommended clinically for years. Formerly** it was recommended as a bland diet that would not exacerbate peptic ulcer disease.
- **It is now known that these diets are heavily calcium-laden and probably exacerbate peptic ulcer disease.**

Ans 196: (d) Oral antacid therapy.
Reference: Read the text below
Sol:

- All patients should **undergo nasogastric suction, rehydration, and control of acid secretion.**
- This control of acid secretion requires an H 2 **antagonist since oral antacids are often** inadequate to neutralize the large volume of acid often present in the obstructed stomach.
- Patients with a long history of obstruction are **often nutritionally compromised and need careful nutritional assessment before operative planning.**

Ans-197: (b) Undescended abdominal testis
Ref: Read the text below
Sol :
The exact cause of testicular cancer is unknown. There is no link between vasectomy and testicular cancer. **Factors that may increase a man's risk for testicular cancer include:**

- Abnormal testicle development
- History of testicular cancer
- History of undescended testicle
- Klinefelter syndrome

Other possible causes include exposure to certain chemicals and HIV infection. A family history of testicular cancer may also increase risk.
Testicular cancer is the most common **form of cancer in men between the ages of 15 and 35. It can occur in older men, and rarely, in younger boys.**

Ans-198: (d) Echinococcus granulosus
Ref: Read the text below
Sol :

- Pyogenic **abscesses, such as that with Staphylococcus or Proteus may cause** febrile reactions and can lead to septicemia, but not hypersensitivity reactions.
- **Clonorchis sinensis is an Oriental liver fluke that takes up residence** in the biliary tree, and is a source of inflammatory response, but not anaphylaxis. Amoeba are protozoans that in some zymogen classes not only give rise to colonic inflammation but invade the portal blood stream and can set up hepatic abscess, which when drained does not give **anaphylaxis.**
- **This is not the case with hydatid cyst caused by Echinococcus granulosus. Not only can rupture of the cyst result in implantation and dissemination of daughter cysts, Echinococcus can cause a lethal** hypersensitivity reaction as well if spilled into the peritoneum.

Ans-199: (b) Traumatic splenic laceration in a child with minimum blood loss
Ref: Read the text below
Sol :

- **Thrombocytopenia from idiopathic or other acquired** origins may respond to splenectomy if steroid therapy no longer induces a response in raising platelets. Spherocytosis is a frequent hemolytic **indication for splenectomy as one of the only treatments and with excellent success rate.**
- **Splenic abscess and splenic artery** aneurysm both are treated by splenectomy if simple drainage is inadequate or an exterior splenic artery aneurysmectomy is not possible. In children, **however, splenectomy is to be avoided for trauma unless there is hemodynamic instability and no other way to control the intra-abdominal hemorrhage.**
- With **minimal blood loss and stable vital signs, minimal splenic** disruption can be managed by observation in order that the splenic filtration and immunologic function be preserved. If surgical exploration is undertaken, attempts at repair of minor traumatic splenic **injuries are recommended,**

particularly in children, and splenectomy reserved for unsalvageable disruption or patients with multiple other injuries requiring urgent attention.

Ans-200: (b) Anaplastic carcinoma
Ref: Read the text below
Sol :

- **Anaplastic carcinoma** is essentially an untreatable disease, with nearly uniformly fatal **outcome despite the treatments that have been tried. It spreads quickly and early and is not controlled by radioiodine, radiation or chemotherapy.**
- **Extensive surgical efforts have** resulted in some relief of obstructive disease while tumor spread usually continues unchecked. In order of malignant behavior, medullary thyroid carcinoma would be next worst, followed by follicular, lymphoma (which may **present primarily in the thyroid gland) and papillary with the best prognosis.**

Ans-201: (c) Ankylosing spondylitis (AS)
Ref:Read the text below
Sol:

- AS occurs in 1–6% **of adults inheriting human lymphocyte antigen B27 (HLA-B27).**
- However, the prevalence in B27-positive relatives of patients **with AS is up to 30%. Men are three times more likely to be affected.**

Ans-202: (a) Duodena atresia
Ref: Bailey - 1199
Sol :

- **Congenital atresia is not** common cause of neonatal intestinal obstruction, out of which **duodenal atresia is most leading one.**
  Duodenal atresia
- Atresia at the **level of ampulla of Vater**. 30% babies have associated Down's syndrome.
- Radiograph shows double bubble sign with two air fluid level.
- Treatment – Immediate surgery **after resuscitation. Duodeno jejunostomy is the operation of choice.**

Ans-203: (d) Recurrent dislocation of shoulder
Ref: Maheshwari's -74
Sol :

- A **Hill-Sachs lesion usually** result from recurrent anterior shoulder dislocation with resultant **posterolateral humeral** head compression fracture as the humeral head comes to rest against the **anteroinferior part of the glenoid.**
- It is often associated with a **Bankart lesion of the glenoid (stripping of the glenoidal labrum along with the periosteum from the anterior surface** of the glenoid and scapular neck.

Ans-204: (a) Fat embolism
Ref: Maheshwari-34
Sol :
Early complications :

I. **Local :**
   a. **Vascular injury** causing hemorrhage, internal or external.
   b. Visceral injury causing damage to structures such as brain, lung or bladder.
   c. Damage to surrounding tissue, nerves or skin.
   d. Haemarthrosis.
   e. Compartment syndrome/Volkmann's ischaemia
   f. Wound infection, more common for open fractures.

II. **Systemic :**
   a. Fat embolism
   b. Shock
   c. Pulmonary/venous thromboembolism.

Ans-205: (a) Nasal bones
Ref: Dhingra's- 195
Sol :

- **Nasal fracture is the most common facial fracture** and the third most common fracture of the skeleton overall.
- However, **because many fractures are subclinical and** many others are associated with multiple traumas, a high percentage **are not diagnosed or treated at the time of injury.**
- These often lead to chronic nasal obstruction and account for **many of the septoplasty procedures performed for obstruction and septal deviation.**
- Most facial fractures can be restored to their preoperative **state with proper early intervention.**

Ans 206 : (a) Barium swallow
Ref:Read the text below
Sol:

- Barium swallow is the **diagnostic procedure of choice.**
- Patients with symptomatic disease usually **have a posterior midline pouch greater than** 2 cm in diameter arising just above the cricopharyngeus muscle.
- No other study is required if **no other abnormality is present.**

Ans 207 : (b) High gastric residue
Ref:Read the text below
Sol:

- Ultrasound diagnostic accuracy has **been found to be around 95%**, with diagnostic criteria including **wal thickness >4mm**
- Segment **length >16mm.**

Ans 208 : (d) X-RAY LUMBAR SPINE- AP view
Ref:Read the text below
Sol:

- Although for imaging of **spondylolisthesis usually all are done, AP view appears to be least useful of these choices.**
- However, please remember on AP **view spondylolisthesis can show a sign called as Napolean Hat sign.**
- The lateral view is useful in detecting **spondylolisthesis; it may demonstrate the pars defect.**
- Bilateral oblique views are especially useful in visualizing the pars interarticularis defect, which has the appearance of a Scottie **dog with a collar. Cross sectional imaging including CT and MRI are helpful in further evaluation.**

Ans-209: (b) A higher incidence of systemic hypotension
Ref: Fundamental Principles and Practice of Anesthesia-219,221
Sol :

- The hypotension **produced by epidural anesthesia** being slower in onset than in spinal anesthesia can often be compensated for by fluids alone, but in both cases, a small dose of a **vasopressor agent may be needed.**
- The incidence of dural puncture in experienced hands should be less than 1% for epidural anesthesia.
- In **epidural anesthesia, missed segments or unilateral block may occur in over 2% of patients.**

Ans-210: (d) All of the above
Ref: Lee's Synopsis of Anesthesia, 13th edn. Pg. 101-02.
Sol :
Clinical monitoring

- **Circulation ; Pulse rate**. Rhythm and quality, vein filling, skin elasticity and temperature, and urine output (if catheterized).
- **Respiration; Effort**, pattern, tidal volume, frequency, reservoir bag movement.
- **Oxygenation: Skin,** mucous membrane and blood color.

- **Depth of anesthesia : Pupillary** signs (after Guedel), watering of eyes (lacrimation), sweating, muscle movement.

Ans-211: (b) Use of either is associated with quick induction time
Ref: KD Tripathi, 6th edn. Pg. 371
Sol :
Ether (Diethyl either)

▪ **Pharmacology**	- WTG Morton first used ether in Boston on 16th October 1846. - It is stored in dark bottles with corks/ caps as light may decompose it. If it is taken to high altitude its boiling point is lowered.
▪ **Advantages**	- Ether stimulates respiration and blood flow due to its sympathomimetic effect mediated by adrenaline release. - When too much ether is given respiration becomes depressed before the heart. These effects make ether a "safe" anaesthetic agent. - It is a bronchodilator and produces analgesia. - It may be used as the sole anesthetic agent and is capable of producing good abdominal muscle relaxation. It is the safest anesthetic in unskilled hands. - It is the volatile agent of choice when general anesthesia is needed but no oxygen is available.
▪ **Disadvantages**	- Ether is explosive when mixed with oxygen and is inflammable in air. - Ether is highly soluble in blood – induction is prolonged and unpleasant; recovery is slow; it stimulates salivation; has a pungent odor; postanesthetic nausea, vomiting and retching are marked.

Ans 212: (c) Rapid restoration of the circulating volume
Ref– Read the text below
Sol:

- **Renal dysfunction in shock of any type may be due to prerenal or renal etiologies.**
- **Prerenal renal dysfunction** is due to poor perfusion of the kidney secondary to hypotension.
- If **no intrinsic renal injury occurs**, renal function will improve with restoration of renal blood flow.
- If **hypotension is severe and prolonged**, acute tubular or (if even more severe) cortical necrosis may **produce intrinsic renal failure.**
- **Acute tubular necrosis** is often reversible, but cortical necrosis results in chronic renal insufficiency.

Ans 213: (a) Normalize blood gases
Ref– Read the text below
Sol:

- To **avoid oxygen toxicity, excessive PEEP and PIP, and volutrauma or barotrauma**, blood gases should not be normalized.
- This **principle of respiratory management** has been the most significant improvement in the care of **ARDS in the last 10 years.**

Ans 214: (c) Moro reflex
Ref: Read the text below.
Sol:

- The **moro reflex is initiated by loud noise or sudden motion.**
- It involves abduction of the **extremities and extension of the elbows and knees, followed by flexion.**
- The **Moro reflex** appears at birth and disappears at approximately 4 months of age.
- **If reflex is asymmetric, this suggests extremity fracture or peripheral nerve injury.**

Ans 215: (a) Chromosome translocation that brings together an Ig heavy chain with an oncogene
Ref: Read the text below.
Sol

- **Chromosome translocations may often promote tumors in somatic cells by placing regulatory genes next to promoters that aberrantly increase their expression.**

- **Burkitt's lymphoma, a B cell lymphoma** that usually occurs in childhood, often involves reciprocal translocation of chromosomes 8 and 14.
- The result of this is to place the **c-myc protooncogene from 8q24** into the immunoglobulin **heavy chain locus at 14q32**. Since immunoglobulin genes are actively transcribed, this move alters the normal regulatory control of c-myc.
- Another example is the **Philadelphia chromosome, a shortened chromosome 22** caused by **translocation t(9:22)(q34:q11).** This translocation is seen in almost all patients with **chronic myelogenous leukemia (CML) and in a percentage of patients with acute lymphoblastic leukemia (ALL).**
- The **Philadelphia chromosome** is seen with increased frequency in individuals with Down's syndrome.

Ans 216: (d) Tissue plasminogen activator infusion
Ref: Read the text below.
Sol:

- Many enzymes interact to **regulate blood clotting. Plasmin** is activated by proteolytic cleavage of **its zymogen, plasminogen.**
- The activating protease is called **tissue plasminogen activator (tPA). Plasmin** hydrolyzes fibrin clots to form soluble products, and is used to dissolve clots in coronary arteries that cause myocardial infarction.
- **Platelets, thrombin, and fibrinogen** promote clotting through the intrinsic pathway and would be contraindicated in myocardial infarction.
- **Platelets** form a plug at the site of **bleeding and bind prothrombin** to facilitate its conversion to thrombin. Fibrinogen is the substrate acted upon by thrombin to yield the fibrin mesh of blood clots.
- **Heparin is a mucopolysaccharide that terminates clot formation by interfering with a number of steps in the coagulation cascade.**
- **Heparin** inhibits the formation of clots, but cannot dissolve clots that have already formed.

Ans 217: (c) Reye's syndrome
Ref: Read the text below.
Sol:

a) **Reye's syndrome** shows a very high association with the ingestion of aspirin-containing **medicines during influenza-like illnessews or varicella.**
b) **Reye's syndrome has a biphasic course.**
c) It usually presents in a **previously healthy child who had an upper respiratory infection (90%) or varicella (5%-7%).**
d) After the child seems to have recovered, the symptoms of vomiting, lethargy, and confusion can appear and progress quickly. **Liver enzymes and ammonia are elevated.**
e) Treatment requires **early recognition and control of increased intracranial pressure.** Prognosis depends on **duration of disordered cerebral function.**

Ans 218: (c) Reassure the mother that this is normal
Ref: Read the text below.
Sol

- **Vaginal bleeding, or pseudomenses, may occur in a new born female.**
- In **utero, the vaginal epithelium** is stimulated by circulating maternal estrogens, which diffuse across the placenta.
- **After birth, these hormone levels rapidly fall, which results in endometrial sloughing.**
- There may be a **thick mucoid discharge from the newborn's vagina**, which is sometimes bloody.
- The discharge will usually resolve within **10 days after birth. No testing or treatment is necessary, only reassurance.**

Ans 219: (d) Fragile X syndrome
Ref– Read the text below
Sol:
Fragile X syndrome is a common chromosomal cause of mental retardation in boys. Affected boys have allelic expansion of trinucleotide repeats to more than 200 (normal is 6-54 repeats).

Ans 220: (a) Serum ammonia level

Ref– Read the text below
Sol:

- The child is presenting with **symptoms of Reye syndrome**, which is an acute encephalopathy associated **with high ammonia levels.**
- It most commonly **occurs in young children after a viral illness. Administration of aspirin increases the risk of developing this disorder**.
- The **vomiting is characteristic**. Renal failure leading to uremia is characterized by an increase in the urea nitrogen level.
- However, the **presentation would be more chronic and the patient's presentation would be more indicative of renal failure**.
- **Hypercalcemia can cause mental status** changes and management would include intravenous hydration and furosemide. Again, presentation would be more acute, and a history **of a malignancy, use of thiazides, milk alkali syndrome, or the like, would be elicited**.
- **Opiate intoxication** would cause pinpoint pupils, depressed breathing and obtundation. **Combativeness should not occur.**

Ans-221: (d) Laparoscopic salpingostomy
Ref: Read the text below
Sol :
Laparoscopy is one of the major advancement for tubal and uterine disease. Surgical procedures for managing benign adnexal masses include aspiration, fenestration, ovarian cystectomy, unilateral or bilateral salpingo-oophorectomy and laparoscopically-assisted vaginal hysterectomy (LAVH) with or without unilateral or bilateral salpingo-oophorectomy

For unruptured tubal pregnancy the fallopian tubes is identified and mobilized to minimize bleeding, a 5 to 8 ml diluted solution containing 5 Unit vasopressin in 20 ml of saline is injected with a 20 gauge spinal or laparoscopic needle. It should be injected in the mesosalpinx just below the ectopic and over the antemesentric surface of the tubal segment containing gestational product. The needle must not inserted deep within a blood vessel because intravascular injection may precipitate acute arterial hypertension, bradycardia and sometime it may be fatal.

Ans-222: (d) All of the above
Ref: Read the text below
Sol :

- **Normal cells and tumor cells are dividing cells, constantly** producing genetic material during the cell cycle. DNA synthesis may yield various errors in the replicated DNA, altering the structure **and function of the cells.**
- **A number of these aberrations have been identified in premalignant, malignant, and benign neoplasm.**
- Amplification, point mutations, deletions, and rearrangements are all mechanisms that lead to genetic errors.
- **Amplification is an increase in the copy number of a gene and can enhance gene expression by increasing the amount of template DNA available for** transcription.
- Protooncogene amplification is a common event in gynecologic malignancies. An example of oncogene amplification is erbB2, which **is found in 30% of all ovarian malignancies.**

Ans-223: (d) None of the above
Ref: Read the text below
Sol :

- Although a variety of **tumor-associated antigens such as SCC, CA125, and CEA** have been described in gynecologic malignancy, unfortunately none of these tumor markers are specific for a particular type of cancer.
- Tumor-associated **antigens have been identified using monoclonal antibody techniques.**
- **They are useful markers in following** the progression of the disease and the success of treatment. The combination of different tumor markers, for **example CA 125 and OVXI in ovarian cancer**, may improve the specificity and sensitivity of screening tests.

Ans-224: (b) IIIb
Ref: Shaw's gynaecology 14th ed.page 359 -388
Sol:
The following stages are used for endometrial cancer:
Stage I
In stage I, cancer is found in the uterus only. Stage I is divided into stages IA, IB, and IC, based on **how far the cancer has spread.**

- Stage IA: Cancer is in the endometrium only.
- Stage IB: Cancer has spread into the inner half of the myometrium (muscle layer of the uterus).
- Stage IC: Cancer has spread into **the outer half of the myometrium.**

Stage II
In stage II, cancer has spread from the uterus to the cervix, but has not spread outside the uterus. Stage II is divided into stages IIA and IIB, based on how far the cancer has spread into the cervix.

- Stage IIA: Cancer has spread to the glands where the cervix and uterus meet.
- Stage IIB: Cancer has spread into the connective tissue of the cervix.

Stage III
In stage III, cancer has spread beyond the uterus and cervix, but has not spread beyond the pelvis. Stage III is divided into stages IIIA, IIIB, and IIIC, based on how far the cancer has spread within the pelvis.

- Stage IIIA: Cancer has spread to one or more of the following:
  - the outermost layer of the uterus; or
  - tissue just beyond the uterus; or
  - the peritoneum.

  Stage IIIB: Cancer has spread beyond the uterus and cervix, into the vagina.
  Stage IIIC: Cancer has spread to lymph nodes near the uterus.

Stage IV
In stage IV, cancer has spread beyond the pelvis. Stage IV is divided into stages IVA and IVB, based on how far the cancer has spread.

- Stage IVA: Cancer has spread to the bladder and/or bowel wall.
- Stage IVB: Cancer has spread to other parts of the body beyond the pelvis, including lymph nodes in the abdomen and/or groin.

The following stages are used for cervical cancer:

- Stage 0 - full-thickness involvement of the epithelium without invasion into the stroma (carcinoma in situ)
- **Stage I** - limited to the cervix
  - IA - diagnosed only by microscopy; no visible lesions
    - IA1 - stromal invasion less than 3 mm in depth and 7 mm or less in horizontal spread
    - IA2 - stromal invasion between 3 and 5 mm with horizontal spread of 7 mm or less
  - IB - visible lesion or a microscopic lesion with more than 5 mm of depth or horizontal spread of more than 7 mm
    - IB1 - visible lesion 4 cm or less in greatest dimension
    - IB2 - visible lesion more than 4 cm
- **Stage II** - invades beyond cervix
  - IIA - without parametrial invasion, but involve upper 2/3 of vagina
  - IIB - with parametrial invasion
- **Stage III** - extends to pelvic wall or lower third of the vagina
  - IIIA - involves lower third of vagina
  - IIIB - extends to pelvic wall and/or causes hydronephrosis or non-functioning kidney
- **Stage IV - extends** outside the vagina
- IVA - invades mucosa of bladder or rectum and/or extends beyond true pelvis
- IVB - distant metastasis

OVARIAN CARCINOMA STAGING-

- Stage I - limited to one or both ovaries
  - IA - involves one ovary; capsule intact; no tumor on ovarian surface; no malignant cells in ascites or peritoneal washings

- IB - involves both ovaries; capsule intact; no tumor on ovarian surface; negative washings
- IC - tumor limited to ovaries with any of the following: capsule ruptured, tumor on ovarian surface, positive washings
- Stage II - pelvic extension or implants
  - IIA - extension or implants onto uterus or fallopian tube; negative washings
  - IIB - extension or implants onto other pelvic structures; negative washings
  - IIC - pelvic extension or implants with positive peritoneal washings
- Stage III - microscopic peritoneal implants outside of the pelvis; or limited to the pelvis with extension to the small bowel or omentum
  - IIIA - microscopic peritoneal metastases beyond pelvis
  - IIIB - macroscopic peritoneal metastases beyond pelvis less than 2 cm in size
  - IIIC - peritoneal metastases beyond pelvis > 2 cm or lymph node metastases
- Stage IV - distant metastases to the liver or outside the peritoneal cavity

Para-aortic lymph node metastases are considered regional lymph nodes (Stage IIIC). As there is only one para-aortic lymph node intervening before the thoracic duct on the right side of the body, the ovarian cancer can rapidly spread to distant sites such as the lung.

Ans-225: (b) PPH
Ref: Obstetrics D.C. Dutta 6th ed. page 411,421,422.
Sol:
Both option (2)&(3) seems correct though the uterine inversion is very much acute but still it's very rare condition and on other hand post-partum huge is having a incidence of 1% in hospital deliveries & much-more in non-institutional deliveries so the answer of choice here is PPH.

POSTPARTUM HAEMORRHAGE

DEFINITION-
"Any amount of bleeding from or into the genital tract following birth of the baby upto the end of the puerperium which adversely affects the general condition of the patient evidenced by rise in pulse rate and falling blood pressure is called postpartum haemorrhage".

INCIDENCE-
The incidence widely varies mainly because of lack of uniformity in the criteria used in definition and the extent of the use prophylactic ergometrine. The incidence is about 1% amongst hospital deliveries.

TYPE:
- **Primary**
- Secondary

Primary: Haemorrhage occurs within 24 hours following the birth of the baby. In the majority, haemorrhage occurs within two hours following delivery.
These are of two types:
* **Third stage haemorrhage- Bleeding occurs before expulsion of placenta.**
* **True postpartum haemorrhage-** Bleeding occurs subsequent to expulsion of placenta (majority)

Secondary: Haemorrhage occurs beyond 24 hours and within puerperium, also called delayed or late puerperal haemorrhage.

Ans-226: (b) Bacterial vaginosis
Ref: Read the text below
Sol :
- **Bacterial vaginosis (BV**) has previously been called "nonspecific vaginitis" or Gardnerella vaginitis**. The condition is an alteration of the normal vaginal flora that results in the loss of normal lactobacilli and the associated hydrogen-peroxide production.**
- This situation encourages the overgrowth of the anaerobic bacteria, which normally account for less **than 1% of normal vaginal flora, and produces the infection.**
- It is the most common form of **vaginitis in the developed countries.**
- The fishy odor and the exacerbation **of the condition by coitus are** characteristic of the infection. The vaginal pH is **typically between 4.7 and 5.7. The treatment is typically metronidazole or clindamycin.**

Ans-227: (b) Lung
Ref: Read the text below

Sol :

- The most **common sites of metastases are as follows**; lung 80%; vagina 30%; pelvis 20% liver 10%; brain 10%.
- At the time of presentation. **80% of the patients with metastatic GTT show lung involvement on chest radiographs.**
- **Patients with pulmonary metastases** may have chest pain, cough, hemoptysis, dyspnea, or an asymptomatic lesion on chest radiographs.
- Respiratory symptoms may be **acute or chronic, persisting over many months.**

Ans-228: (d) Interval between the antecedent pregnancy and the occurrence of the GTD
Ref: Read the text below
Sol :

- **Stage of the GTD correlates** with outcome; however, the majority of women with stages I **through III disease, fortunately, are cured. Within** stages II and III, there are several prognostic features that correlate with outcome.
- In addition to **the interval between antecedent** pregnancy and the development of the GTD (the longer the interval, the poorer the prognosis), other risk features include patient age, **level of hCG, ABO blood group, size of tumor, size of metastases, and the number of prior chemotherapy regimens.**

Ans-229: (c) Enlarged adrenal gland
Ref: Dutta 6th -408
Sol:
ANENCEPHALY

- Is the absence **of the cranial vault and cerebral hemispheres.**
- It is the most common type of **neural tube defect.**
- Caused by **failure of colosure of Rostral Neuropore** at an early embryonic stage.
- Base of skull and **facial bones are not affected.**
- Pituitary gland **is either absent or hypoplastic,as a result adrenal gland** is diminished in size.

Ans-230: (a) Giving folic acid to the mother in periconceptional period
Ref: BRS Obs and Gyn 2nd -59
Sol:

- **Prevention of neural tube defects** – Maternal folate supplementation has been shown to decrease the risk of NTDS.
- (1) **For all women of reproductive age** – 0.4 mg daily (1 month before conception and for 1st 3 months of pregnancy.)
- (2) **For high – risk women (i.e. those with diabetes, seizure disorders, and previous history of infant with NTD) – 4mg daily starting 3 months, prior to planned pregnancies.**

Ans-231: (d) Single agent chemotherapy with either methotrexate or actinomycin-D
Ref: Read the text below
Sol :

- Single-agent **chemotherapy is the** preferred treatment in patients with nonmetastatic gestational trophoblastic tumors who desire to retain fertility. Single-agent chemotherapy with either actinomycin-D or methotrexate has achieved comparable and **excellent remission rates in both nonmetastatic and low-risk metastatic GTT.**

Ans-232: (d) She should expect a generally normal reproductive outcome
Ref: Read the text below
Sol :

- Patients with **GTT who are treated successful with chemotherapy can expect normal reproduction in the future.**

Ans-233: (c) Colonization resistance
Ref: Read the text below
Sol :

- Development and **persistence of vaginal** infections with candida species is known as **colonization resistance.**
- **This phenomenon** results from conditions that predispose to the infection, such **as antibiotic use, pregnancy, and diabetes.**
- Lactobacilli normally prevent the **overgrowth of fungi in the vagin**a. With the disruption of the normal flora, an **overgrowth of the fungi occurs.**

Ans-234 : (c) HPV type 16
Ref: Read the text below
Sol :

- The **transformation zone is an area** established as metaplasia advances from the original **squamocolummar junction (SCJ) inward toward** the external so and over the columnar villi.
- The transformation **zone extends from the original SCJ to the physiologically active SCJ.**

Ans-235: (a) Pelvic inflammatory disease
Ref: Novak's - 510-12.
Sol :
RISK OF ECTOPIC PREGNANCY :

Conditions	Risk
▪ After ectopic pregnancy	▪ 7-13-fold increase for subsequent ectopic pregnancy ▪ The chance of subsequent pregnancy will be-intrauterine 50-80%, tubal 10-25% ▪ Chronic inflammatory disease accounts for almost 50% of ectopic pregnancy ▪ Salpingitis is commonest cause of tubal pregnancy
▪ PID	▪ The incidence of tubal obstruction increased with successive episodes of PID – 13% after 1 episode, 35% after 2 episodes, 75% after 3 episodes ▪ Increase of ectopic pregnancy by 6-10 folds.
▪ IUDs	▪ Woman conceiving with IUD is 6-10 times more likely have tubal pregnancy – with CU IUDs 4% Progesterone IUD 17%
▪ Sterilization	▪ Risk for tubal pregnancy after any sterilization procedure 5-16%

Ans-236: (b) Well-differentiated squamous cell carcionoma
Ref: Dutta -318
Sol :
Prognosis of carcinoma of the cervix :

1. Stage of lesion at the **initial therapy-most important factor**.

Stage	5-year survival rate (%)
I	85
II	55
III	38
IV	15

2. **Endocervical tumour-diagnosed late and grows** faster. (Adenocarcinoma develops from endocervical canal)
3. **Depth of tumour** – when < 1 cm, less lymph nodes are involved and improved survival.
4. Tumour size > 4 cm, asso**ciated** with more lymph node metastasis and poor survival.
5. Well-differentiated squamous cell carcinoma grows slowly and metastasis late than the anaplastic type.

Ans-237: (d) Misoprostol
Ref: Read the text below
Sol :
Hormonal medication

- Progesterone or Progestins: Progesterone counteracts estrogen and inhibits the growth of the endometrium. Such therapy can reduce or eliminate menstruation in a controlled and reversible fashion. Progestins are chemical variants of natural progesterone.

- Avoiding products with xenoestrogens, which have a similar effect to naturally produced estrogen and can increase growth of the endometrium.
- Hormone contraception therapy: Oral contraceptives reduce the menstrual pain associated with endometriosis.[47] They may function by reducing or eliminating menstrual flow and providing estrogen support. Typically, it is a long-term approach. Recently Seasonale was FDA approved to reduce periods to 4 per year. Other OCPs have however been used like this off label for years. Continuous hormonal contraception consists of the use of combined oral contraceptive pills without the use of placebo pills, or the use of Nuva Ring or the contraceptive patch without the break week. This eliminates monthly bleeding episodes.
- Danazol (Danocrine) and gestrinone are suppressive steroids with some androgenic activity. Both agents inhibit the growth of endometriosis but their use remains limited as they may cause hirsutism and voice changes.
- Gonadotropin Releasing Hormone (GnRH) agonist: These agents work by increasing the levels of GnRH. Consistent stimulation of the GnRH receptors results in downregulation, inducing a profound hypoestrogenism by decreasing FSH and LH levels. While effective in some patients, they induce unpleasant menopausal symptoms, and over time may lead to osteoporosis. To counteract such side effects some estrogen may have to be given back (add-back therapy). These drugs can only be used for six months at a time.
    - Lupron depo shot is a GnRH agonist and is used to lower the hormone levels in the woman's body to prevent or reduce growth of endometriosis. The injection is given in 2 different doses: a 3 month course of monthly injections, each with the dosage of (11.25 mg); or a 6 month course of monthly injections, each with the dosage of (3.75 mg).[48]
- Aromatase inhibitors are medications that block the formation of estrogen and have become of interest for researchers who are treating endometriosis.[49]

Ans-238: (c) Dermoid
Ref: Read the text below
Sol :
Dermoid is the most common **ovarian tumour to undergo torsion.**
A dermoid, or mature teratoma, is a benign type of ovarian tumor. Dermoids are common, constituting about one-third of all benign ovarian tumors. They are often found in young women. Dermoids rarely become cancerous. Cancer occurs in only 1-2 percent of cases, usually in women over 40. There is a similar tumor called an immature teratoma that is cancerous but rare (accounting for 1 percent of all ovarian cancers). In roughly 10 percent of cases of dermoids, these cysts will be found in both ovaries.

Ans-239: (b) It should be tested by inflating
Ref: Chaudhuri S.K. Practice of Fertility Control- 63
Sol :

- **Direction for use :**

1. The condom should be put on by unrolling into the erect penis after pulling back the foreskin.
2. It should be **used once only.**
3. It should **not be inflated to test, Vaseline, oils, skin lotion**, cold creams, butter or margarine should not be used. If **lubrication is needed, glycerin, K-Y jelly or spermicidal jelly can be used.**
4. **Soon after discharge, the male should** withdraw the penis holding the condom firmly against his body.
5. To increase effectiveness, a **dose of spermicidal cream, jelly or foam tablets may be used at the same time.**

Ans-240: (b) Making endometrium unreceptive
Ref: Read the text below
Sol :
Mechanisms of birth control
The Mirena is intended to initially release a daily dose of 20 micrograms levonorgestrel (a progestin). No single mechanism accounts for the effectiveness of the IUS in preventing pregnancy; it has several effects on the reproductive system:

- Frequency of ovulation is reduced.
- Cervical mucus is changed to obstruct passage of sperm through the cervix.
- The presence of a foreign body in the uterus prompts the release of leukocytes and prostaglandins by the endometrium, substances that are hostile to both sperm and eggs.